Emergency Medicine: Clinical Advances and Challenges in Diagnosis and Treatment

Emergency Medicine: Clinical Advances and Challenges in Diagnosis and Treatment

Editor

Ovidiu Alexandru Mederle

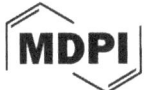

Basel • Beijing • Wuhan • Barcelona • Belgrade • Novi Sad • Cluj • Manchester

Editor
Ovidiu Alexandru Mederle
Department of Surgery
"Victor Babes" University
of Medicine and
Pharmacy Timisoara
Timisoara
Romania

Editorial Office
MDPI
St. Alban-Anlage 66
4052 Basel, Switzerland

This is a reprint of articles from the Special Issue published online in the open access journal *Journal of Personalized Medicine* (ISSN 2075-4426) (available at: https://www.mdpi.com/journal/jpm/special_issues/O3R11NE3X4).

For citation purposes, cite each article independently as indicated on the article page online and as indicated below:

Lastname, A.A.; Lastname, B.B. Article Title. *Journal Name* **Year**, *Volume Number*, Page Range.

ISBN 978-3-7258-1277-6 (Hbk)
ISBN 978-3-7258-1278-3 (PDF)
doi.org/10.3390/books978-3-7258-1278-3

Cover image courtesy of Ovidiu Alexandru Mederle

© 2024 by the authors. Articles in this book are Open Access and distributed under the Creative Commons Attribution (CC BY) license. The book as a whole is distributed by MDPI under the terms and conditions of the Creative Commons Attribution-NonCommercial-NoDerivs (CC BY-NC-ND) license.

Contents

About the Editor vii

Ovidiu Alexandru Mederle, Popa Daian Ionel and Williams Gabriela Carmen
Special Issue: Emergency Medicine: Clinical Advances and Challenges in Diagnosis
and Treatment
Reprinted from: *J. Pers. Med.* **2024**, *14*, 263, doi:10.3390/jpm14030263 1

Rakesh Jalali, Jacek Zwiernik, Ewa Rotkiewicz, Beata Zwiernik, Adam Kern, Jacek Bil, et al.
Predicting Short- and Long-Term Functional Outcomes Based on Serum S100B Protein Levels
in Patients with Ischemic Stroke
Reprinted from: *J. Pers. Med.* **2024**, *14*, 80, doi:10.3390/jpm14010080 6

Rakesh Jalali, Izabela Godlewska, Magdalena Fadrowska-Szleper, Agata Pypkowska, Adam
Kern, Jacek Bil, et al.
Significance of S100B Protein as a Rapid Diagnostic Tool in Emergency Departments for
Traumatic Brain Injury Patients
Reprinted from: *J. Pers. Med.* **2023**, *13*, 1724, doi:10.3390/jpm13121724 16

Daian Popa, Aida Iancu, Alina Petrica, Florina Buleu, Carmen Gabriela Williams,
Dumitru Sutoi, et al.
Emergency Department Time Targets for Interhospital Transfer of Patients with Acute Ischemic
Stroke
Reprinted from: *J. Pers. Med.* **2024**, *14*, 13, doi:10.3390/jpm14010013 26

Hyelin Han, Da Seul Kim, Minha Kim, Sejin Heo, Hansol Chang, Gun Tak Lee, et al.
A Simple Bacteremia Score for Predicting Bacteremia in Patients with Suspected Infection in the
Emergency Department: A Cohort Study
Reprinted from: *J. Pers. Med.* **2024**, *14*, 57, doi:10.3390/jpm14010057 41

Silvia Ioana Musuroi, Adela Voinescu, Corina Musuroi, Luminita Mirela Baditoiu,
Delia Muntean, Oana Izmendi, et al.
The Challenges of The Diagnostic and Therapeutic Approach of Patients with Infectious
Pathology in Emergency Medicine
Reprinted from: *J. Pers. Med.* **2024**, *14*, 46, doi:10.3390/jpm14010046 52

Alina Daginnus, Jan Schmitt, Jan Adriaan Graw, Christian Soost and Rene Burchard
Rate of Complications after Hip Fractures Caused by Prolonged Time-to-Surgery Depends on
the Patient's Individual Type of Fracture and Its Treatment
Reprinted from: *J. Pers. Med.* **2023**, *13*, 1470, doi:10.3390/jpm13101470 65

Marco Di Serafino, Giuseppina Dell'Aversano Orabona, Martina Caruso, Costanza Camillo,
Daniela Viscardi, Francesca Iacobellis, et al.
Point-of-Care Lung Ultrasound in the Intensive Care Unit—The Dark Side of Radiology: Where
Do We Stand?
Reprinted from: *J. Pers. Med.* **2023**, *13*, 1541, doi:10.3390/jpm13111541 76

Cosmin Ioan Faur, Razvan Nitu, Simona-Alina Abu-Awwad, Cristina Tudoran and Ahmed
Abu-Awwad
The Arterial Axis Lesions in Proximal Humeral Fractures—Case Report and Literature Review
Reprinted from: *J. Pers. Med.* **2023**, *13*, 1712, doi:10.3390/jpm13121712 95

Bogdan Anglitoiu, Ahmed Abu-Awwad, Jenel-Marain Patrascu, Jr., Simona-Alina Abu-Awwad, Anca Raluca Dinu, Alina-Daniela Totorean, et al.
Staged Treatment of Posttraumatic Tibial Osteomyelitis with Rib Graft and Serratus Anterior Muscle Autografts—Case Report
Reprinted from: *J. Pers. Med.* **2023**, *13*, 1651, doi:10.3390/jpm13121651 . . . . **108**

Wei-Kai Liao, Ming-Shun Hsieh, Sung-Yuan Hu, Shih-Che Huang, Che-An Tsai, Yan-Zin Chang and Yi-Chun Tsai
Predictive Performance of Scoring Systems for Mortality Risk in Patients with Cryptococcemia: An Observational Study
Reprinted from: *J. Pers. Med.* **2023**, *13*, 1358, doi:10.3390/jpm13091358 . . . . **119**

Mariusz Goniewicz, Anna Włoszczak-Szubzda, Ahmed M. Al-Wathinani and Krzysztof Goniewicz
Resilience in Emergency Medicine during COVID-19: Evaluating Staff Expectations and Preparedness
Reprinted from: *J. Pers. Med.* **2023**, *13*, 1545, doi:10.3390/jpm13111545 . . . . **132**

Adina Maria Marza, Alexandru Cristian Cindrea, Alina Petrica, Alexandra Valentina Stanciugelu, Claudiu Barsac, Alexandra Mocanu, et al.
Non-Ventilated Patients with Spontaneous Pneumothorax or Pneumomediastinum Associated with COVID-19: Three-Year Debriefing across Five Pandemic Waves
Reprinted from: *J. Pers. Med.* **2023**, *13*, 1497, doi:10.3390/jpm13101497 . . . . **144**

Jen-Wen Ma, Sung-Yuan Hu, Ming-Shun Hsieh, Yi-Chen Lee, Shih-Che Huang, Kuan-Ju Chen, et al.
PEAL Score to Predict the Mortality Risk of Cardiogenic Shock in the Emergency Department: An Observational Study
Reprinted from: *J. Pers. Med.* **2023**, *13*, 1614, doi:10.3390/jpm13111614 . . . . **161**

About the Editor

Ovidiu Alexandru Mederle

Ovidiu Alexandru Mederle is a professor at the Victor Babes University of Medicine and Pharmacy, Head of the Emergency Medicine discipline, and Chief of the Emergency Municipal Clinical Hospital in Timisoara. He has also been a member of the University senate since 2012 and a member of the European and Romanian Society of Emergency Medicine and the Romanian Society of Morphology.

He has published 12 books as the principal author or co-author, published 115 ISI/BDI articles as the principal author/co-author, and holds four invention patents.

Professor Mederle's primary areas of academic interest include novel treatment options, long-term sepsis outcomes, and histopathological changes in acute ischemic stroke.

Professor Mederle's current projects include developing simulation-based training programs for ED staff to enhance their collaboration in high-pressure scenarios, evaluating biomarkers of acute neuronal injury in traumatic brain injury and their relationship with pathology, developing a sepsis quality improvement program, and Erasmus "Journey to Balance," a youth exchange initiative in collaboration with six UE partners.

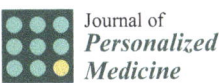

Editorial

Special Issue: Emergency Medicine: Clinical Advances and Challenges in Diagnosis and Treatment

Ovidiu Alexandru Mederle [1,2], Popa Daian Ionel [1,2,*] and Williams Gabriela Carmen [2]

1. Surgery Department, Faculty of Medicine, "Victor Babes" University of Medicine and Pharmacy, E. Murgu Square No. 2, 300041 Timisoara, Romania; mederle.ovidiu@umft.ro
2. Emergency Department, Emergency Clinical Municipal Hospital, Gheorghe Dima Street, Number 5, 300079 Timisoara, Romania; drcarmen.williams@yahoo.com
* Correspondence: daian-ionel.popa@umft.ro; Tel.: +40-746-912-660

1. Introduction

The development of Emergency Medicine brings various challenges. However, this journey offers many opportunities, and with the joint efforts and hard work of medical professionals, continuously updated medical technology and concepts, Emergency Medicine will undergo more historic advancements. The landscape of Emergency Medicine is characterized by its continuous evolution. It has significantly transformed how healthcare professionals respond to emergencies, ensuring the safety of patients in emergencies is still paramount.

This Special Issue entitled "Emergency Medicine: Clinical Advances and Challenges in Diagnosis and Treatment" has attracted 13 high-quality articles contributed by authors from six different countries: Poland, Korea, Taiwan, Romania, Germany, and Italy. These articles highlight the breadth and depth of research in the field, offering insights into the latest advancements and personalized approaches.

2. An Overview of Published Articles

The two studies conducted by Rakesh J. et al. (Contributions 1 and 2) aimed to investigate the usefulness of serum S100B protein levels as a short- and long-term prognostic factor in patients with ischemic stroke and [1] the diagnostic values of S100B in brain damage related to TBI (traumatic brain injury), pointing out that the pivotal role of this protein obtained using these data indicates that S100B may be regarded as a therapeutic target for acute brain injury. Serum biomarker S100B has been explored for its potential role in improving clinical decision-making in the management of patients suffering from ischemic stroke [2].

The detection of high S100B levels in peripheral circulation after acute ischemic stroke and the correlations of S100B levels with infarct size (good) and disability (poor) imply that S100B protein may be used as a peripheral marker in acute ischemic stroke patients. To reduce costs and ED overcrowding and minimize radiation exposure, biomarkers are urgently needed to find patients for whom a CT scan can be avoided. S100B is the most studied astroglia and blood–brain barrier biomarker in traumatic brain injury (TBI). The serum levels of S100B in patients with TBI indicate patient outcomes, where elevated levels correlate with injury severity and mortality. In a parallel effort, authors have initiated the proposal of criteria that utilize serum S100B analysis in the TBI diagnostic process based on NICE guidelines and highlighted the need for more extensive multicenter studies to establish its integration into the clinical algorithm as S100B protein proves to be a promising diagnostic tool [1].

Emergency departments (ED) place a high priority on perfecting the management of acute ischemic stroke. The time-sensitive nature of intervention for stroke patients has been emphasized, with guidelines suggesting the administration of intravenous (IV)

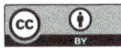

recombinant tissue plasminogen activator (rt-PA) within 4.5 h of symptom onset and the initiation of endovascular procedures "as early as possible" when necessary. According to a study conducted by Daian Popa et al. (Contribution 3), there is potential for improvement in the thrombolysis rate at Municipal Clinical Hospital Timișoara, Romania, despite being relatively favorable compared to global benchmarks. The research revealed a noteworthy association between the highest door-to-CT time and mortality rates for all patients, emphasizing the importance of meeting emergency department (ED) time targets. The findings strongly recommend that hospitals lacking a resolute stroke unit reorganize their acute ischemic stroke (AIS) management protocols to prioritize achieving ED time targets. By doing so, hospitals can enhance their response to AIS cases, ultimately influencing the outcomes of AIS patients and facilitating smoother inter-hospital transfers [3].

Hyelin H. et al. (Contribution 4) focused on developing and confirming a simple tool for predicting bacteremia, a scoring system that helps classify bacteremia risk, stratify patients earlier, and initiate prompt treatment in high-risk patients. Scoring systems can supplement physicians' clinical judgment when deciding whether to perform a blood culture and start treatment. In their retrospective cohort study, conducted over five years, they developed and confirmed a simple bacteremia prediction score. It used only five variables and proved a similar performance to the model with sixteen variables using all laboratory results and vital signs [4].

Antimicrobials are one of the most prescribed drug classes in the ED. The global increase in antimicrobial resistance (AMR) is one of the leading international health threats, reducing the effective treatment of infections, increasing the need for intensive care units (ICUs), the length of stay, healthcare costs, and significantly affecting patient morbidity and mortality. Pathogen resistance develops in response to selective pressure associated with all antibiotic prescribing but is accelerated by inappropriate use. Musuroi S. et al., (Contribution 5) in their retrospective observational study, aimed to evaluate the etiology and antimicrobial resistance (AMR) pattern of community-acquired pathogens, as well as the epidemiological characteristics of patients admitted through the ED, to guide appropriate antibiotic therapy and underlined the imperative introduction of rapid microbiological diagnostic methods in ED to identify AMR strains and improve therapeutic protocols [5].

Hip fracture injuries have been identified as one of the most serious healthcare problems, associated with a high rate of mortality and profound temporary or permanent impairment of quality of life. The effect of delayed surgery on postoperative outcomes has been widely discussed. The demand for early surgery often exceeds available resources, and considerable variability among hospitals in time to surgery has been reported. Confirmation of the clinical consequences of surgical delay on different patient groups could help in the decision-making process when not all patients can be performed on as early as desired. The optimal time for surgery associated with the lowest risk of complications after hip fracture surgery is still under debate. The most controversial factor recognized and examined in multiple studies of hip fractures is the "time-to-surgery" interval, which includes also the time in the emergency department (ED). Authors Daginnus et al. (Contribution 6) analyzed in a study over five years whether the occurrence of complications after the treatment of hip fractures differs according to the patient's type of fractures and the specific treatment procedures. The authors concluded that a 24 h time interval between injury and surgical procedure plays a significant role in extracapsular fractures treated with osteosynthesis but not in intracapsular fractures treated with arthroplasty. Therefore, they recommend reevaluating guidelines on hip fracture surgery according to the patient's case scenario, particularly the individual hip fracture type [6].

Imaging plays a significant role in assessing pulmonary diseases and currently serves as a tool to diagnose lung pathology, check its course, and guide clinical management. Lung ultrasound is a real-time imaging modality that is non-invasive, simple, and free of ionizing radiation. Due to unique features and growing scientific evidence, lung ultrasound (LUS) is an emerging technique for bedside chest imaging in critical care. While the utility of lung ultrasound in the emergency setting is unquestioned, its potential role in the more complex and resource-rich intensive care environment is still under debate. The purpose of this paper by Marco Di Serafino et al. (Contribution 7) is to underline the role of point-of-care LUS in ICUs from a purely radiological point of view as an advanced method in ICU CXR reports to improve the interpretation and monitoring of lung CXR findings [7].

In a study over nine years and a literature review, authors Faur C et al. (Contribution 8) highlighted the importance of early diagnosis and efficient management of axillary arterial injuries associated with proximal humeral fractures, emphasizing the importance of heightened clinical awareness to avoid oversight for these less common injuries. Axillary artery injury due to proximal humerus fracture is rare, although its incidence is uncertain. As the number of inpatient admissions for proximal humerus fractures is on the rise, we are now detecting more axillary artery injuries than we did in the past. Recognition at first presentation can sometimes be complex owing to palpable peripheral pulses and the absence of ischemia. Increased awareness of this injury should be maintained, mainly when paresthesia and concomitant injuries (e.g., brachial plexus or scapula fractures) are present. Accurate physical examination, in combination with a low threshold for Doppler examination or angiography, can set up the diagnosis of axillary artery injury [8].

Authors Anglitoiu B. et al. (Contribution 9) presented a case study detailing the successful staged treatment of posttraumatic tibial osteomyelitis using a unique combination of rib graft and serratus anterior muscle, focusing on wound management, infection control, and limb salvage. The tibia is the most common site of posttraumatic osteomyelitis. In recent years, posttraumatic osteomyelitis has become one of the most essential types of exogenous bone infections. This case report proves that with a careful and comprehensive strategy, patients can achieve positive outcomes despite complex and multifaceted clinical challenges. As the field of orthopedic and trauma surgery continues to progress, the lessons from this case serve as a reminder of the potential for innovation and improvement in patient care, particularly for those facing the daunting prospect of posttraumatic tibial osteomyelitis [9].

Cryptococcemia is a rare, life-threatening fungal infection that can occur in immunocompromised patients. It often presents a diagnostic challenge, given its non-specific clinical manifestation that can mimic other diseases. Cryptococcemia requires early identification and prompt antifungal therapy. Authors Wei-Kai Liao et al. (Contribution 10) presented the first study of applying scoring systems in predicting the mortality risk of patients with cryptococcosis and finding higher scores associated with a significantly higher mortality rate in patients with cryptococcosis. The study offers valuable insights for future guidelines in this area [10].

The COVID-19 pandemic has shown vulnerabilities and brought considerable challenges to medical systems, especially Emergency Medicine. Healthcare personnel need regular, up-to-date information and communication to be protected from chronic stress and poor mental health so they can have a better ability to fulfill their roles. The research of Goniewicz et al. (Contribution 11) was performed online from 2021 to 2022 and included medical professionals from diverse healthcare settings, with the survey link in four provinces of Poland. The study highlighted the importance of adaptive, agile, compassionate, and supportive organizational structures, especially during global health emergencies. While many aspects of the pandemic crisis are still being researched, healthcare organizations must be on the frontline. They must play vital functions by updating and following strict infection prevention and control practices. Smart, targeted investments in health system resilience are needed to improve health and ensure the next shock is less disruptive and costly [11].

The retrospective analysis conducted by Marza A. et al. (Contribution 12) offers exciting insights into the uncommon clinical manifestations, such as spontaneous pneumomediastinum (SPM) and spontaneous pneumothorax (SP) associated with COVID-19, from 2020 to 2022 across five pandemic waves, highlighting the importance of early recognition and management of each SPM/SP case. As COVID-19 has become one of the world's deadliest pandemics known in history, new knowledge has been gained about the virus and its possible complications. The main finding of this analysis shows that the risks associated with mortality, mechanical ventilation, and ICU admission in patients with

SP-SPM are greatly influenced by the presence of COVID-19, extensive lung damage, and a higher number of comorbidities. This holds regardless of patient age and the severity of different strains during a pandemic outbreak [12,13].

Mortality prediction in critically ill patients with cardiogenic shock can guide triage and selection of potentially high-risk treatment options. Authors Jen-Wen Ma et al. (Contribution 13) developed a prediction model to assess the mortality risk and provide guidance on treatment for patients with cardiogenic shock based on four parameters: platelet counts, left ventricular ejection fraction, age, and lactate (PEAL). The study between 2014 and 2019 focused on patients with cardiogenic shock in the emergency department, where clinical outcomes and risk factors for 30-day mortality were evaluated. The model is the first risk score incorporating the number of platelet counts at presentation and showed good predictive performance for all-cause mortality at 30 days in all patients. This score can assess the impact of treatment strategies on expected mortality, enable the design of future clinical trials, and serve as a model for developing future risk scores in cardiology [14].

To conclude, the published papers in this Special Issue covered a wide range of topics. We want to express our gratitude to these authors for their invaluable contributions and dedicated efforts to research. The knowledge and perspectives they have shared have the incredible ability to influence the trajectory of Emergency Medicine, propelling the concept of tailored healthcare. We urge readers to explore the articles and embrace the revolutionary impact of groundbreaking interventions as they strive to elevate the quality of patient care.

Author Contributions: Conceptualization, O.A.M. and W.G.C.; methodology, P.D.I. and W.G.C.; software, O.A.M.; validation, O.A.M., W.G.C. and P.D.I.; formal analysis, O.A.M.; investigation, W.G.C.; resources, P.D.I.; data curation, O.A.M.; writing—original draft preparation, O.A.M., W.G.C. and P.D.I.; writing—review and editing, W.G.C. and P.D.I.; visualization, O.A.M.; supervision, O.A.M. All authors have read and agreed to the published version of the manuscript.

Acknowledgments: The Guest Editors would like to thank the authors who contributed to this Special Issue and the reviewers who dedicated their time to providing the authors with valuable and constructive recommendations.

Conflicts of Interest: The authors declare no conflicts of interest.

List of Contributions:

1. Jalali, R.; Zwiernik, J.; Rotkiewicz, E.; Zwiernik, B.; Kern, A.; Bil, J.; Jalali, A.; Manta, J.; Romaszko, J. Predicting Short- and Long-Term Functional Outcomes Based on Serum S100B Protein Levels in Patients with Ischemic Stroke. *J. Pers. Med.* **2024**, *14*, 80. https://doi.org/10.3390/jpm14010080.
2. Jalali, R.; Godlewska, I.; Fadrowska-Szleper, M.; Pypkowska, A.; Kern, A.; Bil, J.; Manta, J.; Romaszko, J. Significance of S100B Protein as a Rapid Diagnostic Tool in Emergency Departments for Traumatic Brain Injury Patients. *J. Pers. Med.* **2023**, *13*, 1724. https://doi.org/10.3390/jpm13121724.
3. Popa, D.; Iancu, A.; Petrica, A.; Buleu, F.; Williams, C.G.; Sutoi, D.; Trebuian, C.; Tudor, A.; Mederle, O.A. Emergency Department Time Targets for Interhospital Transfer of Patients with Acute Ischemic Stroke. *J. Pers. Med.* **2024**, *14*, 13. https://doi.org/10.3390/jpm14010013.
4. Han, H.; Kim, D.S.; Kim, M.; Heo, S.; Chang, H.; Lee, G.T.; Lee, S.U.; Kim, T.; Yoon, H.; Hwang, S.Y.; et al. A Simple Bacteremia Score for Predicting Bacteremia in Patients with Suspected Infection in the Emergency Department: A Cohort Study. *J. Pers. Med.* **2024**, *14*, 57. https://doi.org/10.3390/jpm14010057.
5. Musuroi, S.I.; Voinescu, A.; Musuroi, C.; Baditoiu, L.M.; Muntean, D.; Izmendi, O.; Jumanca, R.; Licker, M. The Challenges of The Diagnostic and Therapeutic Approach of Patients with Infectious Pathology in Emergency Medicine. *J. Pers. Med.* **2024**, *14*, 46. https://doi.org/10.3390/jpm14010046.
6. Daginnus, A.; Schmitt, J.; Graw, J.A.; Soost, C.; Burchard, R. Rate of Complications after Hip Fractures Caused by Prolonged Time-to-Surgery Depends on the Patient's Individual Type of Fracture and Its Treatment. *J. Pers. Med.* **2023**, *13*, 1470. https://doi.org/10.3390/jpm13101470.
7. Di Serafino, M.; Dell'Aversano Orabona, G.; Caruso, M.; Camillo, C.; Viscardi, D.; Iacobellis, F.; Ronza, R.; Sabatino, V.; Barbuto, L.; Oliva, G.; et al. Point-of-Care Lung Ultrasound in the Intensive Care Unit—The Dark Side of Radiology: Where Do We Stand? *J. Pers. Med.* **2023**, *13*, 1541. https://doi.org/10.3390/jpm13111541.

8. Faur, C.I.; Nitu, R.; Abu-Awwad, S.-A.; Tudoran, C.; Abu-Awwad, A. The Arterial Axis Lesions in Proximal Humeral Fractures—Case Report and Literature Review. *J. Pers. Med.* **2023**, *13*, 1712. https://doi.org/10.3390/jpm13121712.
9. Anglitoiu, B.; Abu-Awwad, A.; Patrascu, J.-M., Jr.; Abu-Awwad, S.-A.; Dinu, A.R.; Totorean, A.-D.; Cojocaru, D.; Sandesc, M.-A. Staged Treatment of Posttraumatic Tibial Osteomyelitis with Rib Graft and Serratus Anterior Muscle Autografts—Case Report. *J. Pers. Med.* **2023**, *13*, 1651. https://doi.org/10.3390/jpm13121651.
10. Liao, W.-K.; Hsieh, M.-S.; Hu, S.-Y.; Huang, S.-C.; Tsai, C.-A.; Chang, Y.-Z.; Tsai, Y.-C. Predictive Performance of Scoring Systems for Mortality Risk in Patients with Cryptococcemia: An Observational Study. *J. Pers. Med.* **2023**, *13*, 1358. https://doi.org/10.3390/jpm13091358.
11. Goniewicz, M.; Włoszczak-Szubzda, A.; Al-Wathinani, A.M.; Goniewicz, K. Resilience in Emergency Medicine during COVID-19: Evaluating Staff Expectations and Preparedness. *J. Pers. Med.* **2023**, *13*, 1545. https://doi.org/10.3390/jpm13111545.
12. Marza, A.M.; Cindrea, A.C.; Petrica, A.; Stanciugelu, A.V.; Barsac, C.; Mocanu, A.; Critu, R.; Botea, M.O.; Trebuian, C.I.; Lungeanu, D. Non-Ventilated Patients with Spontaneous Pneumothorax or Pneumomediastinum Associated with COVID-19: Three-Year Debriefing across Five Pandemic Waves. *J. Pers. Med.* **2023**, *13*, 1497. https://doi.org/10.3390/jpm13101497.
13. Ma, J.-W.; Hu, S.-Y.; Hsieh, M.-S.; Lee, Y.-C.; Huang, S.-C.; Chen, K.-J.; Chang, Y.-Z.; Tsai, Y.-C. PEAL Score to Predict the Mortality Risk of Cardiogenic Shock in the Emergency Department: An Observational Study. *J. Pers. Med.* **2023**, *13*, 1614. https://doi.org/10.3390/jpm13111614.

References

1. Wang, K.K.; Yang, Z.; Zhu, T.; Shi, Y.; Rubenstein, R.; Tyndall, J.A.; Manley, G.T. An update on diagnostic and prognostic biomarkers for traumatic brain injury. *Expert Rev. Mol. Diagn.* **2018**, *18*, 165–180. [CrossRef] [PubMed]
2. Weglewski, A.; Ryglewicz, D.; Mular, A.; Juryńczyk, J. Zmiany stezenia białka S100B w surowicy krwi w udarze niedokrwiennym i krwotocznym mózgu w zaleznosci od wielkosci ogniska udarowego [Changes of protein S100B serum concentration during ischemic and hemorrhagic stroke in relation to the volume of stroke lesion]. *Neurol. Neurochir. Pol.* **2005**, *39*, 310–317. (In Polish) [PubMed]
3. Stubblefield, J.J.; Lechleiter, J.D. Time to Target Stroke: Examining the Circadian System in Stroke. *Yale J. Biol. Med.* **2019**, *92*, 349–357. [PubMed]
4. Su, C.; Tsai, I.-T.; Lai, C.-H.; Lin, K.-H.; Chen, C.; Hsu, Y.-C. Prediction of 30-Day Mortality Using the Quick Pitt Bacteremia Score in Hospitalized Patients with *Klebsiella pneumoniae* Infection. *Infect. Drug Resist.* **2023**, *16*, 4807–4815. [CrossRef] [PubMed]
5. Monari, C.; Onorato, L.; Allegorico, E.; Minerva, V.; Macera, M.; Bosso, G.; Calò, F.; Pagano, A.; Russo, T.; Sansone, G.; et al. The impact of a non-restrictive Antimicrobial Stewardship Program in the emergency department of a secondary-level Italian hospital. *Intern. Emerg. Med.* **2023**. [CrossRef] [PubMed]
6. Simunovic, N.; Devereaux, P.J.; Bhandari, M. Surgery for hip fractures: Does surgical delay affect outcomes? *Indian J. Orthop.* **2011**, *45*, 27–32. [CrossRef] [PubMed]
7. Mojoli, F.; Bouhemad, B.; Mongodi, S.; Lichtenstein, D. Lung Ultrasound for Critically Ill Patients. *Am. J. Respir. Crit. Care Med.* **2019**, *199*, 701–714, Erratum in *Am. J. Respir. Crit. Care Med.* **2020**, *201*, 1015; Erratum in *Am. J. Respir. Crit. Care Med.* **2020**, *201*, 1454. [CrossRef] [PubMed]
8. Karita, Y.; Kimura, Y.; Sasaki, S.; Nitobe, T.; Tsuda, E.; Ishibashi, Y. Axillary artery and brachial plexus injury secondary to proximal humeral fractures: A report of 2 cases. *Int. J. Surg. Case Rep.* **2018**, *50*, 106–110. [CrossRef] [PubMed]
9. Arshad, Z.; Lau, E.J.-S.; Aslam, A.; Thahir, A.; Krkovic, M. Management of chronic osteomyelitis of the femur and tibia: A scoping review. *EFORT Open Rev.* **2021**, *6*, 704–715. [CrossRef] [PubMed]
10. Jean, S.-S.; Fang, C.; Shau, W.; Chen, Y.; Chang, S.; Hsueh, P.; Hung, C.; Luh, K. Cryptococcaemia: Clinical features and prognostic factors. *QJM Int. J. Med.* **2002**, *95*, 511–518. [PubMed]
11. Shah, Z.; Singh, V.; Supehia, S.; Mohan, L.; Gupta, P.K.; Sharma, M.; Sharma, S. Expectations of healthcare personnel from infection prevention and control services for preparedness of healthcare organization in view of COVID-19 pandemic. *Med. J. Armed Forces India* **2021**, *77* (Suppl. 2), S459–S465. [CrossRef] [PubMed]
12. Nieves-Ortiz, A.A.; Fonseca-Ferrerm, V.; Hernández-Moyam, K.; Ramirezm, K.M.; Ayala-Rivera, J.; Delgado, M.; Garcia-Puebla, J.; Fernández-Medero, R.L.; Fernández-González, R. Spontaneous pneumomediastinum associated with COVID-19: Rare complication of 2020 pandemic. *J. Pulmonol. Respir. Res.* **2020**, *4*, 018–020.
13. Talwar, A.; Esquire, A.; Sahni, S.; Verma, S.; Grullon, J.; Patel, P. Spontaneous pneumomediastinum: Time for consensus. *N. Am. J. Med. Sci.* **2013**, *5*, 460–464. [CrossRef] [PubMed]
14. Kalra, S.; Ranard, L.S.; Memon, S.; Rao, P.; Garan, A.R.; Masoumi, A.; O'Neill, W.; Kapur, N.K.; Karmpaliotis, D.; Fried, J.A.; et al. Risk Prediction in Cardiogenic Shock: Current State of Knowledge, Challenges and Opportunities. *J. Card. Fail.* **2021**, *27*, 1099–1110. [CrossRef] [PubMed]

Disclaimer/Publisher's Note: The statements, opinions and data contained in all publications are solely those of the individual author(s) and contributor(s) and not of MDPI and/or the editor(s). MDPI and/or the editor(s) disclaim responsibility for any injury to people or property resulting from any ideas, methods, instructions or products referred to in the content.

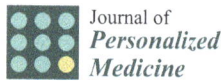

Article

Predicting Short- and Long-Term Functional Outcomes Based on Serum S100B Protein Levels in Patients with Ischemic Stroke

Rakesh Jalali [1,2,*], Jacek Zwiernik [3], Ewa Rotkiewicz [1], Beata Zwiernik [3], Adam Kern [4], Jacek Bil [5], Anita Jalali [6], Joanna Manta [1,2] and Jerzy Romaszko [7]

[1] Department of Emergency Medicine, School of Medicine, Collegium Medicum, University of Warmia and Mazury, 10-082 Olsztyn, Poland; ewarotkiewicz@wp.pl (E.R.)
[2] Clinical Emergency Department, Regional Specialist Hospital, 10-561 Olsztyn, Poland
[3] Department of Neurology, School of Medicine, Collegium Medicum, University of Warmia and Mazury, 10-082 Olsztyn, Poland; jacek.zwiernik@uwm.edu.pl (J.Z.); beata.zwiernik@uwm.edu.pl (B.Z.)
[4] Department of Cardiology and Internal Medicine, School of Medicine, Collegium Medicum, University of Warmia and Mazury, 10-082 Olsztyn, Poland; adam.kern@uwm.edu.pl
[5] Department of Invasive Cardiology, Centre of Postgraduate Medical Education, 01-813 Warsaw, Poland; jacek.bil@cmkp.edu.pl
[6] Students' Research Group, Medical University of Warsaw, 02-091 Warsaw, Poland; s079559@student.wum.edu.pl
[7] Department of Family Medicine and Infectious Diseases, School of Medicine, Collegium Medicum, University of Warmia and Mazury, 10-082 Olsztyn, Poland; jerzy.romaszko@uwm.edu.pl
* Correspondence: rakesh.jalali@uwm.edu.pl

Abstract: Background: Ischemic stroke is one of the leading causes of mortality and disability. The neuroimaging methods are the gold standard for diagnostics. Biomarkers of cerebral ischemia are considered to be potentially helpful in the determination of the etiology and prognosis of patients with ischemic stroke. Aim: This study aimed to investigate the usefulness of serum S100B protein levels as a short- and long-term prognostic factor in patients with ischemic stroke. Study design and methods: The study group comprised 65 patients with ischemic stroke. S100B protein levels were measured by immunoenzymatic assay. Short-term functional outcome was determined by the NIHSS score on day 1 and the difference in the NIHSS scores between day 1 and day 9 (delta NIHSS). Long-term outcome was assessed by the modified Rankin Scale (MRS) at 3 months after the stroke. At the end of the study, patients were divided into groups based on the NIHSS score on day 9 (0–8 "good" and >8 "poor"), the delta NIHSS ("no improvement" ≤ 0 and >0 "improvement"), and the MRS ("good" 0–2 and >2 "poor"). Differences in S100B levels between groups were analyzed with the ROC curve to establish the optimal cut-off point for S100B. The odds ratio was calculated to determine the strength of association. Correlations between S100B levels at three time points and these variables were evaluated. Results: We revealed a statistically significant correlation between S100B levels at each measurement point (<24 h, 24–48 H, 48–72 h) and the NIHSS score on day 9 (R Spearman 0.534, 0.631, and 0.517, respectively) and the MRS score after 3 months (R Spearman 0.620, 0.657, and 0.617, respectively). No statistically significant correlation was found between S100B levels and the delta NIHSS. Analysis of the ROC curve confirmed a high sensitivity and specificity for S100B. The calculated AUC for the NIHSS on day 9 were 90.2%, 95.0%, and 82.2%, respectively, and for the MRS, 83.5%, 83.4%, and 84.0%, respectively. After determining the S100B cut-off, the odds ratio for beneficial effect (NIHSS ≤ 8 at day 9 or MRS 0–2 after 3 months) was determined for each sampling point. Conclusion: S100B is a useful marker for predicting short- and long-term functional outcomes in patients with ischemic stroke.

Keywords: ischemic stroke; functional outcome; S100B

Citation: Jalali, R.; Zwiernik, J.; Rotkiewicz, E.; Zwiernik, B.; Kern, A.; Bil, J.; Jalali, A.; Manta, J.; Romaszko, J. Predicting Short- and Long-Term Functional Outcomes Based on Serum S100B Protein Levels in Patients with Ischemic Stroke. *J. Pers. Med.* **2024**, *14*, 80. https://doi.org/10.3390/jpm14010080

Academic Editor: Ovidiu Alexandru Mederle

Received: 25 November 2023
Revised: 28 December 2023
Accepted: 4 January 2024
Published: 10 January 2024

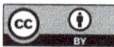

Copyright: © 2024 by the authors. Licensee MDPI, Basel, Switzerland. This article is an open access article distributed under the terms and conditions of the Creative Commons Attribution (CC BY) license (https://creativecommons.org/licenses/by/4.0/).

1. Introduction

Despite advances in diagnosis and treatment, ischemic stroke remains one of the leading causes of mortality and disability [1–3]. The development of diagnostic tools, especially neuroimaging methods, makes it possible to diagnose ischemic stroke with increasing certainty, determine the size of the ischemic area, and introduce more effective treatment. Unfortunately, this is also associated with an increase in costs [4,5]. Determining the size of a stroke lesion has implications for the prognosis of patients' short- and long-term functional improvement. The commonly available computed tomography (CT) is not very sensitive in this regard and often fails to visualize early ischemic lesions. Magnetic resonance imaging (MRI) is more sensitive but has many limitations: it cannot be performed on patients with pacemakers and other metal objects, as well as in anxious patients. It is also less accessible, more time-consuming, and generates higher costs [6–8]. The commonly used National Institutes of Health Stroke Scale (NIHSS) was designed to determine the physical size of the ischemic area. Unfortunately, it is not very sensitive in regard to damage to the right brain hemisphere and the posterior circulation [9,10]. Therefore, in recent decades, biomarkers of cerebral ischemia have been searched for that can assist clinicians in the differential diagnosis, as well as in the determination of the etiology and prognosis of patients with ischemic stroke [11,12]. One of the biomarkers under scrutiny is S100B. It belongs to a group of small proteins with a specific calcium-binding capacity. In the central nervous system (CNS), it is secreted from astrocytes. Its biological role is to stimulate the proliferation and maturation of neurons and to promote the development of astrocytes and oligodendrocytes. In ischemic stroke, S100B is released into the blood and cerebrospinal fluid. Increased S100B levels in the extracellular space promote neuroinflammation, thus exacerbating brain tissue damage [13,14]. Since S100B has a short biological half-life, its presence in the blood indicates an active process that damages brain tissue. Significantly, S100B release appears to take place not in the infarct core (where there is a lack of perfusion that would allow its release into the blood) but in the penumbra area and the area of local brain edema as a response to the presence of adenosine and glutamate. Thus, it is hypothetically possible to control the course of ischemic stroke and formulate a prognosis for the recovery [15,16]. The results of clinical studies conducted in recent years have suggested that patients with ischemic stroke have significantly elevated blood levels of S100B. Some studies have also revealed that S100B levels correlate with the severity of ischemic stroke, as measured by the NIHSS, and may be useful in determining functional prognosis [17–20]. The aim of our study was to investigate the relationship between serum S100B levels and their changes over time and short- and long-term functional outcomes in patients with ischemic stroke.

2. Materials and Methods

Patients were included in the study in years 2018 to 2020 in accordance with the protocol approved by the Bioethics Committee of the Warmia and Mazury Regional Chamber of Physicians and Dentists in Olsztyn (WMIL-KB/266/2018) dated 17 May 2018, and the Clinical Research Committee of the Regional Specialized Hospital in Olsztyn, Poland. The aim of the study was to determine the role of arterial stiffness as a risk factor for ischemic stroke and the usefulness of biomarkers, including S100B protein, in assessing early and late prognosis. After obtaining consent to participate in the study, established procedures were performed for each patient. To determine S100B levels, blood was drawn three times—on admission, on the second day, and on the third day. Blood samples were collected in biochemical tubes. Then, 10 min after collection, samples were centrifuged for 20 min with a frequency of 3000 revolutions per minute. Briefly, 1 mL of the obtained serum was transferred to Eppendorf tubes and frozen to $-20\ °C$. Samples are durable for up to 3 months in this temperature. Prior to analysis, tubes were thawed and brought to a temperature of 20–$25\ °C$. Samples with visible turbidity were centrifuged.

All recognized procedures for treating ischemic stroke, including thrombolytic therapy, mechanical thrombectomy, or a combination of both, were performed, depending on the indication. Stroke severity was determined with the NIHSS score and was assessed on admission and on the ninth day. The change in the NIHSS scores during that time was considered to be an indicator for the short-term functional outcome. The long-term functional outcome was assessed three months following the stroke with the Modified Rankin Scale (MRS). As in other similarly designed studies, in order to facilitate a better comparison of the obtained results, patients were arbitrarily categorized into two groups based on the NIHSS score on the ninth day: NIHSS 0–8 (mild to moderate ischemic stroke) and NIHSS >8 (moderate to severe stroke). For the same reasons, patients were divided according to the MRS score after 3 months: 0–2 (no residual symptoms to slight disability) and >2 (from slight to severe disability). A routine medical history was taken, including risk factors for ischemic stroke. The type of ischemic stroke was determined with the Trial of Org 10,172 in Acute Stroke Treatment (TOAST) classification.

Serum concentrations of S100B were determined by the electrochemiluminescence immunoassay (ECLIA) method on the Cobas 6000 device, which was calibrated with S100 CalSet. The Roche Elecsys® S100 kit (Roche, Mannheim, Germany) with detection limits between 0.005 and 39 µg/L was used according to the manufacturer's instructions. PerciControl Universal PCU1 and PCU2 were used for controlling the accuracy of measurements.

Qualitative data were expressed in percentages (%) and numbers (n). Quantitative data were expressed as mean and standard deviation (SD). Statistical analyses were performed with Statistica software12. Mean S100B values in two groups were compared with Student's t-test for paired data. Analysis of variance was used for a larger number of groups. The correlation between variables was determined with Spearman's rank correlation coefficient, or Pearson's linear correlation coefficient. A p-value ≤ 0.05 was considered as statistically significant. The bivariate tables were analyzed with Chi-square, V-square, and Chi-square with Yates' correction. McNemar's test was used for paired data. ROC curves were analyzed with pROC package for R. The Youden Index was used to determine the optimal cut-off point for a continuous variable. DeLong's test for correlated curves was used to compare two AUCs. Power calculations were performed for each ROC curve separately.

3. Results

In total, 65 patients were included in the study. The average age was 67 years; women constituted 52% of the study group. Demographic characteristics of the group are presented in Table 1.

Changes in the NIHSS score between admission and day 9, which are the basis for further calculations, are presented in Table 2.

When correlating the S100B level < 24 h with the short-term functional outcome as measured by the NIHSS on day 9, a significant correlation between them was revealed, similarly to the remaining time points—24–48 h and 48–72 h. When correlating the S100B level < 24 h with the long-term functional outcome as measured by MRS after 3 months, a significant correlation between them was revealed, similarly to the remaining time points—24–48 h and 48–72 h. However, there was no significant correlation between the S100B level and delta NIHSS (Table 3).

At the end of the study, patients were divided into groups based on their NIHSS score on day 9 (0–8 "good" and >8 "poor"), the delta NIHSS ("no improvement" ≤ 0 and >0 "improvement"), and the MRS ("good" 0–2 and >2 "poor"). The ROC curve analysis revealed that the cut-off value of S100B in each sampling point was 0.100 µg/L. For the ROC curve to determine the sensitivity and specificity of S100B at different time points, predicting the outcome measured as "good" (NIHSS 0–8) and "poor" (NIHSS > 8), the AUC was 95.0% (89.3–100.0%) for time point 24–48 h (sensitivity 82.1, specificity 100.0%). For other sampling points, the AUC was 90.2% (<24 h) and 82.2% (>48 h), respectively (Figure 1).

Table 1. Baseline characteristic and stroke risk factors.

Factor	Total Patients ($n = 65$)
Sex (female)	34 (52.31%)
Age (years)	67.43 ± 13.08 *
Risk factors:	
Hypertension	45 (69.23%)
Diabetes	23 (35.38%)
Dyslipidemia	26 (40.00%)
Atrial fibrillation	28 (43.08%)
Smoking	32 (49.23%)
Thrombectomy only	5 (7.70%)
Thrombolysis only	20 (30.77%)
Thrombolysis and thrombectomy	10 (15.40%)
TOAST:	
Large artery atherosclerosis (LAA)	13 (20.00%)
Small artery occlusion (SAO)	12 (18.46%)
Cardio embolism (CE)	20 (30.77%)
Stroke of undetermined etiology (SUE)	20 (30.77%)
Stroke of other determined etiology	0 (0.00%)

* mean and SD.

Table 2. Comparison of NIHSS groups.

NIHSS on Admission	NIHSS on Day 9		Total
	0–8	>8	
0–8	38	0	38
>8	15	12	27
Total	53	12	65
$p < 0.001$		McNemary test (A/D)	

Table 3. Correlation between S100B < 24 h and 24–48 h and 48–72 h with NIHSS, delta NIHSS, and MRS.

		NIHSS on Day 9	Delta NIHSS	MRS after 3 Months
S100B < 24 h	R(p)	0.534 (0.000)	−0.039 (0.761)	0.620 (0.000)
S100B 24 h–48 h	R(p)	0.631 (0.000)	0.127 (0.899)	0.657 (0.000)
S100B > 48 h	R(p)	0.517 (0.000)	−1.176 (0.245)	0.617 (0.000)

For the ROC curve to determine the sensitivity and specificity of S100B at different time points predicting the short-term outcome measured as "no improvement" (delta NIHSS ≤ 0) and "improvement" (delta NIHSS > 0), the AUC was 74.2% (51.4–97.0%) for time point >48 h (sensitivity 48.0, specificity 100.0%). For other sampling points, the AUC was 65.8% (<24 h) and 64.7% (24–48 h), respectively (Figure 2).

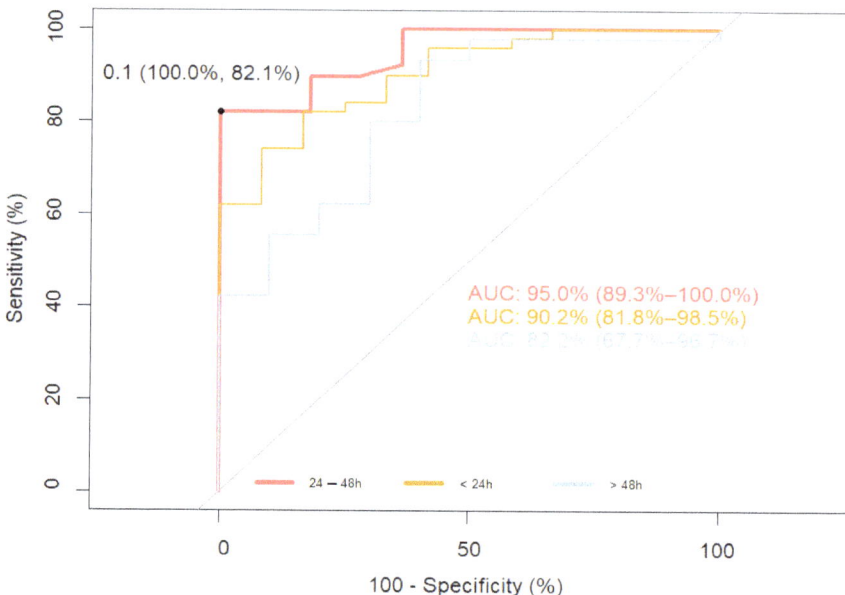

Figure 1. ROC curve to determine the sensitivity and specificity of S100B at different time points, predicting the outcome measured as "good" (NIHSS 0–8) and "poor" (NIHSS > 8). The bootstrap method was used to determine confidence intervals. The Youden Index was used for setting optimal thresholds.

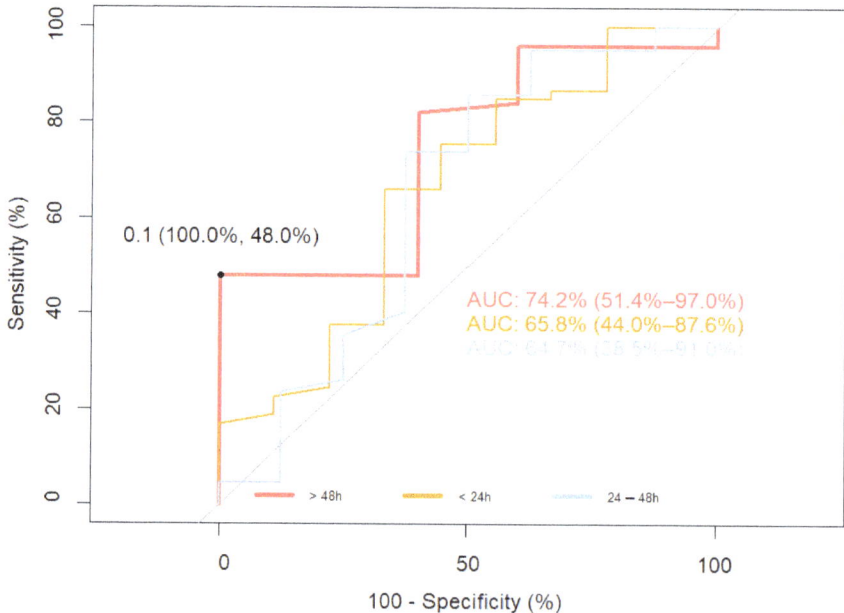

Figure 2. ROC curve to determine the sensitivity and specificity of S100B at different time points, predicting the short-term outcome measured as "no improvement" (delta NIHSS $\leq$ 0) and "improvement" (delta NIHSS > 0). The bootstrap method was used to determine confidence intervals. The Youden Index was used for setting optimal thresholds.

For the ROC curve to determine the sensitivity and specificity of S100B at different time points, predicting the long-term outcome measured as "good" (MRS 0–2) and "poor" (MRS ≥ 3), the AUC was 83.4% (71.3–95.5%) for time point 24–48 h (sensitivity 80.0%, specificity 80.0%). For other sampling points, the AUC was 83.5% (73.3–93.8%) (<24 h) (sensitivity 80.0%, specificity 80.0%) and 84.0% (73.8–94.1%) (24–48 h), respectively (Figure 3).

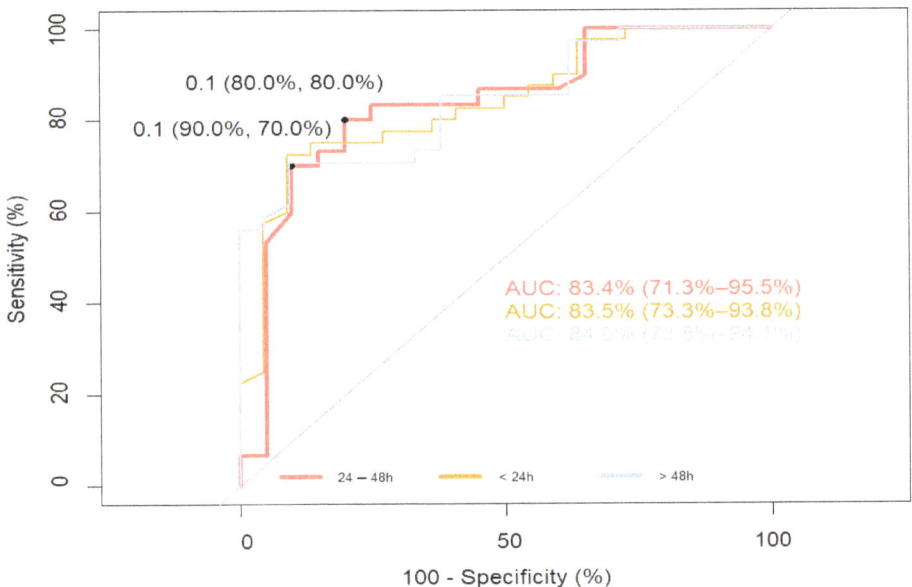

Figure 3. ROC curve to determine the sensitivity and specificity of S100B at different time points, predicting the long-term outcome measured as "good" (MRS 0–2) and "poor" (MRS ≥ 3). The Youden Index was used for setting optimal thresholds.

According to the ROC curve analysis, we used the cut-off 0.100 µg/L and then categorized the subjects into two groups. The first group included subjects with a serum S100B level of 0.100 µg/L or less, and the second group consisted of subjects with a S100B level of 0.100 µg/L or above. We found out that this cut-off threshold was useful in defining groups with better prognoses in terms of early and late disability. Results of this analysis are provided in Tables 4 and 5.

Table 4. OR for a chance to achieve a better functional result—MRS 0–2 after 3 months.

	Cut-Off, µg/L	MRS 0–2 OR	p
S100B < 24 h	0.1	4.78 (95% CI: 1.47; 15.55)	0.009
S100B 24 h–48 h	0.1	OR = 9.35 (95% CI: 3.04; 28.77)	0.001
S100B 48 h–72 h	0.1	OR = 4.26 (95% CI: 1.42; 12.8)	0.01

Table 5. OR for a chance to achieve a better functional result—NIHSS 0–8 on day 9.

	Cut-Off	NIHSS 0–8 OR	p
S100B < 24 h	0.1	13.51 (95% CI: 3.24; 56.36)	0.001
S100B 24 h–48 h	0.1	15.35 (95% CI: 4.06; 58)	0.001
S100B 48 h–72 h	0.1	4.48 (95% CI: 1.12; 17.92)	0.034

Analysis of variance did not reveal any statistically significant differences in the mean levels of S100B between various subtypes of ischemic stroke—LAA, SAO, CE, and SUC (stroke of undetermined etiology), with the p-values of 0.911, 0.369, 0.262, and 0.693, respectively.

No statistically significant differences were also revealed in the mean levels of S100B between patients who had undergone recanalization (thrombolytic therapy, mechanical thrombectomy, or the combination of both) and patients treated conservatively. The p-value was 0.649, 0.245, and 0.837, respectively (see Figures S1–S7, Supplementary Files).

4. Discussion

The main finding supporting the validity of our study is that serum S100B levels in patients with ischemic stroke, measured on day 1, 2 and 3, are strongly correlated with the short-term functional outcomes determined with the NIHSS on day 9 after the stroke, as well as with the long-term outcomes, which were assessed with the MRS after 3 months (Figures 1 and 3).

Our interest in the S100B protein stems from several reasons. Despite the development of diagnostic methods, there is still no way to continuously, non-invasively, and inexpensively monitor the changes in brain tissue that occur as a result of ischemia. S100B, unlike other proteins in the S100 family, is more specific to brain tissue and appears in the blood when the brain is damaged rather than other organs [21]. Perfusion is necessary for this protein to appear in the blood, so its presence is not related to the infarct core but to the penumbra and the developing cytotoxic cerebral edema. Moreover, once released from the cell, it promotes inflammation and increases cytotoxic edema. These properties, further supported by clinical studies, make S100B an excellent marker for stroke severity regarding active metabolic responses [13,14,22]. Given the short half-life of this protein and renal clearance, serum S100B levels illustrate the course of ischemic stroke in real-time [15,16]. It seems that these suppositions are in line with clinical observations. Elting et al. compared changes in S100B levels in patients with ischemic stroke, transient ischemic attack (TIA), and traumatic brain injury (TBI). In patients with ischemic stroke, peak levels of S100B were most often observed on day 3 or 4 after the stroke (during the formation of cytotoxic edema), whereas in patients with TBI, peak levels were observed on day 1 or 2 after the injury [15]. The same results were obtained by Weglewski et al. who studied 57 patients and observed peak levels of S100B on day 3 after ischemic stroke [23]. An important question is whether short- and long-term functional outcomes can be predicted based on the changes in S100B levels. Our study revealed that S100B levels measured on days 1, 2 and 3 were significantly correlated with the NIHSS scores on day 9 and the MRS scores after 3 months (Table 3). In addition, ROC curve analysis confirmed a high sensitivity and specificity of S100B in predicting functional outcomes (Figures 1 and 3). The power computation for ROC curves was confirmed by the results obtained for the odds ratio. These results do not fully match those obtained by other researchers. Selcuk et al. searched for correlations between S100B levels measured on days 1, 3, 5 and the MRS score after 1 month. They revealed only a weak correlation with S100B measured on day 3. However, it should be remembered that their study was conducted on a very small group of patients ($n = 26$), and the time points for the functional assessment with the MRS were different from those in our study [24]. Abdel et al. determined the serum S100B levels in a group of 40 patients on day 1 and 3 and then correlated the results with the NIHSS and MRS on day 14. They found a strong correlation on day 3, but not on day 1. The AUC calculated based on the ROC curve was characterized by a high sensitivity and specificity (91.0% and 80.0%, respectively) and was similar to our results [25]. The lack of correlation on day 1 may be due to the methodology as the measurement of the S100B level can vary in time up to several minutes. Presently, there are no universally adopted standards regarding the time for collecting samples. Moreover, researchers use different time points to assess the outcome and different clinical scales. This can be confirmed by the results obtained by Singapore researchers because their study was designed similarly to ours. In order to determine S100B levels, blood was collected on days 1 and 3, and the assessment with the MRS was performed after 1 and 3 months. A strong correlation between S100B levels and the functional outcome after 3 months was revealed. A very interesting finding of that study was the relationship between the functional outcome and the rate of the decrease of S100B levels over time [26]. Branco et al. studied, in the same way as we did, a group of 131 patients only with ischemic stroke [27]. They determined biomarker levels (CRP, D-dimer, and fibrinogen) on admission, while blood was collected 48 h later to measure S100B levels. The results obtained were compared with the MRS scores after 48 h and 12 weeks following the stroke. The authors revealed an evident correlation between S100B levels and the MRS scores after 12 weeks. Their results are in line with our findings. Also, the cut-off point for S100B in that study (140 ng/L) was the same as ours. However, no association was found between the other biomarkers tested and the functional outcome. Retnaningsih et al. arrived at interesting findings [28]. In their study conducted on 42 patients with ischemic stroke, they measured S100B levels on day 3 after the stroke. Stroke severity was assessed with the NIHSS on days 3 and 7. Then, the patients were divided into two groups: with improvement according to the NIHSS score and without improvement. The ROC curve was analyzed to establish the cut-off point for S100B. This parameter was employed to determine the odds ratio for clinical improvement and, consequently, for a good functional outcome. For the cut-off point at the level of 608 ng/mL and below, the odds ratio for the improved outcome was six-fold higher than for the value of S100B above 608 ng/mL (26). In our study, we also attempted to determine the odds ratio for clinical improvement. Our results in this regard were not satisfactory due to the small number of measurements (Figure 2). However, our calculations for the beneficial outcome showed the strength of the ROC curve (Tables 4 and 5). Although we did not reveal significant differences in S100B levels between patients who had recanalization performed, in our view, this is not inconsistent with the latest study by Luger et al. In their study involving 171 patients, they demonstrated that the S100B level assessed on the second day following thrombectomy is an independent prognostic factor in the long-term functional outcome of ischemic stroke. Unfortunately, they did not compare the results they obtained with the group without recanalization [29]. In another study, Hawash et al. assessed the prognostic usefulness of S100B in a group of 80 patients with ischemic stroke. Their analyses indicate that S100B alone is a significant prognostic factor, but the performed thrombolysis does not influence its prognostic strength [17]. Our results, similarly to the aforementioned studies, suggest that the statistical strength of S100B in determining long-term functional outcome in ischemic stroke is similar for all patients, irrespective of the introduced treatment (Figures S5–S7). As in the case of treatment methods, we also did not find significant correlations between ischemic stroke subtypes and S100B levels. This is intriguing because S100B is an indicator of the size of the infarct core, and so we had expected to find at least a correlation between S100B levels and ischemic stroke caused by large artery atherosclerosis (LAA). Nevertheless, other researchers obtained similar results. Foerch et al. assessed the usefulness of S100B in predicting malignant course of infarction resulting from the occlusion of the middle cerebral artery (MCA). They revealed that the occlusion of MCA is as frequent in the course of LAA as in the cardio embolism subtype [30]. Analogous results were obtained by Yoruk Hazar et al., who examined 50 patients with ischemic stroke and compared the results with those of healthy volunteers [18]. Researchers from Singapore arrived at even more far-reaching conclusions. Sakdejayont et al. revealed that the level of S100B allows for the determination of long-term functional outcomes and severity of the course of ischemic stroke, irrespective of its mechanism. S100B levels were measured before the treatment was commenced (thrombolysis, thrombectomy, antiplatelet therapy) and after 72 h. The difference between these levels was also determined. Stroke severity was established based on the NIHSS score, and the outcome was measured with the Ranking Scale after 30 and 90 days. Although their study group had different characteristics than our study (small artery occlusion was the dominating subtype), the relation of groups with LAA occlusion and cardio embolism vs. small artery occlusion and EUS was similar. The conducted analyses revealed that the S100B level after 72 h and the change in the levels between the measurement points are the optimal prognostic factors for the adverse outcome irrespective of the stroke type [26]. This seems to be easily explained: prognosis depends on the size of the ischemic area and not on the stroke etiology. We believe that our results, which confirm those obtained by other researchers, will consolidate knowledge in this area (Figures S1–S4). We are aware of the limitations of our study. A major drawback is the lack of a control group due to financial constraints. The small group of patients included in the study did not allow us to conduct reliable statistical analyses to independently evaluate other risk factors affecting the course of the disease. In particular, we regret that we were unable to determine the usefulness of S100B in monitoring permanent recanalization because this might potentially make this molecule a cheap and non-invasive marker.

5. Conclusions

Ultimately, we suggest that serum S100B protein levels can predict the course of ischemic stroke in the context of short- and long-term functional outcomes.

Supplementary Materials: The following supporting information can be downloaded at https://www.mdpi.com/article/10.3390/jpm14010080/s1, Figure S1. Distribution of S100B levels over time according to stroke subtype—LAA. Figure S2. Distribution of S100B levels over time according to stroke subtype—SAO. Figure S3. Distribution of S100B levels over time according to stroke subtype—CE. Figure S4. Distribution of S100B levels over time according to stroke subtype—SUE. Figure S5. Distribution of S100B levels over time according to stroke treatment—thrombolysis vs. no recanalisation. Figure S6. Distribution of S100B levels over time according to stroke treatment—thrombectomy vs. no recanalisation. Figure S7. Distribution of S100B levels over time according to stroke treatment—thrombolysis with thrombectomy vs. no recanalisation.

Author Contributions: Conceptualization, R.J.; methodology, R.J. and J.Z.; software, J.Z.; formal analysis, R.J. and J.Z.; investigation, R.J. and J.Z.; resources, R.J.; data curation, R.J., J.Z., E.R., J.B., A.K., A.J. and J.M.; writing—original draft, R.J. and J.Z.; writing—review and editing, R.J., J.Z., E.R., J.B., A.K., B.Z., A.J., J.M. and J.R.; visualization, R.J., J.Z. and B.Z.; supervision, R.J. and J.R.; project administration, R.J. All authors have read and agreed to the published version of the manuscript.

Funding: The research was financially supported by the Statutory research funding from the University of Warmia and Mazury, Decision Nr 25.014.002-25.620.024-300.

Institutional Review Board Statement: Patients were included in the study in accordance with the protocol approved by the Bioethics Committee of the Warmia and Mazury Regional Chamber of Physicians and Dentists in Olsztyn (WMIL-KB/266/2018) dated 17 May 2018.

Informed Consent Statement: Informed consent was obtained from the subjects included in the study.

Data Availability Statement: The data that support the findings of this study are available on request from the corresponding author.

Conflicts of Interest: Authors declare no conflict of interest.

References

1. Feigin, V.L.; Stark, B.; Johnson, C. GBD 2019 Stroke Collaborators Global, regional, and national burden of stroke and its risk factors, 1990–2019: A systematic analysis for the Global Burden of Disease Study 2019. *Lancet Neurol.* **2021**, *20*, 795–820. [CrossRef] [PubMed]
2. Luengo-Fernandez, R.; Violato, M.; Candio, P.; Leal, J. Economic burden of stroke across Europe: A population-based cost analysis. *Eur. Stroke J.* **2020**, *5*, 17–25. [CrossRef] [PubMed]
3. Pu, L.; Wang, L.; Zhang, R.; Zhao, T.; Jiang, Y.; Han, L. Projected Global Trends in Ischemic Stroke Incidence, Deaths and Disability-Adjusted Life Years from 2020 to 2030. *Stroke* **2023**, *54*, 1330–1339. [CrossRef]
4. Burke, J.F. Cost and utility in the diagnostic evaluation of stroke. *Contin. Lifelong Learn. Neurol.* **2014**, *20*, 436. [CrossRef]
5. Girotra, T.; Lekoubou, A.; Bishu, K.G.; Ovbiagele, B. A contemporary and comprehensive analysis of the costs of stroke in the United States. *J. Neurol. Sci.* **2020**, *410*, 116643. [CrossRef]
6. Latchaw, R.E.; Alberts, M.J.; Lev, M.H.; Connors, J.J.; Harbaugh, R.E.; Higashida, R.T.; Hobson, R.; Kidwell, C.S.; Koroshetz, W.J.; Mathews, V. Recommendations for imaging of acute ischemic stroke: A scientific statement from the American Heart Association. *Stroke* **2009**, *40*, 3646–3678. [CrossRef] [PubMed]

7. Nukovic, J.J.; Opancina, V.; Ciceri, E.; Muto, M.; Zdravkovic, N.; Altin, A.; Altaysoy, P.; Kastelic, R.; Velazquez Mendivil, D.M.; Nukovic, J.A. Neuroimaging Modalities Used for Ischemic Stroke Diagnosis and Monitoring. *Medicina* **2023**, *59*, 1908. [CrossRef]
8. Simonsen, C.Z.; Madsen, M.H.; Schmitz, M.L.; Mikkelsen, I.K.; Fisher, M.; Andersen, G. Sensitivity of diffusion-and perfusion-weighted imaging for diagnosing acute ischemic stroke is 97.5%. *Stroke* **2015**, *46*, 98–101. [CrossRef]
9. Marsh, E.B.; Lawrence, E.; Gottesman, R.F.; Llinas, R.H. The NIH Stroke Scale has limited utility in accurate daily monitoring of neurologic status. *Neurohospitalist* **2016**, *6*, 97–101. [CrossRef]
10. Ramachandran, K.; Radha, D.; Gaur, A.; Kaliappan, A.; Sakthivadivel, V. Is the National Institute of Health Stroke Scale a valid prognosticator of the aftermath in patients with ischemic stroke? *J. Fam. Med. Prim. Care* **2022**, *11*, 7185.
11. Gkantzios, A.; Tsiptsios, D.; Karatzetzou, S.; Kitmeridou, S.; Karapepera, V.; Giannakou, E.; Vlotinou, P.; Aggelousis, N.; Vadikolias, K. Stroke and emerging blood biomarkers: A clinical prospective. *Neurol. Int.* **2022**, *14*, 784–803. [CrossRef] [PubMed]
12. Huang, Y.; Wang, Z.; Huang, Z.-X.; Liu, Z. Biomarkers and the outcomes of ischemic stroke. *Front. Mol. Neurosci.* **2023**, *16*, 1171101. [CrossRef] [PubMed]
13. Bianchi, R.; Giambanco, I.; Donato, R. S100B/RAGE-dependent activation of microglia via NF-κB and AP-1: Co-regulation of COX-2 expression by S100B, IL-1β and TNF-α. *Neurobiol. Aging* **2010**, *31*, 665–677. [CrossRef] [PubMed]
14. Donato, R. Intracellular and extracellular roles of S100 proteins. *Microsc. Res. Tech.* **2003**, *60*, 540–551. [CrossRef]
15. Elting, J.-W.; de Jager, A.E.; Teelken, A.W.; Schaaf, M.J.; Maurits, N.M.; van der Naalt, J.; Sibinga, C.T.S.; Sulter, G.A.; De Keyser, J. Comparison of serum S-100 protein levels following stroke and traumatic brain injury. *J. Neurol. Sci.* **2000**, *181*, 104–110. [CrossRef]
16. Jönsson, H.; Johnsson, P.; Höglund, P.; Alling, C.; Blomquist, S. Elimination of S100B and renal function after cardiac surgery. *J. Cardiothorac. Vasc. Anesth.* **2000**, *14*, 698–701. [CrossRef]
17. Hawash, A.M.A.; Zaytoun, T.M.; Helmy, T.A.; El Reweny, E.M.; Galeel, A.M.A.A.; Taleb, R.S.Z. S100B and brain ultrasound: Novel predictors for functional outcome in acute ischemic stroke patients. *Clin. Neurol. Neurosurg.* **2023**, *233*, 107907. [CrossRef]
18. Hazar, T.Y.; Nazliel, B.; Gurses, A.A.; Caglayan, H.B.; Irkec, C. High Serum S-100B Protein Levels within the First 36 Hours of Acute Ischemic Stroke Predicts High NIHSS Scores. *Ann. Med. Res.* **2022**, *27*, 1675–1680. [CrossRef]
19. Park, S.-Y.; Kim, M.-H.; Kim, O.-J.; Ahn, H.-J.; Song, J.-Y.; Jeong, J.-Y.; Oh, S.-H. Plasma heart-type fatty acid binding protein level in acute ischemic stroke: Comparative analysis with plasma S100B level for diagnosis of stroke and prediction of long-term clinical outcome. *Clin. Neurol. Neurosurg.* **2013**, *115*, 405–410. [CrossRef]
20. Rahmati, M.; Azarpazhooh, M.R.; Ehteram, H.; Ferns, G.A.; Ghayour-Mobarhan, M.; Ghannadan, H.; Mobarra, N. The elevation of S100B and downregulation of circulating miR-602 in the sera of ischemic stroke (IS) patients: The emergence of novel diagnostic and prognostic markers. *Neurol. Sci.* **2020**, *41*, 2185–2192. [CrossRef]
21. Lisachev, P.D.; Shtark, M.B.; Sokolova, O.O.; Pustylnyak, V.O.; Salakhutdinova, M.Y.; Epstein, O.I. A comparison of the dynamics of S100B, S100A1, and S100A6 mRNA expression in hippocampal CA1 area of rats during long-term potentiation and after low-frequency stimulation. *Cardiovasc. Psychiatry Neurol.* **2010**, *2010*, 720958. [CrossRef] [PubMed]
22. Beer, C.; Blacker, D.; Bynevelt, M.; Hankey, G.J.; Puddey, I.B. Systemic markers of inflammation are independently associated with S100B concentration: Results of an observational study in subjects with acute ischaemic stroke. *J. Neuroinflamm.* **2010**, *7*, 1–5. [CrossRef] [PubMed]
23. Weglewski, A.; Ryglewicz, D.; Mular, A.; Juryńczyk, J. Changes of protein S100B serum concentration during ischemic and hemorrhagic stroke in relation to the volume of stroke lesion. *Neurol. I Neurochir. Pol.* **2005**, *39*, 310–317.
24. Selçuk, Ö.; Yayla, V.; Cabalar, M.; Güzel, V.; Uysal, S.; Gedikbaşi, A. The relationship of serum S100B levels with infarction size and clinical outcome in acute ischemic stroke patients. *Nöro Psikiyatr. Arşivi* **2014**, *51*, 395. [CrossRef] [PubMed]
25. Abdel-Ghaffar, W.E.; Ahmed, S.; Elfatatry, A.; Elmesky, M.; Hashad, D. The role of s100b as a predictor of the functional outcome in geriatric patients with acute cerebrovascular stroke. *Egypt. J. Neurol. Psychiatry Neurosurg.* **2019**, *55*, 1–5. [CrossRef]
26. Sakdejayont, S.; Pruphetkaew, N.; Chongphattararot, P.; Nanphan, P.; Sathirapanya, P. Serum S100β as a predictor of severity and outcomes for mixed subtype acute ischaemic stroke. *Singap. Med. J.* **2020**, *61*, 206. [CrossRef]
27. Branco, J.P.; Oliveira, S.; Sargento-Freitas, J.; Costa, J.S.; Cordeiro, L.; Cunha, L.; Gonçalves, A.F.; Pinheiro, J. S100β protein as a predictor of poststroke functional outcome: A prospective study. *J. Stroke Cerebrovasc. Dis.* **2018**, *27*, 1890–1896. [CrossRef]
28. Retnaningsih Retnaningsih, B.A.P. Windri Kartikasari, Christina Roseville Lasma Aritonang, Amin Husni, Santoso Jaeri, The Association Between Serum Biomarker Levels and Clinical Outcomes among Acute Ischemic Stroke Patients. *Acta Sci. Neurol.* **2021**, *4*, 15–21.
29. Luger, S.; Koerbel, K.; Martinez Oeckel, A.; Schneider, H.; Maurer, C.J.; Hintereder, G.; Wagner, M.; Hattingen, E.; Foerch, C. Role of S100B serum concentration as a surrogate outcome parameter after mechanical thrombectomy. *Neurology* **2021**, *97*, e2185–e2194. [CrossRef]
30. Foerch, C.; Otto, B.; Singer, O.C.; Neumann-Haefelin, T.; Yan, B.; Berkefeld, J.; Steinmetz, H.; Sitzer, M. Serum S100B predicts a malignant course of infarction in patients with acute middle cerebral artery occlusion. *Stroke* **2004**, *35*, 2160–2164. [CrossRef]

Disclaimer/Publisher's Note: The statements, opinions and data contained in all publications are solely those of the individual author(s) and contributor(s) and not of MDPI and/or the editor(s). MDPI and/or the editor(s) disclaim responsibility for any injury to people or property resulting from any ideas, methods, instructions or products referred to in the content.

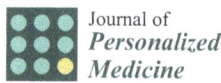

Article

Significance of S100B Protein as a Rapid Diagnostic Tool in Emergency Departments for Traumatic Brain Injury Patients

Rakesh Jalali [1,2,*], Izabela Godlewska [1], Magdalena Fadrowska-Szleper [1], Agata Pypkowska [1], Adam Kern [3], Jacek Bil [4], Joanna Manta [1,2] and Jerzy Romaszko [5]

1. Department of Emergency Medicine, School of Medicine, Collegium Medicum, University of Warmia and Mazury, 10-082 Olsztyn, Poland; iza.gdlwsk@gmail.com (I.G.); magdafadrowska@gmail.com (M.F.-S.); pypkowska.agata@gmail.com (A.P.)
2. Clinical Emergency Department, Regional Specialist Hospital, 10-561 Olsztyn, Poland
3. Department of Cardiology and Internal Medicine, School of Medicine, Collegium Medicum, University of Warmia and Mazury, 10-082 Olsztyn, Poland; adam.kern@uwm.edu.pl
4. Department of Invasive Cardiology, Centre of Postgraduate Medical Education, 01-813 Warsaw, Poland; jacek.bil@cmkp.edu.pl
5. Department of Family Medicine and Infectious Diseases, School of Medicine, Collegium Medicum, University of Warmia and Mazury, 10-082 Olsztyn, Poland; jerzy.romaszko@uwm.edu.pl
* Correspondence: rakesh.jalali@uwm.edu.pl

Abstract: Traumatic brain injuries (TBIs) are not only the leading cause of death among people below 44 years of age, but also one of the biggest diagnostic challenges in the emergency set up. We believe that the use of serum biomarkers in diagnosis can help to improve patient care in TBI. One of them is the S100B protein, which is currently proposed as a promising diagnostic tool for TBI and its consequences. In our study, we analyzed serum biomarker S100B in 136 patients admitted to the Emergency Department of the Regional Specialist Hospital in Olsztyn. Participants were divided into three groups: patients with head trauma and alcohol intoxication, patients with head trauma with no alcohol intoxication and a control group of patients with no trauma or with injury in locations other than the head. In our study, as compared to the control group, patients with TBI had a significantly higher S100B level (both with and without intoxication). Moreover, in both groups, the mean S100B protein level was significantly higher in patients with pathological changes in CT. According to our study results, the S100B protein is a promising diagnostic tool, and we propose including its evaluation in routine regimens in patients with TBI.

Keywords: emergency department; traumatic brain injury (TBI); S100B protein; alcohol; diagnostic process

1. Introduction

Injuries are the leading cause of death among people below 44 years of age [1]. According to the CDC (Centers for Disease Control and Prevention), more than 82,700 traumatic brain injury (TBI)-related hospitalizations were recorded in the USA in 2001, and the number almost tripled in 2020 [2,3]. However, deaths are only the tip of the iceberg. Among 223,135 TBI incidents recorded in the USA in 2019, it was the cause of death of 60,611 patients, whereas thousands of people became disabled [3]. TBIs lead to severe socio-economic consequences via reducing the quality of life, not only of patients but also their families, and generating costs of billions of dollars annually [4]. According to Brazinova et al., the TBI incidence rate in Europe ranges between 47.3 (Spain) and 849 (Italy) per 100,000 people per year [5].

It is possible to identify specific groups with a higher risk of TBI. For example, people over 75 years of age have the highest risk of hospitalization and death related to TBI [3]. TBI is more frequent among homeless people and marginally housed individuals due to alcohol and drug dependence, mental health problems, suicide attempts, and sociological problems [6,7]. TBI usually results from direct trauma or acceleration–deceleration forces in road traffic accidents or violence. Brain tissue is vulnerable to the effects of trauma because of its high metabolism and low ability to function without a continuous energy supply.

TBIs can be classified into focal brain injuries and diffuse injuries. The first type can be identified in diagnostic imaging; therefore, basic diagnostic tools are used in emergency departments (EDs), especially computed tomography (CT). Nevertheless, indiscriminate CT use generates excessive costs and increases the risk of radiation exposure. Studies have shown that a third of malignant tumors found in patients with CT performed between 35 and 54 years of age result from this procedure [8]. Considering repeatedly occurring mild TBIs in groups of patients with a tendency to fall, such as elderly patients, alcohol addicts, or homeless people, precluding unnecessary CT scanning can significantly reduce its side effects. National Institute for Health and Care Excellence (NICE) Guidelines scales are one of the tools made for assessing the utility of obtaining CT scans and are used worldwide [9]. According to NICE Guidelines, the need for diagnostic imaging should be assessed mainly based on patients' clinical state, Glasgow Coma Scale (GCS) score, age, mechanism of injury, and medication. Moreover, it has been reported that CT imaging shows negative results in the vast majority of mild TBI cases with patients who have a GCS score between 13 and 15 [10].

When dealing with TBI, not only is treating the primary brain damage important, but the prevention of secondary brain damage is also essential. Although the exact mechanisms of brain tissue response to stress and injury are yet to be discovered, we believe that it is possible to establish diagnostic tools with the employment of serum protein biomarkers. Many serum proteins such as glial fibrillary acidic protein, ubiquitin C-terminal hydrolase L1, neuron-specific enolase, and S100B are under investigation for their possible role as a marker for TBI (reviewed in [11]). Among these serum proteins, S100B has been extensively investigated for its use as a biomarker for TBI [12,13]. Its automated assays are readily available and easy to use.

Establishing a new diagnostic standard that would include TBI biomarkers could not only prevent unnecessary radiation in some groups of patients and thus its side effects but also help to estimate the possible injury outcome. The use of serum biomarkers in diagnostics can help to improve care in TBI in two ways. These markers can be a useful tool in assessing the necessity for diagnostic imaging and estimating the extensiveness of injury, which, consequently, can contribute to choosing the right therapeutic pathway.

In our study, we analyzed serum biomarker S100B, a calcium-binding protein mainly found in the astroglia and Schwann cells of the central nervous system (CNS). The aim of this study was to evaluate a correlation between CT with evidence of brain injury (positive CT) and serum S100B and assess the possible use of the S100B protein to determine a need for CT in two groups of patients: with and without alcohol intoxication at the time of injury.

Our study focused on alcohol-intoxicated patients, a group often admitted to the ED due to TBI. Furthermore, we wanted to determine whether alcohol intoxication affected the S100B serum level. The S100B protein test could help choose the right treatment pathway and verify the severity of the injury. Moreover, collecting information from and evaluating the clinical state of alcohol-intoxicated patients is difficult, making it harder to assess risk factors for severe injury (for example, mechanism of injury) and CT scan necessity.

2. Materials and Methods

The present observational study, approved by the local ethical committee of the University of Warmia and Mazury (approval reference number 21/2016 dated 18 May 2016), was based on a retrospective analysis of medical records of patients hospitalized in the Clinical Emergency Department of the Regional Specialist Hospital in Olsztyn, Poland. Patients' medical records were provided to researchers with names and surnames being substituted for codes (anonymized), and all the data collection methods were in compliance with the Helsinki Declaration.

One hundred thirty-six patients admitted to the ED of the Regional Specialist Hospital between 2016 and 2018 in Olsztyn were included in this study. Participants were divided into three groups: patients with head trauma and alcohol intoxication (TrAlc; $n = 49$), patients with head trauma with no alcohol intoxication (NonTrAlc; $n = 58$), and the control group, which included patients with no trauma or with injury in locations other than the head ($n = 29$). Alcohol intoxication was defined as a blood alcohol concentration ≥ 50 mg/dL. We adopted the definition of TBI according to the NICE guidelines where, mild, moderate, and severe TBI are defined by the GCS ranges of 13–15, 9–12, and 8 or less, respectively [14].

Exclusion criteria were as follows: age under 18, neurosurgical intervention in past medical history, brain tumor, severe hypoxia, carbon monoxide intoxication, body temperature over 38.5 °C, malignant melanoma, and cardiac arrest caused by brain injury.

On admission, serum alcohol and S100B level was tested in all groups. CT of the head was performed in the TrAlc and NonTrAlc groups. To evaluate neurological status, the Glasgow Coma State (GCS) was used. In addition, we considered demographic and clinical variables including age, sex, comorbidities, medications, and the need for analgosedation, intubation or craniotomy, as well as the use of tranexamic acid or catecholamines.

3. Sample Processing and Protein Measurement

Blood samples were collected in biochemical tubes without anti-coagulants, and 10 min after collection, samples were centrifuged for 20 min at 3000 revolutions per minute (centrifuge MPW 352 R). Next, 1 mL of serum was transferred to 1 mL Eppendorf tubes and frozen to −20 °C. Samples are durable for up to 3 months at this temperature. Prior to analysis, tubes were thawed and brought to a temperature of 20–25 °C. Samples with visible turbidity were re-centrifuged.

Serum concentrations of S100B were determined by the electrochemiluminescence immunoassay (ECLIA) method on the cobas 6000 device calibrated with S100 CalSet. The Roche Elecsys® S100 kit (Roche, Germany) with detection limits between 0.005 and 39 µg/L was used according to the manufacturer's instructions. The cut-off value used was >0.1 µg/L. PerciControl Universal (PCU)1 and PCU2 were used for controlling the accuracy of measurements.

4. Statistical Analysis

The obtained data were analyzed using the Statistica 12 statistical package.

The Shapiro–Wilk test was used to examine the normal distribution of variables measurable with interval or ratio scales. The assessment of the equality of variances was based on Levene's test. When the distribution of variables did not meet the assumptions of normal distribution, the non-parametric Mann–Whitney U test (for two analyzed groups) or the Kruskal–Wallis test (for three analyzed groups) were performed. The relationships between variables with nominal scales were estimated with the Chi^2 test. Because multiple comparisons were conducted, we applied Bonferroni correction, dividing the assumed significance level of 0.05 by the number of comparisons. Hence, a statistically significant p-value was 0.0083.

5. Results

Patient management on admission.

Out of 107 patients (test group including TrAlc and NonTrAlc patients), 13 needed analgosedation and 12 patients required intubation. In one of the four patients with CT-confirmed intracranial hematoma, craniotomy was performed, and three of them died (on the 1st, 2nd, and 6th day, respectively). Only one patient was admitted to the Intensive Care Unit (ICU). A total of seven patients with TBI who were included in this study died. Abnormalities in CT were found in 10 patients in the TrAlc group and 7 patients in the NonTrAlc group. Patient characteristics are summarized in Table 1.

Table 1. Characteristics of patients included in this study.

	All (n = 136)	NonTrAlc (n = 58)	TrAlc (n = 49)	Control (n = 29)	p
Percentage (n)	100% (136)	42.65% (58)	36.03% (49)	21.32% (29)	
Sex F [% (n)]	32.09% (43)	50.00% (29)	6.12% (3)	40.74% (11)	<0.001
Age (X_{mean}/SD)	50.99/21.40	55.84/23.41	44.86/16.06	51.67 ± 23.26	0.038
No comorbidities	44.70% (59)	42.86% (24)	46.94% (23)	44.44% (12)	0.915
Comorbidities — Alcohol addiction syndrome	43.42% (33)	15.15% (5)	100% (26)	11.76% (2)	<0.001
Comorbidities — Cardiovascular	44.74% (34)	60.61% (20)	11.54% (3)	64.71% (11)	<0.001
Comorbidities — Metabolic	19.74% (15)	27.27% (9)	7.69% (2)	23.53% (4)	0.181
Comorbidities — Nephrological	4.00% (3)	6.25% (2)	0.00% (0)	5.88% (1)	0.555
Comorbidities — Oncological	5.33% (4)	9.38% (3)	0.00% (0)	5.88% (1)	0.407
Comorbidities — Coagulation disorders	12.00% (9)	21.88% (7)	0.00% (0)	11.76% (2)	0.062
Comorbidities — Neurological/psychiatric	10.67% (8)	15.63% (5)	0.00% (0)	17.65% (3)	0.122
Comorbidities — Pulmonary	7.89% (6)	12.50% (4)	3.70% (1)	5.88% (1)	0.537

In the test group of $n = 107$ (TrAlc + NonTrAlc), 53 patients had other injuries besides TBI. The two highest levels of S100B in the entire analysis were found in patients with additional injuries, with the highest result of 32.46 μg/L in a TBI patient with spleen rupture and the second, 8.35 μg/L, in a TBI patient with bone fractures.

We analyzed the use of anticoagulants in the test group: four patients had been taking vitamin K antagonists (VKAs) and six patients had been receiving oral anticoagulants (NOACs) prior to admission to the ED. In only one patient treated with VKAs was a subdural hematoma diagnosed based on the CT scan, and the S100B level was 0.585 μg/L. In other patients in this group, no signs of TBI were found.

The comparison of S100B between the control group and patients after head trauma (TrAlc + NonTrAlc) revealed that the serum marker level was higher in the latter group (0.092 vs. 0.99 μg/L), and the difference was statistically significant ($p < 0.001$) (Figure 1). However, 36 out of 107 patients with a history of injury had a lower S100B protein level than the average level in the control group.

TrAlc and NonTrAlc groups were further analyzed based on the occurrence of abnormalities revealed in CT. CT-positive groups (patients showing abnormalities in CT scans) were separately compared to the control group.

In both groups, TrAlc CT-positive and NonTrAlc CT-positive, the S100B level was significantly higher in comparison to the control group. A plasma S100B protein concentration of 1.84 μg/L ($p < 0.00008$) in the TrAlc CT-positive group and 7.592 μg/L ($p < 0.000003$) in the NonTrAlc CT-positive group as compared to control (0.092 μg/L) was observed.

The comparison of mean S100B levels in the TrAlc group with a positive CT scan versus a negative CT scan revealed a significantly higher level in the first group (1.836 μg/L vs. 0.395 μg/L; $p = 0.0062$). In the NonTrAlc group, differences were even greater. Among CT-positive patients, the mean S100B level was 7.592 μg/L, and among CT-negative patients, it was 0.373 μg/L ($p = 0.000067$).

To evaluate differences between patients after alcohol intoxication and those with no intoxication, an analysis of patients with confirmed pathology in CT in NonTrAlc and TrAlc groups was performed. It revealed a higher S100B serum level in the NonTrAlc group (7.59 μg/L vs. 1.83 μg/L, Figure 2). Although the increase in the protein levels in the NonTrAlc group was over 4-fold higher than in the TrAlc group, the difference was not statistically significant ($p = 0.088$).

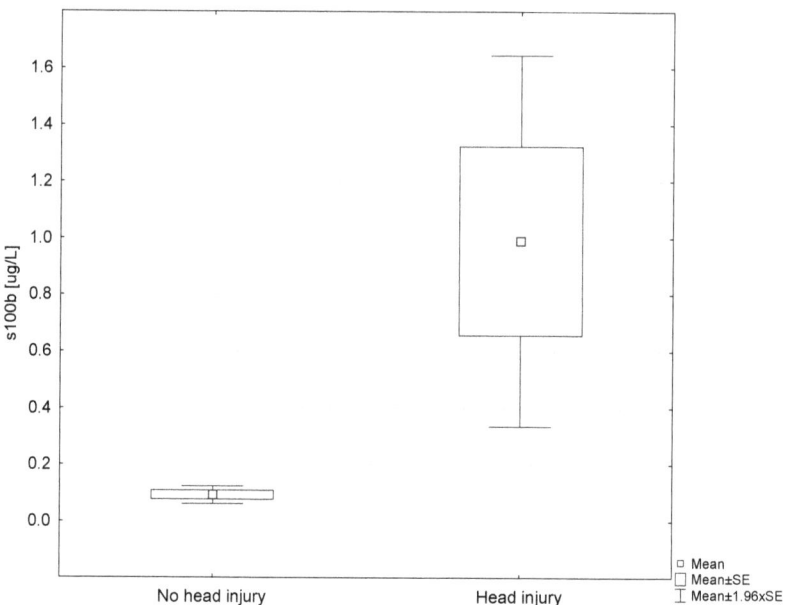

Figure 1. Comparison of S100B protein level between the control group and patients after head trauma.

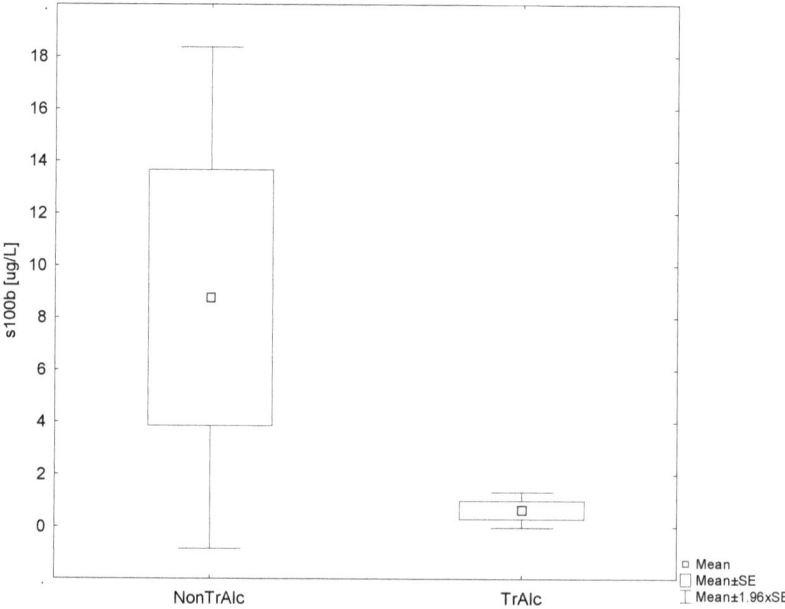

Figure 2. Comparison of S100B level between the NonTrAlc group and the TrAlc group (pathology in CT confirmed).

6. Discussion

S100B is a calcium-binding protein found in astroglia and other glial cells, including Schwann cells, ependymal cells, and oligodendrocytes in the CNS. It has also been found in definite neuron subpopulations [15–17]. The less significant fraction of S100B, referred to as an extracranial fraction, is present in striated muscle cells, heart, kidneys, and malignant melanoma cells [18,19]. The presence of S100B in tissues other than the brain tissue may contribute to the test's low specificity in confirming TBI [20]. It is possible to measure the level of the S100B protein in the cerebrospinal fluid, and, according to Mokuno et al., it can be a promising tool for predicting the recovery of patients with neurological diseases such as Guillain–Barré syndrome [21].

Our results indicate, with high statistical significance, that S100B protein level is much higher in patients with TBI with or without alcohol intoxication as compared to the controls. Since S100B cannot be an alternative for CT, we hope the establishment of S100B as a TBI biomarker helps in the decision making process in regard to the patients who require, e.g., a delayed CT scan [22] or no CT scan in case of patients with no loss of consciousness and fulfilling other exclusion criteria as are depicted in the algorithm below [Figure 3]. However, this approach needs to be further verified in a large group of patients.

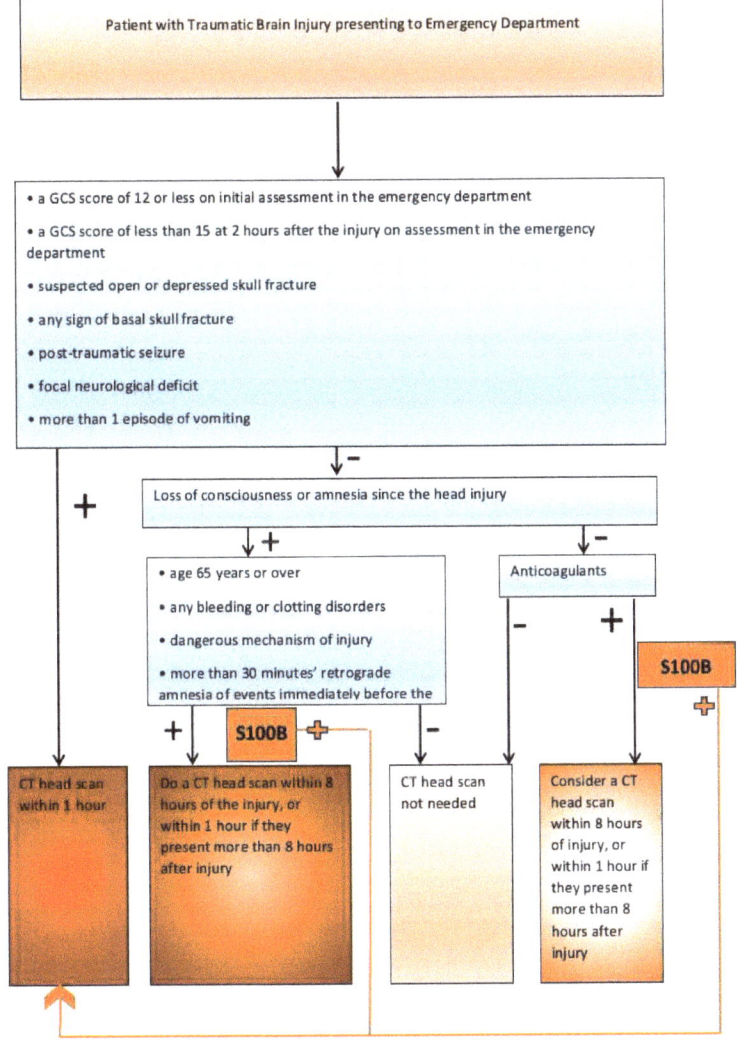

Figure 3. Schematic for use of serum S100B protein levels in TBI diagnosis based on NICE guidelines.

An elevated S100B level is not specific to TBI, and it can occur in many pathologies of the CNS, such as neurogenerative diseases and congenital disorders [15,21]. Also, S100B levels can be increased due to its extracranial fraction, especially because of its presence in adipose and muscle tissues, in patients with trauma in other body regions than the head [19]. The impact of alcohol intoxication on the S100B serum level is unclear [16,23,24]. Chronic alcohol dependence can lead to higher S100B protein serum levels, and this is correlated with the amount of alcohol consumption [25]. According to Brin et al., an elevated serum level can also be an effect of acute intoxication in groups with head trauma but also among those with no trauma at all [26]. However, according to other researchers, acute alcohol intoxication should not affect the S100B serum level [16,24,27]. In a recent study, involving healthy young individuals, moderate alcohol intoxication had no effect on serum S100B levels [28]. In our study, as compared to the control group, patients with TBI had a significantly higher S100B level. Moreover, in both the TrAlc and NonTrAlc groups, the mean S100B level was higher in patients with abnormalities identified in CT, and the difference was statistically significant. In our study, we observed a decreased serum s100B in TrAlc patients (Figure 2). However, although concentrations of S100B differed between alcohol-intoxicated patients and those with no alcohol consumption, these differences were not statistically significant. Our results are consistent with the previous report where intoxicated patients with definitive TBI had lower S100B levels as compared to the sober patients [23]. This is an interesting observation, and since patients under the influence of alcohol are a large group of individuals admitted to EDs owing to head injuries, more research is necessary to determine the relationship between alcohol intake and the S100B protein level. In our opinion, this thread in the discussion is perhaps the most important for the future of assessing the usefulness of S100B protein in patients with TBI and alcohol intoxication. Its confirmation in a study with a larger sample size, or finding a cut-off point with the concentration of alcohol in the patient's blood, may influence the recommendations regarding the use of S100B protein assays. We are planning such a study in a larger group of patients.

Despite its limitations, Scandinavian Neurotrauma Committee Guidelines included testing the S100B protein level as an addition to the clinical evaluation in patients with head trauma [27]. Data analysis suggested that incorporating this biomarker into the diagnostic algorithm enables practitioners to discharge a large proportion of patients after mild head trauma without performing CT, which can be cost-saving [27,29,30].

Establishing a TBI biomarker, potentially the S100B protein, could possibly decrease the number of unnecessary CT scans performed for patients after head trauma and economize hospital costs [31]. Our study does not include a cost–effectiveness analysis, but each biochemical test performed serially is cheaper than an imaging test. The economic aspect requires further evaluation, but the results of this study give hope for its positive development. According to Ruane et al., use of biomarkers lowers hospital costs in two situations: in medical institutions where the proportion of mild TBI patients being scanned exceeds 78% or when obtaining final CT scan results requires significantly more time than the wait for blood test results [30]. However, using the S100B protein as a pre-CT screen in other situations than those previously mentioned does not lower hospital costs due to its low specificity [4].

Another important limitation of the S100B protein as a biomarker is its changes in serum levels over time [32]. Its concentration is highest directly after head trauma and lowers over time [12]. The most significant decline in its serum level occurs 24–48 h after trauma. It returns to the normal ranges within 72 h following trauma. Therefore, when treating patients with an unknown time of trauma, the S100B test may not be useful.

The available literature provides strong evidence of an association between S100B serum levels and the probability of detecting abnormalities in CT scans after head trauma [11,33]. Therefore, it is possible to include this biomarker in already existing diagnostic algorithms, thus reducing the number of unnecessarily performed CT scans. Subsequent analyses will allow researchers to evaluate the effectiveness of this parameter. The use of biomarkers can save time and reduce diagnostic costs. However, establishing the S100B protein as a new TBI biomarker has potential limitations. First, its specificity is low [34]. Another problem is the non-apparent effect of alcohol intoxication, which is likely to influence the S100B serum level.

When treating a specific group of patients, it is not easy to decide whether diagnostic imaging should be performed. This includes cases of elderly people after falls and pregnant women. With regard to pregnant women, many guidelines indicate the assessment of maternal benefit and fetal risk. As radiation doses raise concerns, in the future, biomarkers in diagnosing mild head trauma may be considered, especially in medical centers with poor availability of MR. Patients who cannot have a CT scan without having anesthesia, for example, children and those with mental disorders, would also benefit from including biomarkers in the diagnostic process, which could help prevent unnecessary CT scans and anesthesia.

We propose a criterion that utilizes serum S100B analysis in the TBI diagnostic process based on the NICE guidelines (Figure 3).

In clinical situations, when, according to the newest NICE guidelines, a CT scan is advised but must be postponed, we suggest the S100B protein be included in the diagnostic process while waiting for imaging diagnosing [9]. The relevant group of patients can be described as follows: patients without loss of consciousness, without risk factors for severe head injury, 65 or older, with bleeding or clotting disorder, dangerous mechanism of injury, more than 30 minutes' retrograde amnesia, or taking anticoagulant or antiplatelets. A high S100B level could indicate oligosymptomatic traumatic brain injury and, therefore, speed up the diagnostic process by performing CT immediately. We also strongly encourage considering testing S100B levels in the group of patients mentioned earlier, in whom a CT scan is essentially performed under general anesthesia. In many clinical cases, this may fill the gap in the diagnostic process.

7. Conclusions

The S100B protein is a promising diagnostic tool. There is a need for larger multicenter studies to establish its integration into clinical algorithms and therefore improvement of the patient care in EDs as regards radiation risks, costs, and time. Until this procedure becomes a standard, the issue of alcohol (a potential confounding factor) must be solved. Although results are promising, this analysis has limitations due to the relatively small study group. Therefore, to confirm the obtained results, more research involving a more extensive group of patients should be performed.

Author Contributions: Conceptualization, R.J.; methodology and investigation, R.J. and I.G.; validation and formal analysis, R.J. and I.G.; resources, R.J.; data curation, R.J., M.F.-S., A.P., A.K., J.M. and J.B.; writing—original draft preparation, R.J., M.F.-S. and A.P.; writing—review and editing, R J.; visualization, R.J., A.K., J.B., J.M. and J.R.; supervision, R.J. and J.K.; project administration, R.J.; funding acquisition, R.J. All authors have read and agreed to the published version of the manuscript.

Funding: The research was financially supported by the Statutory research funding from the University of Warmia and Mazury, Decision Nr 25.620.015-300 and 25.014.002-25.620.024-300.

Institutional Review Board Statement: The study was conducted in accordance with the Declaration of Helsinki, and approved by the Ethics Committee of the University of Warmia and Mazury (approval reference number 21/2016 dated 18 May 2016).

Informed Consent Statement: Informed consent was obtained from the subjects included in the study.

Data Availability Statement: All data are included in the study.

Conflicts of Interest: Authors declare no conflict of interest.

References

1. CDC. Injuries and Violence Are Leading Causes of Death. Available online: https://www.cdc.gov/injury/wisqars/animated-leading-causes.html (accessed on 26 August 2022).
2. CDC. Surveillance of Tbi-Related Emergency Department Visits, Hospitalizations, and Deaths. Available online: https://www.cdc.gov/traumaticbraininjury/pdf/TBI-Data-Archive-Report_Final_links_508.pdf (accessed on 25 August 2022).
3. CDC. Traumatic Brain Injury & Concussion. Available online: https://www.cdc.gov/traumaticbraininjury/index.html (accessed on 25 August 2022).
4. Gustavsson, A.; Svensson, M.; Jacobi, F.; Allgulander, C.; Alonso, J.; Beghi, E.; Dodel, R.; Ekman, M.; Faravelli, C.; Fratiglioni, L. Cost of disorders of the brain in Europe 2010. *Eur. Neuropsychopharmacol.* **2011**, *21*, 718–779. [CrossRef] [PubMed]
5. Brazinova, A.; Rehorcikova, V.; Taylor, M.S.; Buckova, V.; Majdan, M.; Psota, M.; Peeters, W.; Feigin, V.; Theadom, A.; Holkovic, L. Epidemiology of traumatic brain injury in Europe: A living systematic review. *J. Neurotrauma* **2021**, *38*, 1411–1440. [CrossRef] [PubMed]
6. Romaszko, J.; Kuchta, R.; Opalach, C.; Bertrand-Bucińska, A.; Romaszko, A.M.; Giergielewicz-Januszko, B.; Buciński, A. Socioeconomic characteristics, health risk factors and alcohol consumption among the homeless in north-eastern part of Poland. *Cent. Eur. J. Public Health* **2017**, *25*, 29–34. [CrossRef] [PubMed]
7. Stubbs, J.L.; Thornton, A.E.; Sevick, J.M.; Silverberg, N.D.; Barr, A.M.; Honer, W.G.; Panenka, W.J. Traumatic brain injury in homeless and marginally housed individuals: A systematic review and meta-analysis. *Lancet Public Health* **2020**, *5*, e19–e32. [CrossRef]
8. De González, A.B.; Mahesh, M.; Kim, K.-P.; Bhargavan, M.; Lewis, R.; Mettler, F.; Land, C. Projected cancer risks from computed tomographic scans performed in the United States in 2007. *Arch. Intern. Med.* **2009**, *169*, 2071–2077. [CrossRef]
9. Davis, T.; Ings, A. Head injury: Triage, assessment, investigation and early management of head injury in children, young people and adults (NICE guideline CG 176). *Arch. Dis. Child.-Educ. Pract.* **2015**, *100*, 97–100. [CrossRef]
10. Isokuortti, H.; Iverson, G.L.; Silverberg, N.D.; Kataja, A.; Brander, A.; Öhman, J.; Luoto, T.M. Characterizing the type and location of intracranial abnormalities in mild traumatic brain injury. *J. Neurosurg.* **2018**, *129*, 1588–1597. [CrossRef]
11. Amoo, M.; Henry, J.; O'Halloran, P.J.; Brennan, P.; Husien, M.B.; Campbell, M.; Caird, J.; Javadpour, M.; Curley, G.F. S100B, GFAP, UCH-L1 and NSE as predictors of abnormalities on CT imaging following mild traumatic brain injury: A systematic review and meta-analysis of diagnostic test accuracy. *Neurosurg. Rev.* **2022**, *45*, 1171–1193. [CrossRef]
12. Di Battista, A.P.; Buonora, J.E.; Rhind, S.G.; Hutchison, M.G.; Baker, A.J.; Rizoli, S.B.; Diaz-Arrastia, R.; Mueller, G.P. Blood biomarkers in moderate-to-severe traumatic brain injury: Potential utility of a multi-marker approach in characterizing outcome. *Front. Neurol.* **2015**, *6*, 110. [CrossRef]
13. Abboud, T.; Rohde, V.; Mielke, D. Mini review: Current status and perspective of S100B protein as a biomarker in daily clinical practice for diagnosis and prognosticating of clinical outcome in patients with neurological diseases with focus on acute brain injury. *BMC Neurosci.* **2023**, *24*, 38. [CrossRef]
14. Hodgkinson, S.; Pollit, V.; Sharpin, C.; Lecky, F. Early management of head injury: Summary of updated NICE guidance. *BMJ* **2014**, *348*, g104. [CrossRef] [PubMed]
15. Michetti, F.; D'Ambrosi, N.; Toesca, A.; Puglisi, M.A.; Serrano, A.; Marchese, E.; Corvino, V.; Geloso, M.C. The S100B story: From biomarker to active factor in neural injury. *J. Neurochem.* **2019**, *148*, 168–187. [CrossRef] [PubMed]
16. Rahimian, S.; Potteiger, S.; Loynd, R.; Mercogliano, C.; Sigal, A.; Short, A.; Donato, A. The utility of S100B level in detecting mild traumatic brain injury in intoxicated patients. *Am. J. Emerg. Med.* **2020**, *38*, 799–805. [CrossRef] [PubMed]
17. Rickmann, M.; Wolff, J. S100 protein expression in subpopulations of neurons of rat brain. *Neuroscience* **1995**, *67*, 977–991. [CrossRef] [PubMed]
18. Karonidis, A.; Mantzourani, M.; Gogas, H.; Tsoutsos, D. Serum S100B levels correlate with stage, N status, mitotic rate and disease outcome in melanoma patients independent to LDH. *Small* **2017**, *20*, 1296–1302.
19. Wang, K.K.; Yang, Z.; Zhu, T.; Shi, Y.; Rubenstein, R.; Tyndall, J.A.; Manley, G.T. An update on diagnostic and prognostic biomarkers for traumatic brain injury. *Expert Rev. Mol. Diagn.* **2018**, *18*, 165–180. [CrossRef] [PubMed]
20. Ion, A.; Stafie, C.; Mitu, O.; Ciobanu, C.E.; Halitchi, D.I.; Costache, A.D.; Bobric, C.; Troase, R.; Mitu, I.; Huzum, B. Biomarkers utility: At the borderline between cardiology and neurology. *J. Cardiovasc. Dev. Dis.* **2021**, *8*, 139. [CrossRef] [PubMed]
21. Mokuno, K.; Kiyosawa, K.; Sugimura, K.; Yasuda, T.; Riku, S.; Murayama, T.; Yanagi, T.; Takahashi, A.; Kato, K. Prognostic value of cerebrospinal fluid neuron-specific enolase and S-100b protein in Guillain-Barré syndrome. *Acta Neurol. Scand.* **1994**, *89*, 27–30. [CrossRef]
22. Palmieri, M.; Frati, A.; Santoro, A.; Frati, P.; Fineschi, V.; Pesce, A. Diffuse axonal injury: Clinical prognostic factors, molecular experimental models and the impact of the trauma related oxidative stress. An extensive review concerning milestones and advances. *Int. J. Mol. Sci.* **2021**, *22*, 10865. [CrossRef]
23. Lange, R.T.; Iverson, G.L.; Brubacher, J.R. Clinical utility of the protein S100B to evaluate traumatic brain injury in the presence of acute alcohol intoxication. *J. Head Trauma Rehabil.* **2012**, *27*, 123–134. [CrossRef]
24. Li, Z.; Zhang, J.; Halbgebauer, S.; Chandrasekar, A.; Rehman, R.; Ludolph, A.; Boeckers, T.; Huber-Lang, M.; Otto, M.; Roselli, F. Differential effect of ethanol intoxication on peripheral markers of cerebral injury in murine blunt traumatic brain injury. *Burn. Trauma* **2021**, *9*, tkab027. [CrossRef] [PubMed]

25. Liappas, I.; Tzavellas, E.O.; Kariyannis, C.; Piperi, C.; Schulpis, C.; Papassotiriou, I.; Soldatos, C.R. Effect of alcohol detoxification on serum S-100B levels of alcohol-dependent individuals. *In Vivo* **2006**, *20*, 675–680. [PubMed]
26. Brin, T.; Borucki, K.; Ambrosch, A. The influence of experimental alcohol load and alcohol intoxication on S100B concentrations. *Shock* **2011**, *36*, 356–360. [CrossRef] [PubMed]
27. Calcagnile, O.; Anell, A.; Undén, J. The addition of S100B to guidelines for management of mild head injury is potentially cost saving. *BMC Neurol.* **2016**, *16*, 200. [CrossRef]
28. Stollhof, L.E.; Obertacke, U.; Eschmann, D.; Proba, S.; Bühler, M.; Neumeier, M.; Bludau, F. S100B Serum Level is Independent of Moderate Alcohol Intoxication. *Z. Orthopädie Unfallchirurgie* **2020**, *158*, 201–207. [CrossRef]
29. Asadollahi, S.; Heidari, K.; Taghizadeh, M.; Seidabadi, A.M.; Jamshidian, M.; Vafaee, A.; Manoochehri, M.; Shojaee, A.H.; Hatamabadi, H.R. Reducing head computed tomography after mild traumatic brain injury: Screening value of clinical findings and S100B protein levels. *Brain Inj.* **2016**, *30*, 172–178. [CrossRef]
30. Ruan, S.; Noyes, K.; Bazarian, J.J. The economic impact of S-100B as a pre-head CT screening test on emergency department management of adult patients with mild traumatic brain injury. *J. Neurotrauma* **2009**, *26*, 1655–1664. [CrossRef]
31. Haselmann, V.; Schamberger, C.; Trifonova, F.; Ast, V.; Froelich, M.F.; Strauß, M.; Kittel, M.; Jaruschewski, S.; Eschmann, D.; Neumaier, M. Plasma-based S100B testing for management of traumatic brain injury in emergency setting. *Pract. Lab. Med.* **2021**, *26*, e00236. [CrossRef]
32. Murillo-Cabezas, F.; Muñoz-Sánchez, M.Á.; Rincón-Ferrari, M.D.; Martín-Rodríguez, J.F.; Amaya-Villar, R.; García-Gómez, S.; León-Carrión, J. The prognostic value of the temporal course of S100 β protein in post-acute severe brain injury: A prospective and observational study. *Brain Inj.* **2010**, *24*, 609–619. [CrossRef]
33. Heidari, K.; Vafaee, A.; Rastekenari, A.M.; Taghizadeh, M.; Shad, E.G.; Eley, R.; Sinnott, M.; Asadollahi, S. S100B protein as a screening tool for computed tomography findings after mild traumatic brain injury: Systematic review and meta-analysis. *Brain Inj.* **2015**, *29*, 1146–1157. [CrossRef]
34. Anderson, R.E.; Hansson, L.-O.; Nilsson, O.; Dijlai-Merzoug, R.; Settergren, G. High serum S100B levels for trauma patients without head injuries. *Neurosurgery* **2001**, *48*, 1255–1260. [PubMed]

Disclaimer/Publisher's Note: The statements, opinions and data contained in all publications are solely those of the individual author(s) and contributor(s) and not of MDPI and/or the editor(s). MDPI and/or the editor(s) disclaim responsibility for any injury to people or property resulting from any ideas, methods, instructions or products referred to in the content.

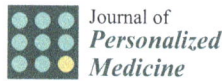

Article

Emergency Department Time Targets for Interhospital Transfer of Patients with Acute Ischemic Stroke

Daian Popa [1], Aida Iancu [2,*], Alina Petrica [1], Florina Buleu [3], Carmen Gabriela Williams [4], Dumitru Sutoi [1], Cosmin Trebuian [1], Anca Tudor [5] and Ovidiu Alexandru Mederle [1,6]

[1] Department of Surgery, Emergency Discipline, "Victor Babes" University of Medicine and Pharmacy, 300041 Timisoara, Romania; daian-ionel.popa@umft.ro (D.P.); alina.petrica@umft.ro (A.P.); dumitru.sutoi@umft.ro (D.S.); trebuian.cosmin@umft.ro (C.T.); mederle.ovidiu@umft.ro (O.A.M.)
[2] Department of Radiology, "Victor Babes" University of Medicine and Pharmacy, E. Murgu Square no. 2, 300041 Timisoara, Romania
[3] Department of Cardiology, "Victor Babes" University of Medicine and Pharmacy, E. Murgu Square no. 2, 300041 Timisoara, Romania; buleu.florina@gmail.com
[4] Emergency Municipal Clinical Hospital, 300254 Timisoara, Romania; drcarmen.williams@yahoo.com
[5] Department of Functional Sciences, "Victor Babes" University of Medicine and Pharmacy, E. Murgu Square no. 2, 300041 Timisoara, Romania; atudor@umft.ro
[6] Department of Surgery, Multidisciplinary Center for Research, Evaluation, Diagnosis and Therapies in Oral Medicine, "Victor Babes" University of Medicine and Pharmacy Timisoara, Eftimie Murgu Square 2, 300041 Timisoara, Romania
* Correspondence: aida.parvu@umft.ro; Tel.: +40-720-174-595

Abstract: *Background and objectives*: Although the intravenous tissue plasminogen activator (rt-PA) has been shown to be effective in the treatment of acute ischemic stroke (AIS), only a small proportion of stroke patients receive this drug. The low administration rate is mainly due to the delayed presentation of patients to the emergency department (ED) or the lack of a stroke team/unit in most of the hospitals. Thus, the aim of this study is to analyze ED time targets and the rate of rt-PA intravenous administration after the initial admission of patients with AIS in an ED from a traditional healthcare center (without a neurologist or stroke team/unit). *Methods:* To analyze which factors influence the administration of rt-PA, we split the general sample (n = 202) into two groups: group No rt-PA (n = 137) and group rt-PA (n = 65). This is based on the performing or no intravenous thrombolysis. *Results:* Analyzing ED time targets for all samples, we found that the median onset-to-ED door time was 180 min (IQR, 120–217.5 min), door-to-physician time was 4 min (IQR, 3–7 min), door-to-CT time was 52 min (IQR, 48–55 min), and door-in-door-out time was 61 min (IQR, 59–65 min). ED time targets such as door-to-physician time (p = 0.245), door-to-CT time (p = 0.219), door-in-door-out time (p = 0.24), NIHSS at admission to the Neurology department (p = 0.405), or NIHSS after 24 h (p = 0.9) did not have a statistically significant effect on the administration or no rt-PA treatment in patients included in our study. Only the highest door-to-CT time was statistically significantly correlated with the death outcome. *Conclusion:* In our study, the iv rt-PA administration rate was 32.18%. A statistically significant correlation between the highest door-to-CT time and death outcome was found.

Keywords: emergency department; ED time targets; acute ischemic stroke; rt-PA; thrombolysis

Citation: Popa, D.; Iancu, A.; Petrica, A.; Buleu, F.; Williams, C.G.; Sutoi, D.; Trebuian, C.; Tudor, A.; Mederle, O.A. Emergency Department Time Targets for Interhospital Transfer of Patients with Acute Ischemic Stroke. *J. Pers. Med.* **2024**, *14*, 13. https://doi.org/10.3390/jpm14010013

Academic Editor: Konstantinos Tziomalos

Received: 13 November 2023
Revised: 13 December 2023
Accepted: 20 December 2023
Published: 21 December 2023

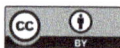

Copyright: © 2023 by the authors. Licensee MDPI, Basel, Switzerland. This article is an open access article distributed under the terms and conditions of the Creative Commons Attribution (CC BY) license (https://creativecommons.org/licenses/by/4.0/).

1. Introduction

Globally, stroke remains the second leading cause of death (11.6% of total deaths) and the third-leading cause of death and disability combined (5.7% of total disability-adjusted life-years), worldwide. The prevalence of strokes is on the rise worldwide and is primarily driven by the expanding elderly demographic. Also, there are associated expenses linked to this medical condition [1]. According to the stroke statistics report from 2015, Romania emerged as the European country with the highest incidence of new strokes and death outcomes resulting from strokes [2].

Although the intravenous (iv) recombinant tissue plasminogen activator (rt-PA) is effective in the treatment of acute ischemic stroke (AIS) by administration within the first 4.5 h of the symptoms' onset [3], only a small proportion of stroke patients receive this drug [4]. The low administration rate is mainly due to the delayed presentation of patients to the emergency department (ED) or lack of a stroke team/unit in most of the hospitals [4].

The current guidelines and local protocols for the early management of these patients highlight the importance of the recognition of stroke symptoms and signs as early as possible by the prehospital services. Moreover, utilizing prehospital emergency medical services was associated with earlier admission to the emergency department (<3 h), faster clinical assessment, shorter door-to-imaging time (<25 min), and faster administration of rt-PA (<60 min), thus increasing the number of patients eligible for the administration of thrombolytics [5,6].

Despite this knowledge, there is a lack of implementation and awareness of medical staff regarding ED time targets in the initial admission of AIS patients to a hospital emergency department without a stroke team or unit. Therefore, it is crucial to explore ways to increase the rate of rt-PA administration, especially in Romania, a developing country, as revealed by the national stroke registry established in 2018 by the board of the Romanian Neurology Society [7,8], and where the rate thrombolysis is around 5.4%, with a notable increase in the last 5 years from 0.8% [9].

For this reason, it is imperative that stroke programs are also performance-evaluated at the ED level to identify which areas need improvement. Thus, the objective of this study is to analyze ED time targets and the rate of rt-PA intravenous administration after the initial admission of patients with AIS in an ED from a traditional healthcare center (without a neurologist or stroke team/unit).

2. Materials and Methods

2.1. Study Population, Inclusion, and Exclusion Criteria

This is an observational study with a retrospective cohort design that included patients with the code stroke activated in our Emergency Department located in a hospital without neurologists or a stroke unit. The study was carried out in Timisoara, Romania, at the Emergency Municipal Clinical Hospital, the second-largest hospital in the county with about 30,000 annual ED patient admissions and access to CT imaging possible 24/7.

Consecutive patients, in whom all medical records (electronic and paper) were available with an ED diagnosis of acute ischemic stroke, were identified ($n = 270$), and only 202 patients that met the inclusion criteria were included in the time of thrombolysis (according to the local protocol [6]). The thrombolysis with intravenous rt-PA (alteplase) was initiated only when the time interval from the first symptoms of stroke is less than 4.5 h to the time of administration. The study data were collected from January 2019 to December 2022. In order to analyze which factors influence the administration of iv rt-PA, we split the sample into two groups: group No rt-PA ($n = 137$) and group rt-PA ($n = 65$). This is based on the performing or no intravenous thrombolysis.

Patients under the ages of 18 years and/or with an initial diagnosis of intracerebral hemorrhage and/or a brain tumor were excluded from this study. Patients who address our ED after more than 3 h from the onset of stroke symptoms were also excluded from this study. We included only patients with less than 3 h from the onset of stroke symptoms in order for the performing or absent intravenous thrombolysis to not be influenced by their initial admission to an ED from a hospital with no stroke team or unit, as well as the interhospital transfer time.

At admission to the ED, the time of the onset of stroke-related symptoms and the time of arrival at the hospital were recorded. The time of the onset of symptoms was defined as the time when the first stroke-related symptoms were noticed according to the patients or their relatives. If the symptoms were experienced during sleep, the time of the onset of symptoms was defined as the last time when they were without symptoms. The time of registration at the ED triage office was the time of arrival at the ED. The door-in-door-out time was calculated as the interval between the hospital arrival and transfer out of our emergency department to the hospital with a neurologist and where the thrombolysis was or was not performed. The time when the cerebral computed tomography (CT) examination results was received was noted. All times analyzed were measured in minutes and relative to the following ED time targets:

- Onset-to-ED door time $\leq$ 3 h (not $\leq$4.5 h, as recommend);
- Door-to-physician < 10 min;
- Door-to-CT < 25 min;
- Door-to-CT-results < 45 min;
- Door-in-door-out time $\leq$ 120 min.

The Joint Commission and Brain Attack Coalition have recommended a target door-in-door-out time of less than 120 min for patients' transfer to a hospital with a stroke team, but limited data have been available on this important process metric [10]. Our local protocol [6] recommend the same time targets for stroke management.

2.2. Evaluation of Stroke

As soon as possible after admission to our Emergency Department, a cerebral computed tomography examination with or without contrast, complete blood count, International normalized ratio (INR), prothrombin time, partial prothrombin time, blood glucose, and electrolytes test was performed for all patients. We did not include patients without medical data. A major advantage was represented by the collaboration between the emergency medicine physician who conducted the clinical examination, as well as the radiologist who performed brain imaging to determine the location, severity, and subtype of the stroke.

All patients in a time of thrombolysis (according to our local protocol—symptoms onset < 4.5 h [6]) were immediately transferred to the largest nearby county hospital with stroke teams but no dedicated stroke unit and where thrombolysis was performed. The distance between both hospitals is 3.5 km and around 7–10 min by ambulance.

Based on The World Health Organization definition of stroke (introduced in 1970 and still used), stroke is defined as a "rapidly developing clinical signs of focal (or global) disturbance of cerebral function, lasting more than 24 h or leading to death (unless interrupted by surgery or medication), with no apparent cause other than that of vascular origin"; this was made the diagnosis of AIS [11,12].

At the time of admission to the Neurology Department, the neurological deficit was assessed by the neurologist and categorized using the National Institutes of Health Stroke Scale (NIHSS) at 1 h, 2 h, and at 24 h. The stroke was classified based on symptoms: no stroke (NIHSS = 0), minor strokes (NIHSS = 1–4), moderate strokes (NIHSS = 5–15), moderate/severe strokes (NIHSS = 16–20), and severe strokes (NIHSS = 21–42) [13].

2.3. Data Analysis

Data analysis was performed using IBM SPSS Statistics version 26.0 (IBM Corp, Armonk, NY, USA). Continuous variables were presented as the mean and standard deviation or median and interquartile range (IQR), and categorical variables were presented as frequency and percentages. To check the distribution of continuous variables, we employed the Shapiro–Wilk test. To compare patient's characteristics with and without thrombolysis, we employed the unpaired t-test or Mann–Whitney U test (in the numeric variable cases) and Chi-square test (for the nominable variables). A p-value < 0.05 was considered statistically significant. Kaplan–Meier curves was made for the 2 compared groups (with the Log-Rank test), considering the days of hospitalization as a survival period.

3. Results

3.1. Baseline Characteristics of Patients Who Arrived at the Emergency Department

As observed in the study flowchart represented in Figure 1, a total of 270 patients with less than 3 h from the onset of stroke symptoms were screened for eligibility to receive intravenous reperfusion therapy. Only patients $n = 202$ were included in the final sample of this study. Sixty-eight patients were excluded. Of these, nine patients had brain tumors at the CT examination, six patients had incorrect diagnostics of AIS, and 53 patients did not meet the national and international criteria for the fibrinolytic and/or endovascular treatment of acute stroke. Among the 202 consecutive patients included in the final sample, 65 received intravenous thrombolytic therapy (rt-PA group) and 137 patients did not receive intravenous thrombolytic therapy (No rt-PA group).

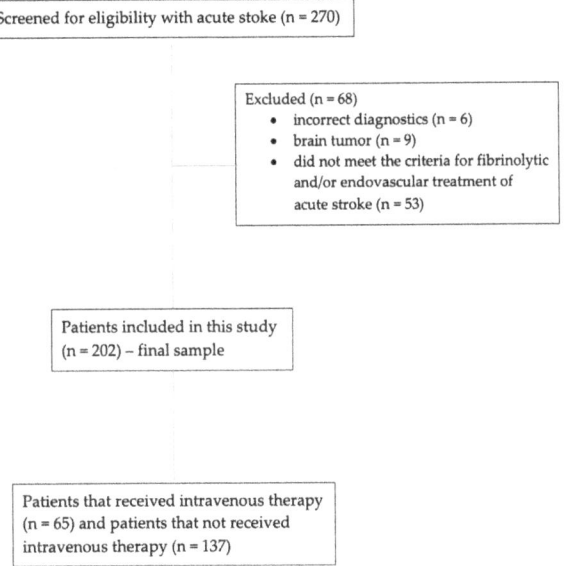

Figure 1. Study flowchart.

The study cohort consisted of 202 patients with acute stroke, 51.98% ($n = 105$) of whom were women and 60.40% ($n = 122$) had an urban origin. The median age was 74 years with an interquartile range of 62–81 years. The systolic blood pressure had a mean of 160 mmHg with an interquartile range of 140–190 mmHg; the diastolic blood pressure had a mean of 90 mmHg with an interquartile range of 80–100 mmHg. INR had an interquartile range of 1.03–1.4 with a mean of 1.13 (Table 1).

Table 1. Baseline characteristics of patients at the time of admission to the ED.

Variable	Mean ±/− Std. Deviation	Median (IQR)
Patient Characteristics		
Age, years	70.93 ± 12.04	74 (62–81)
SBP, mmHg	162.92 ± 32.53	160 (140–190)
DBP, mmHg	89.36 ± 20.35	90 (80–100)
Sp02, %	95.69 ± 4.09	97 (95–98)
Platelet count ($\times 10^9$/L)	198.95 ± 77.37	195 (158–247.75)
Partial thromboplastin time, seconds	30.57 ± 16.33	26.3 (24–30.425)
Prothrombin time, seconds	17.76 ± 19.74	13.3 (12.4–14.9)
INR	1.72 ± 1.8	1.13 (1.03–1.4)

Table 1. Cont.

Variable	Mean ±/− Std. Deviation	Median (IQR)
ED Time Targets (minutes)		
Onset-to-ED door time	173.96 ± 64.84	180 (120–217.5)
Door-to-physician time	5.35 ± 4.66	4 (3–7)
Door-to-CT time	51.05 ± 5.92	52 (48–55)
Door-in-door-out time	61.68 ± 6.62	61 (59–65)
Stroke Severity Scale and Hospitalization Duration		
Hospital stay period, days (SD)	10.69 ± 7.78	8 (5–14)
NIHSS at admission to stroke team	13.62 ± 5.56	13.5 (10–18)
NIHSS at 24 h	11.83 ± 8.74	11 (4–18)
Variable	Number	Percentage
Male	97	48.02
Female	105	51.98
Thrombolysis (yes)	65	32.18
Origin		
Urban	122	60.40
Rural	80	39.60
Arrival Mode		
Ambulance with assistant/paramedic	35	17.33
Ambulance with doctor	138	68.32
Private vehicle	29	14.36
Acute Stroke Symptoms (yes)		
Aphasia	47	23.27
Dysarthria	46	22.77
Headache	7	3.47
Coma	15	7.43
Fatigue	14	6.93
Left hemiparesis	64	31.68
Right hemiparesis	71	35.14
Risk Factors (yes)		
Obesity	12	5.94
Smoking	37	18.32
Alcohol	33	16.34
Dyslipidemia	22	10.98
Arterial Hypertension	166	82.18
Diabetes Mellitus	54	26.73
Anticoagulant treatment	36	17.82
Previous stroke/TIA	25	12.38
Outcomes (yes)		
Dependent disability	10	4.95
Death	71	35.15
Independent (absence of disability)	121	59.90

SBP, systolic blood pressure; DBP, diastolic blood pressure; SpO2, oxygen saturation; INR, international-normalized ratio; TIA, transient ischemic attack. Values were expressed as mean ± standard deviation (SD); by median (interquartile range); or by number (%).

When analyzing ED time targets, we found that the median onset-to-ED door time was 180 min (IQR, 120–217.5 min), door-to-physician time was 4 min (IQR, 3–7 min), door-to-CT time was 52 min (IQR, 48–55 min), and door-in-door-out time was 61 min (IQR, 59–65 min). NIHSS at admission to the stroke team was 13.5 (IQR, 10–18) and at 24 h was 11 (IQR, 4–18). Only 32.18% (n = 65) performed thrombolysis. The most frequent symptom of AIS was right hemiparesis, present in 35.14% (n = 71) of patients, and the rarest symptom was a headache, present in only 7 patients (3.47%). Arterial hypertension (82.18% of patients) was the most frequent risk factor for stroke, followed by diabetes mellitus (26.73% of patients) and smoking (18.32% of patients). About 14.39% arrived by private vehicle at the ED, while the most of the patients (68.32%) arrived by ambulance with a doctor and 17.33% arrived by ambulance with an assistant/paramedic. From all patients with AIS, 35.15% (n = 71) died during hospitalization, 4.95% (n = 10) remained with a dependent disability and 59.90% (n = 121) were discharged with the absence of a disability (Table 1).

3.2. Analysis of Patients' Characteristics between the Two Groups

By applying the Mann–Whitney U Test, we observed that age ($p = 0.525$), INR values ($p = 0.328$), ED time targets such as door-to physician time ($p = 0.245$), door-to-CT time ($p = 0.219$), door-to-transfer ($p = 0.24$), NIHSS at admission to the Neurology department ($p = 0.405$), or NIHSS after 24 h ($p = 0.9$) did not have a statistically significant effect on the administration or no rt-PA treatment in patients included in our study (Table 2).

Table 2. Association of performed or no iv rt-PA treatment with patients' characteristics (n = 202).

Variable	Group	Valid	Mean ±/− Std. Deviation	Median (IQR)	p—Mann–Whitney U Test
Age, years	No rt-PA	137	70.4 ± 12.6	72 (62–81)	0.525
	rt-PA	65	72.05 ± 10.77	75 (65–80)	
Onset-to-ED door time, minutes	No rt-PA	137	203.5 ± 54.87	210 (180–240)	<0.001
	rt-PA	65	111.69 ± 31.6	120 (90–120)	
Door-to-physician time, minutes	No rt-PA	137	5.23 ± 4.98	4 (2–6)	0.245
	rt-PA	65	5.6 ± 3.92	5 (3–7)	
Door-to-CT time, minutes	No rt-PA	137	50.66 ± 6.18	51 (47–55)	0.219
	rt-PA	65	51.88 ± 5.27	53 (49–55)	
Door-in-door-out time, minutes	No rt-PA	137	62.07 ± 6.84	61 (59–67)	0.24
	rt-PA	65	60.86 ± 6.11	59 (59–65)	
Platelet count ($\times 10^9$/L)	No rt-PA	137	192.77 ± 82.09	189 (137–247)	0.044
	rt-PA	65	211.99 ± 65	207 (168–252)	
Partial thromboplastin time, seconds	No rt-PA	137	30.71 ± 16.56	25.9 (23.8–29.9)	0.418
	rt-PA	65	30.27 ± 15.94	26.4 (24.3–31.1)	
Prothrombin time, seconds	No rt-PA	137	17.18 ± 18.13	13.2 (12.5–14.4)	0.279
	rt-PA	65	18.97 ± 22.89	13.7 (12.1–15.1)	
INR	No rt-PA	137	1.77 ± 1.71	1.13 (1.03–1.58)	0.328
	rt-PA	65	1.59 ± 1.97	1.12 (1–1.31)	
Hospitalization period, days (SD)	No rt-PA	137	10.95 ± 7.42	11 (5–14)	0.151
	rt-PA	65	10.15 ± 8.51	8 (5–13)	
NIHSS at admission to Neurology Department	No rt-PA	137	13.86 ± 5.71	14 (10–18)	0.405
	rt-PA	65	13.12 ± 5.25	13 (10–17)	
NIHSS at 24 h	No rt-PA	137	11.66 ± 8.32	12 (5–17)	0.9
	rt-PA	65	12.17 ± 9.63	10 (3–19)	

INR, international-normalized ratio. Values were expressed as mean ± standard deviation (SD); Mann–Whitney U Test for continue variable without Gaussian distribution—data represented by median (interquartile range).

Only the high platelet count ($p = 0.044$) and lower onset-to-ED door time were statistically significant correlated with the administration of rt-PA treatment ($p < 0.001$) (Figure 2A,B).

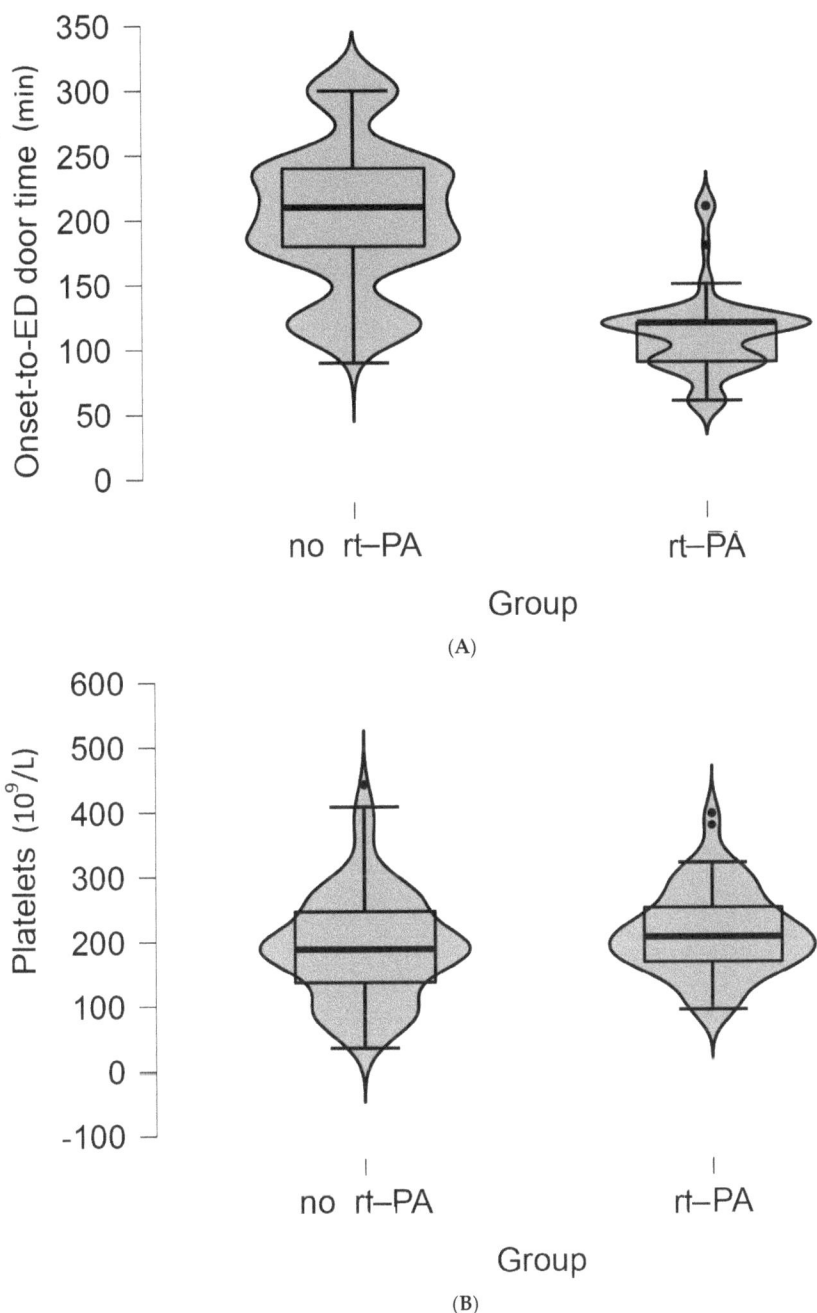

Figure 2. (**A**) Violin plot of the values of the onset-to-ED door time (minutes) between the two groups of patients. The boxplot inside violin represents the median and interquartile range. (**B**) Violin plot of the values of platelet count ($\times 10^9$/L) between the two groups of patients. The boxplot inside violin represents the median and interquartile range.

3.3. Analysis of Outcomes and Factors' Frequency Associated with Administration of Intravenous rt-PA between the Two Groups

Table 3 showed the outcomes and factors frequency between the two groups. No statistically significant correlation was found between the two groups regarding the arrival mode type at ED ($p = 0.958$) or risk factor, like the presence of obesity ($p = 0.755$), smoking ($p = 0.971$), alcohol ($p = 0.068$), arterial hypertension ($p = 0.237$), diabetes mellitus ($p = 0.866$), or atrial fibrillation ($p = 0.308$).

Table 3. Outcomes and factors' frequency between two groups.

Variable	No rt-PA ($n = 137$)	rt-PA ($n = 65$)	p Chi^2 Test
Arrival Mode			
Ambulance with assistant/paramedic (yes)	24 (17.5%)	11 (15.9%)	
Ambulance with doctor (yes)	94 (68.6%)	44 (67.7%)	0.958
Private vehicle (yes)	19 (13.9%)	10 (15.4%)	
Risk factors			
Obesity (yes)	9 (75.0%)	3 (25.0%)	0.755
Smoking (yes)	25 (67.6%)	12 (32.4%)	0.971
Alcohol (yes)	27 (81.8%)	6 (18.2%)	0.068
Arterial hypertension (yes)	116 (69.9%)	50 (30.1%)	0.237
Diabetes mellitus (yes)	36 (66.7%)	18 (33.3%)	0.866
Atrial fibrillation (yes)	40 (74.1%)	14 (25.5%)	0.308
Vitamin K antagonists' treatment (yes)	27 (75.0%)	9 (25.0%)	0.334
Outcomes			
Dependent (disability)	6 (4.4%)	4 (6.2%)	
Death	46 (33.6%)	25 (38.5%)	0.636
Independent (absence of disability)	36 (55.4%)	85 (62.0%)	

Chi^2 Test for nominal variables—data represented by number (%).

In total, seventy-one patients (33.6% patients from the no rt-PA group and 38.5% from the rt-PA group) died. A total of ten patients, six patients from the no rt-PA group (4.4%) and four patients from the rt-PA group (6.2%) remained with a disability after the hospitalization period. After comparing outcomes between groups, no statistically significant correlation ($p = 0.636$) was observed.

3.4. The Association between Administration or Absence of rt-PA Treatment with Hospitalization Days and Length of Survival

In the context of analyzing patient survival, we compare the cum survival curves of those who received intravenous rt-PA and those who did not; we found that the mean of hospitalization days is insignificantly higher for the no rt-PA group ($p = 0.455$) (Figure 3 and Table 4).

Table 4. Mean survival time between the two groups.

	Means and Medians for Survival Time							
	Mean				Median			
Group	Estimate	Std. Error	95% Confidence Interval		Estimate	Std. Error	95% Confidence Interval	
			Lower Bound	Upper Bound			Lower Bound	Upper Bound
No rt-PA	23.100	2.190	18.807	27.393	21.000	0.506	20.008	21.992
rt-PA	22.313	2.766	16.893	27.734	20.000	6.010	8.220	31.780
Overall	23.364	1.744	19.946	26.782	21.000	1.407	18.241	23.759

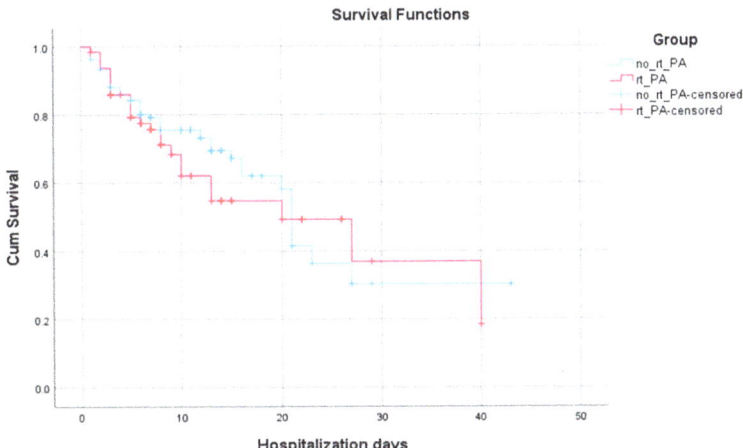

Figure 3. The Kaplan–Meier survival curves for patients with AIS admitted in an ED from a hospital with no stroke team/unit according to administration or absence of intravenous thrombolysis after interhospital transfer.

3.5. Correlation of ED Time Targets with Death Outcome

Analyzing ED time targets, we found that the median onset-to-ED door time was 180 min (IQR, 120–210 min for living patients vs. 120–240 min for deceased patients, $p = 0.016$), and door-to-physician time ($p = 0.281$) was 5 min (IQR, 3–7 min for living people) vs. 4 min (IQR, 2.5–6 min for deceased people). The median of door-to-CT time ($p = 0.037$) (Figure 4) was 50 min (IQR, 47–54 min for living patients) vs. 53 min (IQR, 2.5–6 min for deceased people), and door-in-door-out time was 60 min (IQR, 59–64 min for living people) vs. 62 min (IQR, 59–67 min for deceased people) (Table 5).

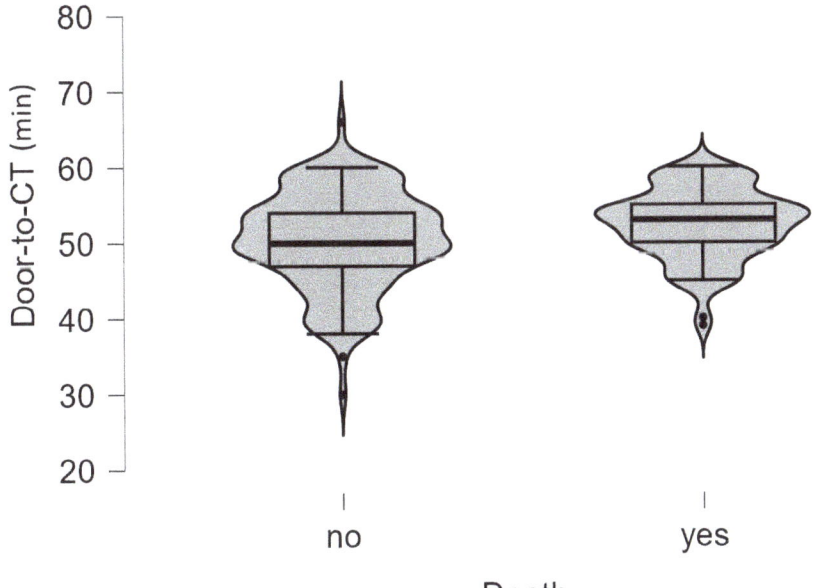

Figure 4. Violin plot of the values of the door-to-CT time (minutes) between the two groups of patients. The boxplot inside violin represents the median and interquartile range.

Table 5. Correlation between ED time targets with death outcome.

Variable	Death	Valid	Mean +/− Std. Deviation	Median (IQR)	p—Mann–Whitney U Test
Onset-to-ED door time	No	131	173.21 ± 63.76	180 (120–210)	0.016
	Yes	71	175.35 ± 67.23	180 (120–240)	
Door-to-physician time	No	131	5.68 ± 5.19	5 (3–7)	0.281
	Yes	71	4.75 ± 3.44	4 (2.5–6)	
Door-to-CT time	No	131	50.38 ± 6.42	50 (47–54)	0.037
	Yes	71	52.28 ± 4.65	53 (50–55)	
Door-in-door-out time	No	131	61.32 ± 6.59	60 (59–64)	0.321
	Yes	71	62.35 ± 6.68	62 (59–67)	

4. Discussion

In this study of acute ischemic stroke patients admitted to our ED, only 32.18% ($n = 65$) received intravenous thrombolysis, which was a lower rate than expected based on the study design (onset of symptoms was under three h, patients were eligible for IV thrombolysis, and there was a distance of 3.5 km from a hospital with a neurologist and stroke team). Internationally, the administration of rt-PA remains largely underutilized, with only 10–20% of all eligible patients estimated by recent studies to receive the treatment [14]. However, the mean value of the last report from Romania according to the National Program of Priority Actions in the Interventional Treatment of Patients with Acute Cerebral Vascular Accident (PA-CVA) registry [7,8], was lower than 10% (around 5.4%) [9]. Compared to other national values, our study founding rate is increased.

Moreover, a low rate of national thrombolysis for AIS was reported by China, at almost 2.4%, with the rate of intravenous rt-PA usage being only about 1.6% [15]. Similarly, 68.7% of patients with acute ischemic stroke from a study conducted in Iran did not arrive at the hospital early enough for intravenous thrombolysis, which was administered to only 3.1% of patients [16]. Aguiar de Sousa et al. performed an analysis of data reported by 44 national stroke societies in Europe, including Romania, and found that, overall, at the European level, only 7.3% of stroke patients with ischemic stroke received intravenous thrombolysis, with only 1.9% received an endovascular treatment; the highest country rates were 20.6% (Netherlands) and 19.6% (Denmark). The proportion of stroke patients with intravenous thrombolysis was reported to be 0.0% in countries like Albania or Georgia [17].

In a retrospective study involving 394 patients with acute ischemic stroke, it was observed that the administration of IV thrombolysis was significantly lower. Out of the total subjects, only 19.8% ($n = 78$) had the stroke code activated, and reperfusion therapy was conducted in 5.3% ($n = 21$) of them. The average time for various steps, such as the arrival of patients, first visit by an emergency medicine resident, presence of a neurology resident in ED, notification of the acute stroke team, and interpretation of the computed tomography scan, was shorter for patients who qualified for iv thrombolysis compared to those who were no longer eligible for fibrinolytic therapy [18].

These low administration rates determined the evaluation of the use of rt-PA in different medical assistance settings and the elaboration of different methods to improve the proportion of patients who received this treatment. To improve ED care, in a study that analyzed all patients who present at the ED in a city for a period of 3 years, it was noted that about 73% of patients with AIS arrive at the ED outside of the treatment window, because they waited to see whether the symptoms will improve on their own [19].

Despite the absence of a stroke team, most of the recommendations [20] that are adopted by stroke unit centers in developed countries to achieve good outcomes in acute stroke care were also adopted in our ED. These include "the availability and interpretation of CT scans 24/7 and the rapid performance of laboratory tests, in addition to administrative support, strong leadership and continuing education".

Among the factors associated with not receiving rt-PA in our study, no statistically significant correlation was found between the two groups regarding the arrival mode type at the ED ($p = 0.958$), or the presence of risk factors for stroke. Referring to the data from the literature, there are different proportions of the arrival mode type or risk factors between groups, such as arriving during the night shift ($p < 0.0001$) and not arriving with the emergency medical system ($p = 0.0080$) [21], and about 18.1% reported arriving at the ED by ambulance, while the majority arrived by private car [22]; considering the fact that the proportion of risk factors and arrival mode are statistically insignificant between our study groups, we find these to be strengths in this study, because we can better analyze the impact of ED time targets on the received or absence of rt-PA treatments in patients with AIS.

Therefore, our study sought to analyze the factors that influence ED time targets in patients with AIS. The data show that for all sample patients, the median onset-to-ED door time was 180 min (IQR, 120–217.5 min), door-to-physician time was 4 min (IQR, 3–7 min), door-to-CT time was 52 min (IQR, 48–55 min), and door-in-door-out time was 61 min (IQR, 59–65 min). ED time targets such as door-to physician time ($p = 0.245$), door-to-CT time ($p = 0.219$), door-to-transfer ($p = 0.24$), NIHSS at admission to Neurology department ($p = 0.405$), or NIHSS after 24 h ($p = 0.9$) did not have a statistically significant effect on the administration or absence of rt-PA treatment in patients included in our study. Only the high platelet count ($p = 0.044$) and the lower onset-to-ED door time were statistically significantly correlated with the administration of rt-PA treatment ($p < 0.001$). The mean door-to-CT time of 52 min in our study is double the target time recommended of < 25 min. Almost the same value of the door-to-CT time (49.4 min) was registered in a study from Lebanon [23]. When Stamm et al. [10] evaluated door-in-door-out times for acute stroke transfers among 108913 patients (mean age, 66.7 years; 71.7% non-Hispanic White; 50.6% male) transferred from 1925 hospitals, the median door-in-door-out time was 174 min, a value that was almost triple compared to the door-in-door-out time from the present study that found a mean of 61 min (IQR, 59–65 min). In another study of over 46 months, a total of 133 AIS patients were transferred from a primary metropolitan stroke center to undergo mechanical thrombectomy. This retrospective analysis found that the mean door-in-door-out time experienced a yearly reduction of 14%. In 2015, the interquartile range for this time frame was 111 min (IQR, 98–142), which decreased to 67 min (IQR, 55–94) by 2018. Based on these findings, the authors concluded that activating the stroke code can achieve a door-in-door-out time target of less than 60 min [24].

When analyzing ED time targets and the death outcome for all study patients, only the highest door-to-CT time (Figure 4) was statistically significantly correlated with this outcome. In the context of analyzing patient survival, we compare the cum survival curves of those who received intravenous rt-PA and those who did not, and we found that the mean of hospitalization days is insignificantly higher for the no rt-PA group ($p = 0.455$). In a study that also analyzed treatment outcomes in hospitals with and without stroke units, the hospitalization time was also similar in both groups ($p = 0.191$), regarding receiving or not receiving the rt-PA treatment. They also did not observe differences between groups in the number of patients presenting a disability at discharge (mRS > 2; $p = 0.986$). However, they did observe a lower rate of disability at discharge among patients who received IV-tPA versus those who did not, in both hospital groups (group A: 19 vs. 30, $p < 0.05$; group B: 2 vs. 41, $p < 0.001$) [25].

In the type 1 (major) ED in England, a study of more than 5 million individual patients admitted over 2 years showed that a total of 433,962 deaths occurred within 30 days. The overall crude all-cause 30-day mortality rate was 8.71%. The most significant change in the standardized all-cause 30-day mortality was an 8% increase in the cohort of patients who waited more than 6 to 8 h from arrival in the ED. The impact of delays becomes evident between 5 and 12 h, resulting in a consistent and proportional effect. When the transfer of admitted patients to inpatient beds is delayed beyond 6 to 8 h from their arrival at the ED, there is an additional death for every 82 patients [26].

Jaffe et al., when examining the relationship between emergency department crowding and the provision of timely emergency care for acute stroke, door-to-imaging time (IQR, 17–52 min), and door-to-needle time (IQR, 31–59 min) for alteplase delivery, found no significant differences during periods of higher ED utilization in bivariate or multivariable testing. Of the 1379 patients who were presented to the ED during the study period, 78% presented during times of normal capacity, 15% during high crowding, and 7% during severe crowding [27]. A single-center cohort of consecutive ischemic stroke patients ($n = 325$) reported that the median emergency department length-of-stay of 5.8 h was inversely associated with the thrombolysis rate ($p = 0.021$) ($n = 67$, 21%) [28].

Last but not least, in the present study, for eligible patients with a symptom onset of less than 3 h, the ED medical team had a favorable clinical performance on ED time targets because the stroke code was activated. However, the rate of thrombolysis was low if we consider the achieved interhospital transfer time. Furthermore, given the current data, there is a clear need for a neurologist at our institution. Because most patients with stroke code activation subsequently became ineligible for intravenous thrombolysis, this demonstrated the need to initiate intravenous thrombolysis performed under the supervision of at least an on-call neurologist as soon as possible if the patient is eligible and the subsequent transfer to a neurology department for continuous supervision afterwards.

Study Limitations

Several limitations should be considered when interpreting these data. As this study was a single hospital-based study conducted on patients belonging to a city where emergency medical systems are trained to activate a stroke code and archive ED time targets, these results may not be generalizable to the entire population due to certain specific characteristics of the group studied. For example, the presence or absence of a team specializing in a stroke code may vary from one health center to another, which could influence transfer times. As another limitation, we mention the impossibility of measuring the effect of prioritizing the care of the patient with a stroke code compared to other patients, which could influence the time for the interhospital transfer of these patients. Finally, we could not control every possible factor of influence, and the observational nature of this design leaves the possibility of residual confounding.

5. Conclusions

In our study, the IV rt-PA administration rate was 32.18% and lower than expected, considering the achievement of almost all of the ED time targets. Although the thrombolysis rate in our hospital is relatively good compared with international standards, there is still room for improvement. A significant correlation for ED time targets was found between the highest door-to-CT time and death outcome for all patients.

Our findings suggest that hospitals without a stroke unit should restructure their AIS management by achieving ED time targets as much as possible to enable a better response in AIS cases; this will impact interhospital transfers and AIS patients' outcome.

Author Contributions: Conceptualization D.P., F.B. and A.I.; methodology, D.P., A.P., D.S., C.G.W., O.A.M., A.T., C.T. and F.B.; software, A.T., F.B. and D.S.; validation, O.A.M., A.I., F.B. and C.G.W.; investigation, A.P., D.P., A.I. and O.A.M.; resources, D.P. and F.B.; writing—original draft preparation, D.P., A.I., C.T. and F.B.; writing—review and editing, F.B., C.G.W., D.S., A.I. and O.A.M.; visualization, O.A.M., D.S., A.P. and A.T.; supervision, O.A.M. and A.I. All authors have read and agreed to the published version of the manuscript.

Funding: This research received no external funding.

Institutional Review Board Statement: The study was conducted in accordance with the Declaration of Helsinki, and approved by the Ethics Committee of Emergency Municipal Clinical Hospital Timisoara (approval number: I-32931/ 20.11.2023).

Informed Consent Statement: Informed consent was obtained from all subjects involved in the study.

Data Availability Statement: The datasets are not publicly available, but de-identified data may be provided upon request from Popa Daian.

Conflicts of Interest: The authors declare no conflict of interest.

References

1. Feigin, V.L.; Stark, B.A.; Johnson, C.O.; Roth, G.A.; Bisignano, C.; Abady, G.G.; Abbasifard, M.; Abbasi-Kangevari, M.; Abd-Allah, F.; Abedi, V.; et al. Global, regional, and national burden of stroke and its risk factors, 1990–2019: A systematic analysis for the Global Burden of Disease Study 2019. *Lancet Neurol.* **2021**, *20*, 795–820. [CrossRef] [PubMed]
2. Stroke Alliance for Europe. The Burden of Stroke in Europe—Challenges for Policy Makers. Available online: https://www.stroke.org.uk/sites/default/files/the_burden_of_stroke_in_europe_-_challenges_for_policy_makers.pdf (accessed on 14 January 2022).
3. Toyoda, K. Intravenous rt-PA therapy for acute ischemic stroke: Efficacy and limitations. *Rinsho Shinkeigaku* **2009**, *49*, 801–803. [CrossRef] [PubMed]
4. Fugate, J.E.; Rabinstein, A.A. Absolute and Relative Contraindications to IV rt-PA for Acute Ischemic Stroke. *Neurohospitalist* **2015**, *5*, 110–121. [CrossRef] [PubMed]
5. Jauch, E.C.; Saver, J.L.; Adams, H.P., Jr.; Bruno, A.; Connors, J.J.; Demaerschalk, B.M.; Khatri, P.; McMullan, P.W., Jr.; Qureshi, A.I.; Rosenfield, K.; et al. Guidelines for the early management of patients with acute ischemic stroke: A guideline for healthcare professionals from the American Heart Association/American Stroke Association. *Stroke* **2013**, *44*, 870–947. [CrossRef] [PubMed]
6. Priority Action for Interventional Treatment of Patients with Acute Stroke. Standard Operating Procedure Regarding the Patient Track and Therapeutic Protocol in Romania. Available online: https://legislatie.just.ro/Public/DetaliiDocument/209994 (accessed on 12 October 2023).
7. Uivarosan, D.; Bungau, S.; Tit, D.M.; Moisa, C.; Fratila, O.; Rus, M.; Bratu, O.G.; Diaconu, C.C.; Pantis, C. Financial Burden of Stroke Reflected in a Pilot Center for the Implementation of Thrombolysis. *Medicina* **2020**, *56*, 54. [CrossRef] [PubMed]
8. Sabau, M.; Bungau, S.; Buhas, C.L.; Carp, G.; Daina, L.-G.; Judea-Pusta, C.T.; Buhas, B.A.; Jurca, C.M.; Daina, C.M.; Tit, D.M. Legal medicine implications in fibrinolytic therapy of acute ischemic stroke. *BMC Med. Ethics* **2019**, *20*, 70. [CrossRef] [PubMed]
9. Tiu, C.; Terecoasă, E.O.; Tuță, S.; Bălașa, R.; Simu, M.; Sabău, M.; Stan, A.; Radu, R.A.; Tiu, V.; Cășaru, B.; et al. Quality of acute stroke care in Romania: Achievements and gaps between 2017 and 2022. *Eur. Stroke J.* **2023**, *8* (Suppl. S1), 44–51. [CrossRef]
10. Stamm, B.; Royan, R.; Giurcanu, M.; Messe, S.R.; Jauch, E.C.; Prabhakaran, S. Door-in-Door-out Times for Interhospital Transfer of Patients With Stroke. *JAMA* **2023**, *330*, 636–649. [CrossRef]
11. Aho, K.; Harmsen, P.; Hatano, S.; Marquardsen, J.; Smirnov, V.E.; Strasser, T. Cerebrovascular disease in the community: Results of a WHO collaborative study. *Bull. World Health Organ.* **1980**, *58*, 113.
12. Sacco, R.L.; Kasner, S.E.; Broderick, J.P.; Caplan, L.R.; Connors, J.J.; Culebras, A.; Elkind, M.S.V.; George, M.G.; Hamdan, A.D.; Higashida, R.T.; et al. An Updated Definition of Stroke for the 21st Century. *Stroke* **2013**, *44*, 2064–2089. [CrossRef]
13. Goldstein, L.B.; Bertels, C.; Davis, J.N. Interrater reliability of the NIH stroke scale. *Arch. Neurol.* **1989**, *46*, 660–662. [CrossRef] [PubMed]
14. de Souza, A.C.; Sebastian, I.A.; Zaidi, W.A.W.; Nasreldein, A.; Bazadona, D.; Amaya, P.; Elkady, A.; Gebrewold, M.A.; Vorasayan, P.; Yeghiazaryan, N.; et al. Regional and national differences in stroke thrombolysis use and disparities in pricing, treatment availability, and coverage. *Int. J. Stroke* **2022**, *17*, 990–996. [CrossRef]
15. Dong, Q.; Dong, Y.; Liu, L.; Xu, A.; Zhang, Y.; Zheng, H.; Wang, Y. The Chinese Stroke Association scientific statement: Intravenous thrombolysis in acute ischaemic stroke. *Stroke Vasc. Neurol.* **2017**, *2*, 147–159. [CrossRef] [PubMed]
16. Ayromlou, H.; Soleimanpour, H.; Farhoudi, M.; Taheraghdam, A.; Sadeghi Hokmabadi, E.; Rajaei Ghafouri, R.; Najafi Nashali, M.; Sharifipour, E.; Mostafaei, S.; Altafi, D. Eligibility assessment for intravenous thrombolytic therapy in acute ischemic stroke patients; evaluating barriers for implementation. *Iran. Red. Crescent. Med. J.* **2014**, *16*, e11284. [CrossRef] [PubMed]
17. Aguiar de Sousa, D.; von Martial, R.; Abilleira, S.; Gattringer, T.; Kobayashi, A.; Gallofré, M.; Fazekas, F.; Szikora, I.; Feigin, V.; Caso, V.; et al. Access to and delivery of acute ischaemic stroke treatments: A survey of national scientific societies and stroke experts in 44 European countries. *Eur. Stroke J.* **2019**, *4*, 13–28. [CrossRef] [PubMed]
18. Hassankhani, H.; Soheili, A.; Vahdati, S.S.; Mozaffari, F.A.; Fraser, J.F.; Gilani, N. Treatment Delays for Patients With Acute Ischemic Stroke in an Iranian Emergency Department: A Retrospective Chart Review. *Ann. Emerg. Med.* **2019**, *73*, 118–129. [CrossRef] [PubMed]
19. Al Khathaami, A.M.; Mohammad, Y.O.; Alibrahim, F.S.; Jradi, H.A. Factors associated with late arrival of acute stroke patients to emergency department in Saudi Arabia. *SAGE Open Med.* **2018**, *6*, 2050312118776719. [CrossRef] [PubMed]
20. Alberts, M.J.; Latchaw, R.E.; Jagoda, A.; Wechsler, L.R.; Crocco, T.; George, M.G.; Connolly, E.S.; Mancini, B.; Prudhomme, S.; Gress, D.; et al. Revised and Updated Recommendations for the Establishment of Primary Stroke Centers. *Stroke* **2011**, *42*, 2651–2665. [CrossRef]
21. Ganti, L.; Mirajkar, A.; Banerjee, P.; Stead, T.; Hanna, A.; Tsau, J.; Khan, M.; Garg, A. Impact of emergency department arrival time on door-to-needle time in patients with acute stroke. *Front. Neurol.* **2023**, *14*, 1126472. [CrossRef]
22. Dimitriou, P.; Tziomalos, K.; Christou, K.; Kostaki, S.; Angelopoulou, S.M.; Papagianni, M.; Ztriva, E.; Chatzopoulos, G.; Savopoulos, C.; Hatzitolios, A.I. Factors associated with delayed presentation at the emergency department in patients with acute ischemic stroke. *Brain Inj.* **2019**, *33*, 1257–1261. [CrossRef]

23. El Sayed, M.J.; El Zahran, T.; Tamim, H. Acute stroke care and thrombolytic therapy use in a tertiary care center in Lebanon. *Emerg. Med. Int.* **2014**, *2014*, 438737. [CrossRef] [PubMed]
24. Choi, P.M.C.; Tsoi, A.H.; Pope, A.L.; Leung, S.; Frost, T.; Loh, P.-S.; Chandra, R.V.; Ma, H.; Parsons, M.; Mitchell, P.; et al. Door-in-Door-Out Time of 60 Minutes for Stroke With Emergent Large Vessel Occlusion at a Primary Stroke Center. *Stroke* **2019**, *50*, 2829–2834. [CrossRef] [PubMed]
25. Masjuan, J.; Gállego Culleré, J.; Ignacio García, E.; Mira Solves, J.J.; Ollero Ortiz, A.; Vidal de Francisco, D.; López-Mesonero, L.; Bestué, M.; Albertí, O.; Acebrón, F.; et al. Stroke treatment outcomes in hospitals with and without stroke units. *Neurologia (Engl. Ed.)* **2020**, *35*, 16–23. [CrossRef] [PubMed]
26. Jones, S.; Moulton, C.; Swift, S.; Molyneux, P.; Black, S.; Mason, N.; Oakley, R.; Mann, C. Association between delays to patient admission from the emergency department and all-cause 30-day mortality. *Emerg. Med. J.* **2022**, *39*, 168–173. [CrossRef]
27. Jaffe, T.A.; Goldstein, J.N.; Yun, B.J.; Etherton, M.; Leslie-Mazwi, T.; Schwamm, L.H.; Zachrison, K.S. Impact of Emergency Department Crowding on Delays in Acute Stroke Care. *West J. Emerg. Med.* **2020**, *21*, 892–899. [CrossRef]
28. Minaeian, A.; Patel, A.; Essa, B.; Goddeau, R.P., Jr.; Moonis, M.; Henninger, N. Emergency Department Length of Stay and Outcome after Ischemic Stroke. *J. Stroke Cerebrovasc. Dis.* **2017**, *26*, 2167–2173. [CrossRef]

Disclaimer/Publisher's Note: The statements, opinions and data contained in all publications are solely those of the individual author(s) and contributor(s) and not of MDPI and/or the editor(s). MDPI and/or the editor(s) disclaim responsibility for any injury to people or property resulting from any ideas, methods, instructions or products referred to in the content.

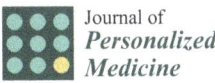

Article

A Simple Bacteremia Score for Predicting Bacteremia in Patients with Suspected Infection in the Emergency Department: A Cohort Study

Hyelin Han [1], Da Seul Kim [1,2], Minha Kim [1], Sejin Heo [1], Hansol Chang [1], Gun Tak Lee [1], Se Uk Lee [1], Taerim Kim [1], Hee Yoon [1], Sung Yeon Hwang [1], Won Chul Cha [1,2,3], Min Sub Sim [1], Ik Joon Jo [1], Jong Eun Park [1,4,*] and Tae Gun Shin [1,2,*]

1. Department of Emergency Medicine, Samsung Medical Center, Sungkyunkwan University School of Medicine, Seoul 06355, Republic of Korea; wc.cha@samsung.com (W.C.C.); minsub01.sim@samsung.com (M.S.S.); ikjoon.jo@samsung.com (I.J.J.)
2. Department of Digital Health, Samsung Advanced Institute for Health Sciences & Technology (SAIHST), Sunkyunkwan University, Seoul 06351, Republic of Korea
3. Digital Innovation, Samsung Medical Center, Seoul 06351, Republic of Korea
4. Department of Emergency Medicine, College of Medicine, Kangwon National University, Chuncheon 20341, Republic of Korea
* Correspondence: jongeun7.park@samsung.com (J.E.P.); taegunshin@skku.edu (T.G.S.); Tel.: +82-2-3410-2053 (J.E.P. & T.G.S.)

Abstract: Bacteremia is a life-threatening condition that has increased in prevalence over the past two decades. Prompt recognition of bacteremia is important; however, identification of bacteremia requires 1 to 2 days. This retrospective cohort study, conducted from 10 November 2014 to November 2019, among patients with suspected infection who visited the emergency department (ED), aimed to develop and validate a simple tool for predicting bacteremia. The study population was randomly divided into derivation and development cohorts. Predictors of bacteremia based on the literature and logistic regression were assessed. A weighted value was assigned to predictors to develop a prediction model for bacteremia using the derivation cohort; discrimination was then assessed using the area under the receiver operating characteristic curve (AUC). Among the 22,519 patients enrolled, 18,015 were assigned to the derivation group and 4504 to the validation group. Sixteen candidate variables were selected, and all sixteen were used as significant predictors of bacteremia (model 1). Among the sixteen variables, the top five with higher odds ratio, including procalcitonin, neutrophil–lymphocyte ratio (NLR), lactate level, platelet count, and body temperature, were used for the simple bacteremia score (model 2). The proportion of bacteremia increased according to the simple bacteremia score in both cohorts. The AUC for model 1 was 0.805 (95% confidence interval [CI] 0.785–0.824) and model 2 was 0.791 (95% CI 0.772–0.810). The simple bacteremia prediction score using only five variables demonstrated a comparable performance with the model including sixteen variables using all laboratory results and vital signs. This simple score is useful for predicting bacteremia-assisted clinical decisions.

Keywords: bacteremia prediction; simple bacteremia score

1. Introduction

Bacteremia is a major cause of morbidity and requires early detection and appropriate antibiotics [1–3]. Blood culture sampling is a mandatory method used to detect bacteremia and it is commonly performed for various patients from less severe infection to septic shock in emergency departments [4,5]. However, the prevalence of bacteremia is 7–20%, with a high rate of false positives, and the indication(s) for performing blood cultures is not well established, and thus remains controversial [6,7]. This results in unnecessary invasive procedures, consumption of resources, increased costs, inappropriate or delayed use of antibiotics, and prolonged hospital admission [8,9]. The rate of false positives in blood cultures or contamination is often the highest in emergency departments (EDs). Robertson et al. reported contamination rates of 11.7% in the ED versus 2.5% in other hospital areas [10].

Several clinical tools have been developed to predict bacteremia using biomarkers and clinical scores [11]. Consequently, prediction tools that enable exclusion of bacteremia are highly desirable to increase the cost effectiveness of microbiological tests [12]. Shapiro et al. suggested indications for blood culture if at least one major or two minor criteria were present among 13 clinical parameters associated with high risk; otherwise, patients are classified as "low risk" and unnecessary blood cultures may be omitted [13,14]. In addition to clinical findings, many studies have suggested that laboratory investigations, such as procalcitonin (PCT) and neutrophil–lymphocyte ratio (NLR), may play a useful role in predicting bacteremia [15,16].

Although many efforts have been made to predict bacteremia, there are no detailed guidelines specifying which patients should undergo blood culture testing, and no simple prediction score for bacteremia has yet been developed. To identify patient groups at low risk for bacteremia and optimize the blood culture practice, we aimed to develop a simple scoring system that has a discriminatory value for predicting bacteremia and can help physicians classify bacteremia risk.

2. Materials and Methods

This large retrospective cohort study was conducted at the Samsung Medical Center, a university-affiliated, tertiary care referral hospital, located in Seoul, South Korea, from 10 November 2014 to 10 November 2019. This study was approved by the Institutional Review Board (IRB, 2023-09-144) of Samsung Medical Center. Given the retrospective nature of the study and the use of anonymized patient data, requirements for informed consent were waived. The study population comprised patients >18 years of age with suspected infection who underwent blood culture sampling and administration of antibiotics at ED admission, excluding those with septic shock [17].

2.1. Study Design

The primary goal was to develop a simple bacteremia score (model 2) and to compare its predictive accuracy with a reference model (model 1).

Data were retrospectively collected from electronic medical records. The population was randomly divided into a derivation cohort (80% of randomly selected samples) and a validation cohort (20% of randomly selected samples) with R statistical programming. The sampling code splits 80% of data selected randomly into the training set and the remaining 20% of samples into the test dataset. The sampling function in R randomly picks 80% of rows from the dataset without replacement. Sixteen candidate variables possibly associated with bacteremia were analyzed, including epidemiological factors, vital signs, and laboratory results, using simple comparison and univariable and multivariable logistic regression analyses of the derivation cohort to identify risk factors using variables with a p value < 0.05. The cut-off values for each variable were determined using the area under the receiver operating characteristic (ROC) curve (AUC) and based on a literature review. A reference model (model 1) was developed using the derivation cohort. Model 1 comprised variables that were found to be risk factors for bacteremia in multivariable logistic regression. Among the variables used in model 1, the top 5 with the highest odds ratio (OR) were selected to develop a simple bacteremia score model (model 2) using a regression coefficient-based scoring method. Predictive factors for bacteremia were identified using multivariable analysis and were assigned a weighted value to each factor using β coefficients that reflect predictive power. The β coefficients were rounded to the nearest whole number. A rounded number for each predictive factor was assigned to the bacteremia score. The overall risk score was calculated as the sum of these scores.

Finally, an ROC curve was generated, and the AUC was used to calculate the performance of the prediction model using the validation cohort. The prediction performances of the two models were compared along with 1 variable (PCT) that exhibited the most potent association with bacteremia.

2.2. Statistical Analysis

Standard descriptive statistics were used for all variables including baseline demographics and outcomes. The results are expressed as the median and interquartile range (IQR) for continuous variables and as the number with percentage for categorical data. Continuous variables were compared using the Wilcoxon rank-sum test. Categorical variables were compared using the chi-squared test. Univariate and multivariate logistic regression analyses were performed to assess variables related to bacteremia. Multivariate analysis using the logistic regression model was used to evaluate independent predictors of bacteremia, as measured by the estimated OR with corresponding 95% confidence interval (CI). Adjusted variables were selected based on their clinical relevance to bacteremia, and significant associations in the univariate analysis were entered into a stepwise logistic regression model. In the stepwise logistic regression model, the p value threshold to enter into the model was set at 0.25, and at 0.1 to be excluded from the model. The goodness-of-fit of the final logistic regression model was assessed using the Hosmer–Lemeshow test. The variables entered into the model were assigned a score based on the ORs to calculate a simple and easy clinical prediction scale. The discrimination performance of the risk index was assessed using the AUC, and the optimum cut-off value was chosen for optimal sensitivity and specificity. DeLong's test was used to compare ROC curves between the models. Differences with $p < 0.05$ were considered to be statistically significant. Statistical analysis was performed using Stata version 18.0 (StataCorp LLC, College Station, TX, USA).

2.3. Definition

The cut-off values for predictors were as follows: age > 65 years; systolic blood pressure (SBP) < 90 mmHg or mean arterial pressure (MAP) $\leq$ 65 mmHg; heart rate (HR) > 130 beats/min; respiratory rate (RR) $\geq$ 22 breaths/min; body temperature (BT) < 36 °C or >38 °C; white blood cell (WBC) count < 4000 or >12,000 cells per microliter; platelet count (PLT) < 150,000 cells per microliter; band neutrophil > 5%, absolute neutrophil count (ANC) < 1.5 or >8.3 cells per microliter; absolute lymphocyte count (ALC) > 2.9 or <0.9 cells per microliter; neutrophil–lymphocyte ratio (NLR, [ANC/ALC]) $\geq$ 10 determined based on previous studies. Five "remnant" variables, including albumin < 3.5 g/dL, creatinine > 1.5 mg/dL, lactate (Lac) > 2 mmol/L [16], C-reactive protein (CRP) > 8 mg/dL, and PCT > 0.5 ng/mL, were determined by the AUC. The outcome variables were bacteremia and positive blood culture results. A positive blood culture was defined as the growth of pathogens compatible with the clinical presentation. Common skin flora (e.g., coagulase-negative staphylococci [CNS], *Corynebacterium* spp., *Cutibacterium* spp., and *Bacillus* spp.) were regarded as contamination and defined as a false-positive blood culture. Two independent physicians assessed "true" blood culture positivity.

3. Results

3.1. Baseline Characteristics

A total of 43,294 patients from the institution registry were assessed for eligibility during the study period. Of these, we excluded a total of 20,775 patients who transferred from another hospital or to another hospital at the ED, who presented with cardiac arrest, who had limitations on invasive care, who had inadequate data such as missing data or non-acquisition of PCT. Ultimately, 22,519 patients were included in the analysis, of whom 18,015 (80%) were randomly assigned to the derivation cohort and 4504 (20%) to the validation cohort (Figure 1).

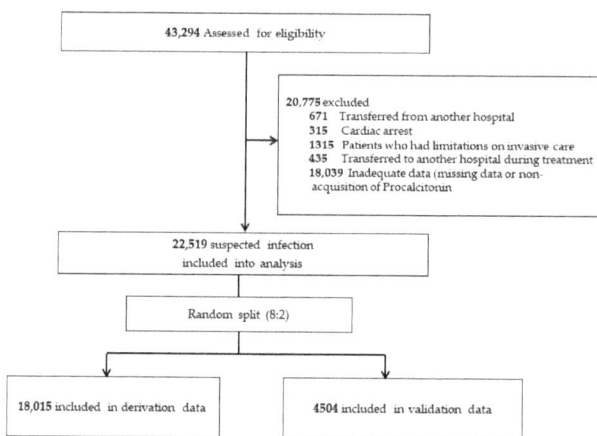

Figure 1. Study flow.

Among the 22,519 patients, 12,232 (54.3%) were male and 9741 (43.3%) were >65 years of age. Additionally, among the 22,519 patients, 174 (0.8%) were contaminated (false positive) and 2701 (12.0%) had bacteremia (true positive). The baseline characteristics of all patients are summarized in Table 1. The total incidence of bacteremia was 12% (n = 2701/22,519), while the proportion of Gram-positive bacteremia (GPB) was 2.8% (n = 693/22,519) and Gram-negative bacteremia (GNB) was 8.6% (n = 1941/22,519). The incidence of bacteremia was 11.9% (n = 2145) in the derivation cohort and 12.3% (n = 556) in the validation cohort. The proportion of GPB was 2.7% (n = 491) and GNB was 8.6% (n = 1551) in the derivation cohort, while the proportion of GPB was 2.9% (n = 132) and GNB was 8.7% (n = 390) in the validation cohort (Table S1). The proportion of bacteremia increased according to the simple bacteremia score in both cohorts (Figure 2).

Table 1. The baseline characteristics of the study population.

	Overall	No Bacteremia	Bacteremia	p Value
	N = 22,519	N = 19,818 (88)	N = 2701 (12)	
Age > 65	9741 (43.3)	8285 (41.8)	1456 (53.9)	<0.001
Gender, Male	12,232 (54.3)	10,771 (54.3)	1461 (54.1)	0.816
Vital Signs				<0.001
Blood pressure				
SBP < 90 or MAP ≤ 65	2047 (9.1)	1535 (7.7)	512 (19.0)	<0.001
HR > 130 beats/min	2557 (11.4)	2090 (10.5)	467 (17.3)	<0.001
RR ≥ 22 cycles/min	4888 (21.7)	4215 (21.3)	673 (24.9)	<0.001
BT (>38 °C or <36 °C)	10,018 (44.5)	8407 (42.4)	1611 (59.6)	<0.001
Laboratories				
WBC (>12,000 or <4000/mm^3)	11,696 (51.9)	10,136 (51.1)	1560 (57.8)	<0.001
PLT < 150,000/mm^3	609 (2.7)	455 (2.3)	154 (5.7)	<0.001
Band Neutrophil > 5%	578 (2.6)	434 (2.2)	144 (5.3)	<0.001
ANC < 1.5 or >8.3	12,563 (55.8)	10,851 (54.8)	1712 (63.4)	<0.001
ALC > 2.9 or <0.9	17,470 (77.6)	15,042 (75.9)	2428 (89.9)	<0.001
Neutrophil–Lymphocyte Ratio	6.9 (3.3–12.9)	6.4 (3.1–11.7)	12.4 (5.9–22.3)	<0.001
Albumin, g/dL	3.7 (3.2–4.1)	3.7 (3.2–4.1)	3.5 (2.9–3.9)	<0.001
Creatinine, mg/dL	0.9 (0.7–1.2)	0.8 (0.7–1.2)	1.1 (0.8–1.7)	<0.001
Lactate, mmol/L	1.7 (1.2–2.5)	1.6 (1.2–2.3)	2.4 (1.6–3.8)	<0.001
CRP, mg/dL	7.5 (2.7–14.9)	7.0 (2.5–14.0)	11.3 (4.8–19.8)	<0.001
Procalcitonin, mg/dL	0.3 (0.1–4.5)	0.2 (0.1–0.8)	2.6 (0.6–14.2)	<0.001

Table 1. Cont.

	Overall	No Bacteremia	Bacteremia	p Value
	N = 22,519	N = 19,818 (88)	N = 2701 (12)	
NLR ≥ 10	7793 (34.6)	6191 (31.2)	1602 (59.3)	<0.001
Lactate > 2 mmol/L	8439 (37.5)	6784 (34.2)	1655 (61.3)	<0.001
Creatinine > 1.5 mg/dL	3881 (17.2)	3074 (15.5)	807 (29.9)	<0.001
Albumin < 3.5 g/dL	8396 (37.3)	7074 (35.7)	1322 (48.9)	<0.001
CRP > 8 mg/dL	10,734 (47.7)	9045 (45.6)	1689 (62.5)	<0.001
PCT > 0.5 mg/dL	8687 (38.6)	6608 (33.3)	2079 (77.0)	<0.001
Vasopressor use	2504 (11.1)	1673 (8.4)	831 (30.8)	<0.001

The data are presented as mean ± standard deviation, median (IQR) or number (%). Abbreviations: IQR, interquartile range; SBP, systolic blood pressure; MAP, mean arterial pressure; HR: heart rate; RR, respiratory rate; BT, body temperature; WBC, white blood cell; PLT, platelet; ANC, absolute neutrophil count; ALC, absolute lymphocyte count; NLR, neutrophil–lymphocyte ratio; CRP, c-reactive protein; PCT, procalcitonin.

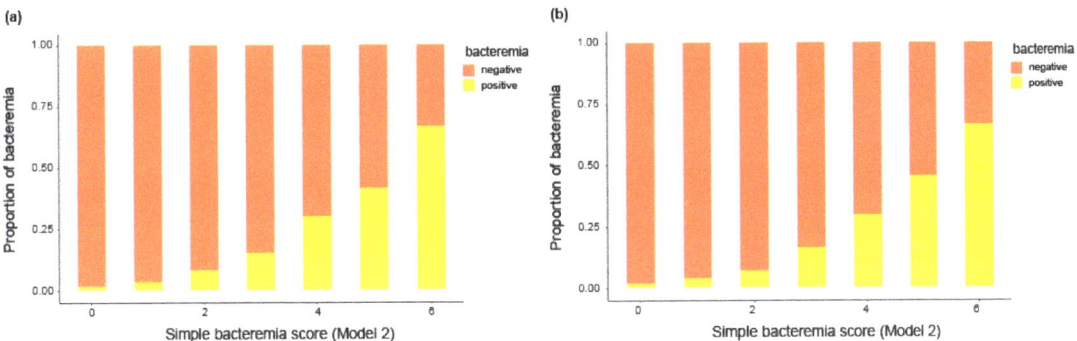

Figure 2. Distribution of bacteremia according to the simple bacteremia score levels in the derivation and validation cohort. (**a**) Derivation cohort. (**b**) Validation cohort.

3.2. Predictors of Bacteremia and Developing a Reference Model (Model 1)

In the analysis comparing the no-bacteremia and bacteremia cohorts, 16 variables were used for multivariable logistic regression analysis. The 16 variables included age > 65 years, SBP < 90 mmHg or MAP ≤ 65 mmHg, HR > 130 beats/min, RR ≥ 22 breaths/min, BT < 36 °C or >38 °C, WBC < 4000 or >12,000 cells per microliter, PLT < 150,000 cells per microliter, band neutrophil > 5%, ANC < 1.5 or >8.3, ALC > 2.9 or <0.9, NLR ≥ 10, albumin < 3.5 g/dL, Creatinine > 1.5 mg/dL, Lac > 2 mmol/L, CRP > 8 mg/dL, and PCT > 0.5 ng/mL. Consequently, all 16 variables were significantly associated with bacteremia in the univariate analysis (all $p < 0.001$) (Supplementary Table S2). This association remained consistently significant after adjusting for confounding factors in the multivariate logistic regression model (Supplementary Table S3). A reference model (model 1) was developed using the derivation cohort.

3.3. Score Development and Developing a Simple Bacteremia Score (Model 2)

Among the sixteen variables, PCT, NLR, Lac, PLT, and BT were the top five variables associated with bacteremia in the derivation cohort. Subsequently, a final logistic regression was performed to develop a simple bacteremia score (model 2) with the top five variables in the derivation cohort (Table 2). More specifically, these top five variables were significantly associated with an increased risk for bacteremia in a multivariable logistic regression: PCT (adjusted odds ratio [aOR] 4.65 [95% confidence interval (CI) 4.16–5.20]; $p < 0.001$); NLR (aOR 2.27 [95% CI 2.05–2.51]; $p < 0.001$); Lac (aOR 2.00 [95% CI 1.81–2.20]; $p < 0.001$); PLT (aOR 2.72 [95% CI 2.15–3.43]; $p < 0.001$); BT (aOR 2.04 [95% CI 1.85–2.25]; $p < 0.001$). The Hosmer–Lemeshow test revealed a goodness-of-fit of 11.18 ($p = 0.131$).

Table 2. Multivariable logistic regression of top five predictors of bacteremia in all variables, derivation cohort, and validation cohort.

Multivariable Predictor Set	(Total) OR	95% CI	p	(Derivation) OR	95% CI	p	(Validation) OR	95% CI	p
PCT > 0.5 mg/dL	4.78	4.33–5.29	<0.001	4.65	4.16–5.20	<0.001	5.33	4.28–6.69	<0.001
NLR ≥ 10	2.25	2.05–2.46	<0.001	2.27	2.05–2.51	<0.001	2.19	1.80–2.67	<0.001
Lactate > 2 mmol/L	1.97	1.80–2.15	<0.001	2.00	1.81–2.20	<0.001	1.87	1.54–2.28	<0.001
PLT < 150,000/mm^3	2.64	2.14–3.25	<0.001	2.72	2.15–3.43	<0.001	2.37	1.48–3.72	<0.001
BT (>38 °C or <36 °C)	2.06	1.89–2.25	0.854	2.04	1.85–2.25	<0.001	2.16	1.78–2.62	<0.001

The p value of goodness-of-fit with the Hosmer–Lemeshow test = 0.131. Abbreviations: OR, odds ratio; CI, confidence interval; PCT, procalcitonin; NLR, neutrophil–lymphocyte ratio; PLT, platelet; BT, body temperature.

Using these top five variables, a simple score was developed. To simplify the assessment of bacteremia risk, we used points-based scoring systems, which enable a rapid decision for risk without the use of computers or electronic devices. To develop point-based scoring systems, the OR (β coefficients) of this model were converted into integer single risk scores by rounding to the nearest whole number. The points associated with each level of each risk factor are defined relative to the points associated with an increase in a specified continuous variable. The calculated points were assigned as independent variables. The simple bacteremia score was developed by summing the computed component variables; the total score ranged from 0 to 6 points (Table 3).

Table 3. Clinical prediction scale (simple bacteremia risk score of the final model).

Risk Factors	Points (Score)
Procalcitonin > 0.5 mg/dL	2
Neutrophil–Lymphocyte Ratio ≥ 10	1
Lactate > 2 mmol/L	1
Platelet < 150,000/mm^3	1
Body Temperature (>38 °C or <36 °C)	1

3.4. Bacteremia Rate According to Score

The rate of bacteremia according to the assigned scores is presented in Figure 3. In the derivation cohort, the rate of bacteremia gradually increased with the simple bacteremia scores: 1.8% at score 0; 3.5% at score 1; 8.2% at score 2; 15.4% at score 3; 30.3% at score 4; 41.5% at score 5; 66.7% at score 6 ($p < 0.01$). This trend in the prevalence of bacteremia was similar in the validation cohort: 1.7% at score 0; 4.0% at score 1; 7.1% at score 2; 16.6% at score 3; 29.9% at score 4; 45.5% at score 5; 66.7% at score 6 ($p < 0.01$).

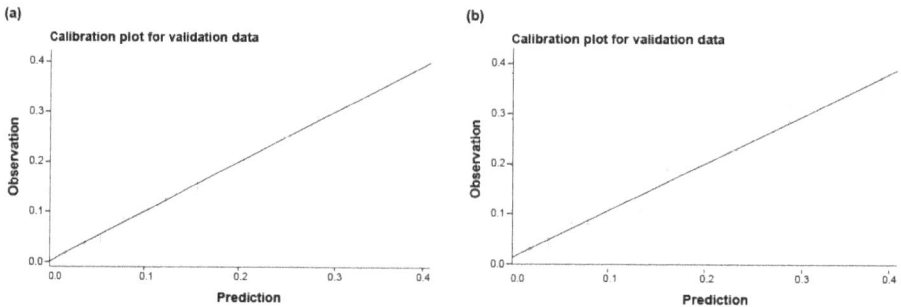

Figure 3. Calibration of simple bacteremia score in the derivation and validation cohort. Calibration plot indicating the agreement between model predictions (predicted probabilities) and observed frequencies. Individual data points are shown for the derivation and validation cohort. (**a**) Derivation cohort. (**b**) Validation cohort.

3.5. Validation

Prediction models were proposed and the performance of each was assessed using ROC curves and calibration plots. In the derivation cohort, the AUC for predicting bacteremia in model 1 was calculated to be 0.803 (95% CI 0.794–0.813), model 2 was 0.790 (95% CI 0.781–0.800), and PCT alone was 0.717 (95% CI 0.708–0.727) ($p < 0.0001$ [DeLong's test]). The predictive accuracy of model 2 (simple bacteremia risk score) was 0.87 (95% CI 0.87–0.88) with sensitivity of 0.958, specificity of 0.215, positive predictive value of 0.900, and negative predictive value of 0.411. Using the validation cohort, an internal validation of the predictive value of PCT versus another prediction rule was performed (model 1, model 2, and PCT alone). A total of 4504 patients were enrolled and analyzed for internal validation. The bacteremia prediction performance of model 1 was 0.805 (95% CI 0.785–0.824), model 2 was 0.791 (95% CI 0.772–0.810), and that of PCT alone was 0.753 (95% CI 0.773–0.774) ($p < 0.0001$ [DeLong's test]) (Table 4, Figure 4). The predictive accuracy of model 2 (simple bacteremia risk score) was 0.86 (95% CI 0.84–0.87) with sensitivity of 0.93, specificity of 0.310, positive predictive value of 0.905, and negative predictive value of 0.389. The constructed model calibration plot is presented in Figure 4, showing that predicted probabilities were close to the observed bacteremia.

Table 4. Area under the receiver operating characteristics curve (AUC) of model 1, simple score, and procalcitonin to predict bacteremia in the derivation and validation data.

Predictor Set	Derivation	Validation
Model 1 (All 16)	0.803 (0.794–0.813)	0.805 (0.785–0.824)
Model 2 (Simple score)	0.790 (0.781–0.800)	0.791 (0.772–0.810)
Procalcitonin	0.717 (0.708–0.727)	0.753 (0.733–0.774)

Model 1: bacteremia predicting model based on 16 predictors associated with bacteremia. Model 2: simple bacteremia score using top five predictors associated with bacteremia among sixteen variables.

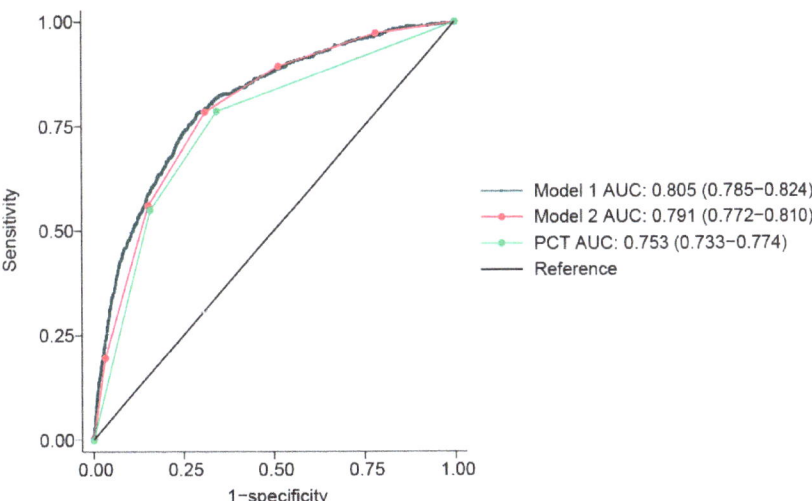

Figure 4. Receiver operating characteristic (ROC) curves of model 1, simple score, and procalcitonin to predict bacteremia in the validation data.

3.6. Subgroup Analysis with Missing Data Imputation

To address missing data, traditional approaches were used by imputing missing values using the median of the observed values. After imputation of missing data, 43,294 patients were enrolled and included in the second analysis. The population was randomly divided into a derivation cohort (n = 30,305 [70% randomly selected sample]) and a validation cohort (n = 12,989 [30% randomly selected sample]). The performances of model 1, model 2, and PCT were 0.797 (95% CI 0.783–0.811), 0.778 (95% CI 0.764–0.793), and 0.706 (95% CI 0.690–0.772), respectively; DeLong's test had a $p < 0.0001$ in the validation cohort (Supplementary Figure S1). In addition, 13,832 had normal PCT within <0.5 ng/mL among 43,294 patients. The proportion of patients with bacteremia was also higher at higher score levels, even in the subgroup with normal PCT (Supplementary Figure S2). The simple bacteremia score was 0.686 (95% CI 0.664–0.709) in the derivation cohort and 0.671 (95% CI 0.624–0.718) in the normal PCT group.

4. Discussion

In this derivation and validation analysis of 22,519 patients with suspected infection, we compared the predictive performance of model 1 comprising 16 variables based on factors associated with bacteremia, model 2 comprising five variables, and PCT which was used alone. This study derived a simple bacteremia prediction score (i.e., model 2) to simplify the prediction of bacteremia, demonstrating a comparable performance to that of model 1. The simple bacteremia score (model 2) demonstrated a similar performance to that of model 1 (AUC of 0.805 vs. 0.791), whereas PCT, as the best individual variable, yielded a weaker AUC of 0.753. The risk for developing bacteremia was proportional to an increase in score.

Strengths of the present study include its large population size with validation, risk stratification guiding blood cultures, applicability to a wide range of populations, including low-risk patients, heterogeneous characteristics of the ED, and simplicity of the score. We identified significant predictors of bacteremia in a large derivation cohort and validated the performance of the model. An increased risk for bacteremia has been an important issue among patients with sepsis; consequently, false-positive blood cultures are associated with prolonged hospital stays and increased costs, with no definitive guidelines for blood cultures [5,7]. Several studies have explored bacteremia prediction tools; however, these have been limited to specific diseases and complexity [18–22]. Therefore, risk stratification of bacteremia using this simple tool may help identify patients who require a blood culture. Conversely, a score of 0 can aid in the direction of not performing a blood culture because the probability of bacteremia was <2% at this score. Miquel et al. established a bacteremia rate < 8% for patients with pneumonia with a score ≤ 1 using six variables [23]. Potentially, the application of our simple bacteremia score (model 2) may better eliminate unnecessary blood cultures and the misuse/abuse of antibiotics.

Moreover, the simplicity of the bacteremia prediction score makes it convenient and useful for clinicians. In a recent study, David et al. used a modified Shapiro score (MSS) ≥ 3 and NLR > 12, which demonstrated an equal ability to predict bacteremia, with AUCs of 0.71 and 0.74, respectively; however, combining MSS and NLR did not increase the predictive performance [24]. Although Chun-Yuan et al. established an AUC of 0.867 (95% CI 0.806–0.928) using a combination of four factors (age ≥ 65 years, involvement area, liver cirrhosis, systemic inflammatory response syndrome); however, this score was limited in patients with cellulitis [22]. Lars et al. reported an AUC of 0.86 (95% CI 0.83–0.89) using a combination of four biomarkers (NLR, CRP, Lac, and PCT) [25]. However, it was likely easier to distinguish bacteremia in the population, which had a relatively high risk for bacteremia because verified bacterial infection reached 55.6% of enrolled patients. However, the present study yielded an AUC of approximately 0.80 using simple variables, even in heterogeneous populations (12% bacteremia). Therefore, our simple bacteremia score would be applicable in a wide range of populations containing low-risk patients and heterogeneous ED characteristics with the advantage of simplicity.

Regarding the risk factors for bacterial infection, the Shapiro score, which was originally developed to rule out patients with a low risk for positive blood cultures, is commonly used [14,26]. Our variables are consistent with the Shapiro scores and the previous literature. Among the variables analyzed in this study, PCT was the most influential independent predictor. Afshan et al. reported that AUCs for PCT were 0.781 and 0.70 [27] in a study by

Sibtain et al. [28], outperforming CRP in both studies. Abderrahim et al. reported that a PCT threshold, ranging from ≤0.4 to ≥0.75 ng/mL, demonstrated high diagnostic accuracies for bacteremia in a cross-sectional study [29]. Marik et al. also suggested PCT < 0.5 ng/mL as an effective screening tool to exclude bacteremia, and NLR as a screening test for bacteremia when PCT is unavailable [30]. The NLR has been described as a predictor of bacteremia [14]. Ratzinger et al. found that neutrophils were the best individual variable to predict bacteremia, with an AUC of 0.694 [31]. Thrombocytopenia has also been known to be a prognostic marker for bacteremia and associated with bacteremia [32–35]. Lac, a prognostic biomarker for sepsis, is not considered to be specific for diagnosing sepsis [36]; however, several studies have shown that Lac is a biomarker for diagnosing bacterial sepsis [25].

Previous studies have proposed several models to predict bacteremia using not only simple predictors but also > 10 variables. In a cross-sectional study, models with 20 and 10 variables were established with AUCs of 0.767 and 0.759, respectively [31]. Paul et al. reported that a computerized decision support system (TREAT) yielded an AUC of 0.68 (95% CI 0.63–0.73) in the first cohort and 0.70 (95% CI 0.67–0.73) in the second cohort in predicting bacteremia [37]. Another study by Ratzinger et al. proposed 29 parameters to predict bacteremia, with an AUC of 0.729 (95% CI 0.679–0.779), whereas PCT exhibited an AUC similar to that reported by machine learning methods that failed to improve the moderate diagnostic accuracy of PCT [38].

Our study had several limitations, the first of which were its single center, cohort design. As a result, the proposed predictive model requires external validation to confirm the fitting of models. Nevertheless, this scoring algorithm enables ease of usability. Second, although we attempted to identify risk factors for bacteremia, other possible confounding factors should be considered, and significant predictors that have clinical validity should be identified. Third, in the subgroup analysis of missing imputations, most single-imputation methods provided biased estimates and incorrect standard errors. Fourth, patients taking antibiotics before their ED visits were not investigated. This could have affected the results of detecting bacteremia, although it could have made the models more practical. Fifth, this study lacks the data such as investigation of underlying disease states including diabetes mellitus or immunosuppression that may impact rates of bacteremia.

5. Conclusions

In this study, we developed and validated a simple bacteremia prediction score, which using only five variables, demonstrated a similar performance to the model with sixteen variables using all laboratory results and vital signs. This simple score is useful in predicting bacteremia and assisting in clinical decisions.

Supplementary Materials: The following supporting information can be downloaded at: https://www.mdpi.com/article/10.3390/jpm14010057/s1. Figure S1: Receiver operating characteristic (ROC) curves of all models, simple score, and procalcitonin to predict bacteremia in the validation data with missing data imputation; Figure S2: Distribution of bacteremia by simple bacteremia score levels in normal procalcitonin level of <0.5; Table S1: Baseline characteristics of the derivation and validation cohort; Table S2: Univariable logistic regression in all 16 variables; Table S3: Multivariable logistic regression in all 16 variables.

Author Contributions: Conceptualization, T.G.S. and S.Y.H.; methodology, T.G.S., H.H. and J.E.P.; software, J.E.P., W.C.C., M.S.S. and I.J.J.; validation, H.Y., G.T.L., T.K. and S.U.L.; formal analysis, T.G.S., H.H. and J.E.P.; investigation, H.C., S.H. and M.K.; resources, D.S.K. and H.H.; data curation, D.S.K. and H.H.; writing—original draft preparation, H.H. and J.E.P.; writing—review and editing, T.G.S. and S.Y.H.; visualization, H.H.; supervision, J.E.P. and T.G.S.; project administration, M.S.S. and T.G.S. All authors have read and agreed to the published version of the manuscript.

Funding: This research received no external funding.

Institutional Review Board Statement: The study was conducted in accordance with the Declaration of Helsinki, and approved by the Institutional Review Board (IRB 2023-09-144) of Samsung Medical Center.

Informed Consent Statement: Patient consent was waived due to the retrospective and anonymous nature of the study.

Data Availability Statement: The datasets used in this work are available upon reasonable request from the corresponding author and are not publicly available.

Conflicts of Interest: The authors declare no conflicts of interest.

References

1. Bearman, G.M.; Wenzel, R.P. Bacteremias: A leading cause of death. *Arch. Med. Res.* **2005**, *36*, 646–659. [CrossRef] [PubMed]
2. Laupland, K.B. Defining the epidemiology of bloodstream infections: The 'gold standard' of population-based assessment. *Epidemiol. Infect.* **2013**, *141*, 2149–2157. [CrossRef] [PubMed]
3. Liu, A.; Yo, C.H.; Nie, L.; Yu, H.; Wu, K.; Tong, H.S.; Hsu, T.C.; Hsu, W.T.; Lee, C.C. Comparing mortality between positive and negative blood culture results: An inverse probability of treatment weighting analysis of a multicenter cohort. *BMC Infect. Dis.* **2021**, *21*, 182. [CrossRef] [PubMed]
4. Park, H.; Shin, T.G.; Kim, W.Y.; Jo, Y.H.; Hwang, Y.J.; Choi, S.H.; Lim, T.H.; Han, K.S.; Shin, J.; Suh, G.J.; et al. A quick Sequential Organ Failure Assessment-negative result at triage is associated with low compliance with sepsis bundles: A retrospective analysis of a multicenter prospective registry. *Clin. Exp. Emerg. Med.* **2022**, *9*, 84–92. [CrossRef] [PubMed]
5. Fabre, V.; Sharara, S.L.; Salinas, A.B.; Carroll, K.C.; Desai, S.; Cosgrove, S.E. Does This Patient Need Blood Cultures? A Scoping Review of Indications for Blood Cultures in Adult Nonneutropenic Inpatients. *Clin. Infect. Dis.* **2020**, *71*, 1339–1347. [CrossRef]
6. van Daalen, F.V.; Kallen, M.C.; van den Bosch, C.M.A.; Hulscher, M.; Geerlings, S.E.; Prins, J.M. Clinical condition and comorbidity as determinants for blood culture positivity in patients with skin and soft-tissue infections. *Eur. J. Clin. Microbiol. Infect. Dis.* **2017**, *36*, 1853–1858. [CrossRef]
7. Coburn, B.; Morris, A.M.; Tomlinson, G.; Detsky, A.S. Does this adult patient with suspected bacteremia require blood cultures? *Jama* **2012**, *308*, 502–511. [CrossRef]
8. Long, B.; Koyfman, A. Best Clinical Practice: Blood Culture Utility in the Emergency Department. *J. Emerg. Med.* **2016**, *51*, 529–539. [CrossRef]
9. Joo, Y.M.; Chae, M.K.; Hwang, S.Y.; Jin, S.C.; Lee, T.R.; Cha, W.C.; Jo, I.J.; Sim, M.S.; Song, K.J.; Jeong, Y.K.; et al. Impact of timely antibiotic administration on outcomes in patients with severe sepsis and septic shock in the emergency department. *Clin. Exp. Emerg. Med.* **2014**, *1*, 35–40. [CrossRef]
10. Robertson, P.; Russell, A.; Inverarity, D.J. The effect of a quality improvement programme reducing blood culture contamination on the detection of bloodstream infection in an emergency department. *J. Infect. Prev.* **2015**, *16*, 82–87. [CrossRef]
11. Barichello, T.; Generoso, J.S.; Singer, M.; Dal-Pizzol, F. Biomarkers for sepsis: More than just fever and leukocytosis-a narrative review. *Crit. Care* **2022**, *26*, 14. [CrossRef] [PubMed]
12. Laukemann, S.; Kasper, N.; Kulkarni, P.; Steiner, D.; Rast, A.C.; Kutz, A.; Felder, S.; Haubitz, S.; Faessler, L.; Huber, A.; et al. Can We Reduce Negative Blood Cultures With Clinical Scores and Blood Markers? Results From an Observational Cohort Study. *Medicine* **2015**, *94*, e2264. [CrossRef] [PubMed]
13. Wyss, G.; Berger, S.; Haubitz, S.; Fankhauser, H.; Buergi, U.; Mueller, B.; Schuetz, P.; Fux, C.A.; Conen, A. The Shapiro-Procalcitonin algorithm (SPA) as a decision tool for blood culture sampling: Validation in a prospective cohort study. *Infection* **2020**, *48*, 523–533. [CrossRef]
14. Shapiro, N.I.; Wolfe, R.E.; Wright, S.B.; Moore, R.; Bates, D.W. Who needs a blood culture? A prospectively derived and validated prediction rule. *J. Emerg. Med.* **2008**, *35*, 255–264. [CrossRef] [PubMed]
15. Ljungström, L.L.; Karlsson, D.; Pernestig, A.; Andersson, R.; Jacobsson, G. Neutrophil to lymphocyte count ratio performs better than procalcitonin as a biomarker for bacteremia and severe sepsis in the emergency department. *Crit. Care* **2015**, *19*, P66. [CrossRef]
16. Kim, S.Y.; Jeong, T.D.; Lee, W.; Chun, S.; Min, W.K. Procalcitonin in the assessment of bacteraemia in emergency department patients: Results of a large retrospective study. *Ann. Clin. Biochem.* **2015**, *52*, 654–659. [CrossRef]
17. Kim, D.S.; Park, J.E.; Hwang, S.Y.; Jeong, D.; Lee, G.T.; Kim, T.; Lee, S.U.; Yoon, H.; Cha, W.C.; Sim, M.S.; et al. Prediction of vasopressor requirement among hypotensive patients with suspected infection: Usefulness of diastolic shock index and lactate. *Clin. Exp. Emerg. Med.* **2022**, *9*, 176–186. [CrossRef]
18. Julián-Jiménez, A.; González Del Castillo, J.; García-Lamberechts, E.J.; Huarte Sanz, I.; Navarro Bustos, C.; Rubio Díaz, R.; Guardiola Tey, J.M.; Llopis-Roca, F.; Piñera Salmerón, P.; de Martín-Ortiz de Zarate, M.; et al. A bacteraemia risk prediction model: Development and validation in an emergency medicine population. *Infection* **2021**, *50*, 203–221. [CrossRef]
19. Kim, B.; Choi, J.; Kim, K.; Jang, S.; Shin, T.G.; Kim, W.Y.; Kim, J.Y.; Park, Y.S.; Kim, S.H.; Lee, H.J.; et al. Bacteremia Prediction Model for Community-acquired Pneumonia: External Validation in a Multicenter Retrospective Cohort. *Acad. Emerg. Med.* **2017**, *24*, 1226–1234. [CrossRef]

20. Washio, Y.; Ito, A.; Kumagai, S.; Ishida, T.; Yamazaki, A. A model for predicting bacteremia in patients with community-acquired pneumococcal pneumonia: A retrospective observational study. *BMC Pulm. Med.* **2018**, *18*, 24. [CrossRef]
21. Oh, W.S.; Kim, Y.S.; Yeom, J.S.; Choi, H.K.; Kwak, Y.G.; Jun, J.B.; Park, S.Y.; Chung, J.W.; Rhee, J.Y.; Kim, B.N. Developing a model to estimate the probability of bacteremia in women with community-onset febrile urinary tract infection. *J. Infect. Dev. Ctries.* **2016**, *10*, 1222–1229. [CrossRef] [PubMed]
22. Lee, C.Y.; Kunin, C.M.; Chang, C.; Lee, S.S.; Chen, Y.S.; Tsai, H.C. Development of a prediction model for bacteremia in hospitalized adults with cellulitis to aid in the efficient use of blood cultures: A retrospective cohort study. *BMC Infect. Dis.* **2016**, *16*, 581. [CrossRef] [PubMed]
23. Falguera, M.; Trujillano, J.; Caro, S.; Menéndez, R.; Carratalà, J.; Ruiz-González, A.; Vilà, M.; García, M.; Porcel, J.M.; Torres, A. A prediction rule for estimating the risk of bacteremia in patients with community-acquired pneumonia. *Clin. Infect. Dis.* **2009**, *49*, 409–416. [CrossRef] [PubMed]
24. Nestor, D.; Andersson, H.; Kihlberg, P.; Olson, S.; Ziegler, I.; Rasmussen, G.; Källman, J.; Cajander, S.; Mölling, P.; Sundqvist, M. Early prediction of blood stream infection in a prospectively collected cohort. *BMC Infect. Dis.* **2021**, *21*, 316. [CrossRef] [PubMed]
25. Ljungström, L.; Pernestig, A.K.; Jacobsson, G.; Andersson, R.; Usener, B.; Tilevik, D. Diagnostic accuracy of procalcitonin, neutrophil-lymphocyte count ratio, C-reactive protein, and lactate in patients with suspected bacterial sepsis. *PLoS ONE* **2017**, *12*, e0181704. [CrossRef] [PubMed]
26. Jessen, M.K.; Mackenhauer, J.; Hvass, A.M.; Ellermann-Eriksen, S.; Skibsted, S.; Kirkegaard, H.; Schønheyder, H.C.; Shapiro, N.I. Prediction of bacteremia in the emergency department: An external validation of a clinical decision rule. *Eur. J. Emerg. Med.* **2016**, *23*, 44–49. [CrossRef]
27. Bibi, A.; Basharat, N.; Aamir, M.; Haroon, Z.H. Procalcitonin as a biomarker of bacterial infection in critically ill patients admitted with suspected Sepsis in Intensive Care Unit of a tertiary care hospital. *Pak. J. Med. Sci.* **2021**, *37*, 1999–2003. [CrossRef]
28. Ahmed, S.; Siddiqui, I.; Jafri, L.; Hashmi, M.; Khan, A.H.; Ghani, F. Prospective evaluation of serum procalcitonin in critically ill patients with suspected sepsis- experience from a tertiary care hospital in Pakistan. *Ann. Med. Surg.* **2018**, *35*, 180–184. [CrossRef]
29. Oussalah, A.; Ferrand, J.; Filhine-Tresarrieu, P.; Aissa, N.; Aimone-Gastin, I.; Namour, F.; Garcia, M.; Lozniewski, A.; Guéant, J.L. Diagnostic Accuracy of Procalcitonin for Predicting Blood Culture Results in Patients With Suspected Bloodstream Infection: An Observational Study of 35,343 Consecutive Patients (A STROBE-Compliant Article). *Medicine* **2015**, *94*, e1774. [CrossRef]
30. Marik, P.E.; Stephenson, E. The ability of Procalcitonin, lactate, white blood cell count and neutrophil-lymphocyte count ratio to predict blood stream infection. Analysis of a large database. *J. Crit. Care* **2020**, *60*, 135–139. [CrossRef]
31. Ratzinger, F.; Dedeyan, M.; Rammerstorfer, M.; Perkmann, T.; Burgmann, H.; Makristathis, A.; Dorffner, G.; Lötsch, F.; Blacky, A.; Ramharter, M. A risk prediction model for screening bacteremic patients: A cross sectional study. *PLoS ONE* **2014**, *9*, e106765. [CrossRef] [PubMed]
32. Tsirigotis, P.; Chondropoulos, S.; Frantzeskaki, F.; Stamouli, M.; Gkirkas, K.; Bartzeliotou, A.; Papanikolaou, N.; Atta, M.; Papassotiriou, I.; Dimitriadis, G.; et al. Thrombocytopenia in critically ill patients with severe sepsis/septic shock: Prognostic value and association with a distinct serum cytokine profile. *J. Crit. Care* **2016**, *32*, 9–15. [CrossRef] [PubMed]
33. Menard, C.E.; Kumar, A.; Houston, D.S.; Turgeon, A.F.; Rimmer, E.; Houston, B.L.; Doucette, S.; Zarychanski, R. Evolution and Impact of Thrombocytopenia in Septic Shock: A Retrospective Cohort Study. *Crit. Care Med.* **2019**, *47*, 558–565. [CrossRef] [PubMed]
34. Schupp, T.; Weidner, K.; Rusnak, J.; Jawhar, S.; Forner, J.; Dulatahu, F.; Brück, L.M.; Hoffmann, U.; Kittel, M.; Bertsch, T.; et al. Diagnostic and prognostic role of platelets in patients with sepsis and septic shock. *Platelets* **2023**, *34*, 2131753. [CrossRef]
35. Péju, E.; Fouqué, G.; Charpentier, J.; Vigneron, C.; Jozwiak, M.; Cariou, A.; Mira, J.P.; Jamme, M.; Pène, F. Clinical significance of thrombocytopenia in patients with septic shock: An observational retrospective study. *J. Crit. Care* **2023**, *76*, 154293. [CrossRef]
36. Fan, S.L.; Miller, N.S.; Lee, J.; Remick, D.G. Diagnosing sepsis—The role of laboratory medicine. *Clin. Chim. Acta* **2016**, *460*, 203–210. [CrossRef]
37. Paul, M.; Andreassen, S.; Nielsen, A.D.; Tacconelli, E.; Almanasreh, N.; Fraser, A.; Yahav, D.; Ram, R.; Leibovici, L. Prediction of bacteremia using TREAT, a computerized decision-support system. *Clin. Infect. Dis.* **2006**, *42*, 1274–1282. [CrossRef]
38. Ratzinger, F.; Haslacher, H.; Perkmann, T.; Pinzan, M.; Anner, P.; Makristathis, A.; Burgmann, H.; Heinze, G.; Dorffner, G. Machine learning for fast identification of bacteraemia in SIRS patients treated on standard care wards: A cohort study. *Sci. Rep.* **2018**, *8*, 12233. [CrossRef]

Disclaimer/Publisher's Note: The statements, opinions and data contained in all publications are solely those of the individual author(s) and contributor(s) and not of MDPI and/or the editor(s). MDPI and/or the editor(s) disclaim responsibility for any injury to people or property resulting from any ideas, methods, instructions or products referred to in the content.

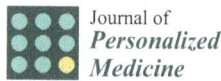

Article

The Challenges of The Diagnostic and Therapeutic Approach of Patients with Infectious Pathology in Emergency Medicine

Silvia Ioana Musuroi [1,2], Adela Voinescu [1,3,4], Corina Musuroi [3,4,*], Luminita Mirela Baditoiu [5], Delia Muntean [3,4], Oana Izmendi [1,3,4], Romanita Jumanca [6] and Monica Licker [3,4]

1. Doctoral School, "Victor Babeș" University of Medicine and Pharmacy, 300041 Timisoara, Romania; silvia.musuroi@umft.ro (S.I.M.)
2. Internal Medicine Department, Municipal Emergency Clinical Hospital, 300254 Timisoara, Romania
3. Microbiology Department, Multidisciplinary Research Center of Antimicrobial Resistance, "Victor Babes" University of Medicine and Pharmacy, 300041 Timisoara, Romania; muntean.delia@umft.ro (D.M.); licker.monica@umft.ro (M.L.)
4. Microbiology Laboratory, "Pius Brinzeu" County Clinical Emergency Hospital, 300723 Timisoara, Romania
5. Epidemiology Department, "Victor Babes" University of Medicine and Pharmacy, 300041 Timisoara, Romania; baditoiu.luminita@umft.ro
6. Romanian and Foreign Languages Department, "Victor Babes" University of Medicine and Pharmacy, 300041 Timisoara, Romania; romanita.jumanca@umft.ro
* Correspondence: corina.musuroi@umft.ro

Abstract: The emergency department (ED) represents an important setting for addressing inappropriate antimicrobial prescribing practices because of the time constraints and the duration of microbiological diagnosis. The purpose of this study is to evaluate the etiology and antimicrobial resistance (AMR) pattern of the community-acquired pathogens, as well as the epidemiological characteristics of patients admitted through the ED, in order to guide appropriate antibiotic therapy. Methods: A retrospective observational study was performed on 657 patients, from whom clinical samples (urine, purulent secretions, blood cultures, etc.) were collected for microbiological diagnosis in the first 3 days after presentation in the ED. The identification of pathogens and the antimicrobial susceptibility testing with minimum inhibitory concentration determination were carried out according to the laboratory protocols. Results: From the 767 biological samples analyzed, 903 microbial isolates were identified. *E. coli* was most frequently isolated (24.25%), followed by *Klebsiella* spp., *S. aureus* (SA), and non-fermentative Gram-negative bacilli. *E. coli* strains maintained their natural susceptibility to most antibiotics tested. In the case of *Pseudomonas* spp. and *Acinetobacter* spp., increased rates of AMR were identified. Also, 32.3% of SA strains were community-acquired MRSA. Conclusions: The introduction of rapid microbiological diagnostic methods in emergency medicine is imperative in order to timely identify AMR strains and improve therapeutic protocols.

Keywords: *Pseudomonas*; *Acinetobacter*; antibiotic

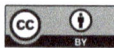

1. Introduction

Antibiotic-resistant bacteria such as methicillin-resistant *S. aureus* (MRSA) or extended-spectrum beta-lactamase (ESBL) producing Gram-negative bacilli (GNB) have emerged and spread from the hospital into the community. Inappropriate antibiotic (AB) use in human and veterinary medicine is the most important preventable cause of antimicrobial resistance (AMR) in both hospital-acquired infection (HAI) and community-acquired infection (CAI). Infections with resistant pathogens are associated with increased morbidity, mortality, and costs, and in addition, represent an important patient safety issue [1,2].

Emergency departments (EDs) are found at the interface between community and hospital and are an important setting concerning the approach of inappropriate antimicrobial prescribing practices, given their frequent use in these areas. ED clinicians routinely prescribe antimicrobials to patients for a wide variety of infections: skin and soft tissue, urinary tract, bloodstream, upper and lower respiratory tract, etc.

Practitioners in this setting have the unique opportunity to have a positive impact on the management of AB in both inpatient and outpatient settings, with important implications for both sectors. There are, for example, observational studies conducted in the ED, reporting significant rates of AB overprescribing in acute bronchitis (over 75% of prescriptions being for broad-spectrum AB, despite a certain improvement in clinical status) [3]. Reducing unnecessary AB administration is imperative, not only for lowering AMR rates in the community, but also for individual patient safety, given the increased rate of allergic reactions and the development of secondary infections associated with antibiotic administration, such as the *C. difficile* infection [4,5].

The literature data underline the importance of correct AB management in the ED and provide practical recommendations drawn from the existing evidence concerning the application of different strategies and tools that could be implemented in the ED: development of clinical guidelines, clinical decision support systems, or implementation of rapid diagnostic methods [6,7].

Antimicrobial stewardship comprises a collection of strategies, policies, and guidelines that aim to provide training and evaluation and collectively result in the optimization of antibiotic prescribing practices. It has been found that when Antimicrobial Stewardship Programs (ASP) are effectively implemented and monitored, they provide a measurable impact across multiple clinical departments: reducing drug costs, duration of treatment, adverse events to antibiotics, and local resistance. However, to date, ASPs have been targeted primarily at the hospital setting and there is a lack of literature data on antimicrobial stewardship strategies in EDs [8,9].

The implementation of ASP in the ED represents a challenge due to the specific conditions of activity in this compartment, such as the large number of patients examined/24 h, the limited time and equipment to support a rapid diagnosis, the decision regarding admission or discharge, and treatment of the patient at home [10].

The purpose of this study was to evaluate the etiology and AMR pattern of the community-acquired pathogens, as well as the epidemiological characteristics of patients admitted through the ED, within the largest tertiary emergency hospital in the western part of the country, in order to guide appropriate antibiotic therapy.

2. Materials and Methods

A retrospective observational study was carried out in the Emergency Department (ED) of the "Pius Brînzeu" Clinical County Emergency Hospital Timișoara (SCJUPBT), over a period of 6 months, from 1 January 2021 to 30 June 2021. This institution is a tertiary teaching hospital, affiliated to the university, with 1174 beds, providing medical care for the western region of Romania. The ED of SCJUPT, the largest and most representative in Western Romania, has 24 workstations (beds), with approximately 80,000 patients per year, an average length of stay of about 4 h, and an admission rate of about 23%.

In accordance with the criteria of the Centers for Disease Control and Prevention, an infection presented on admission to the hospital or developing within 48 h or less from the time of admission was defined as community-acquired [11,12].

Following this definition, the inclusion criteria for CAI-ED patients were as follows:

- The diagnosis of the infection was based on the results of the microbiological tests, corroborated with the symptoms, the clinical examination, and the results of other paraclinical investigations recorded in the database and in the hospital documents.
- The infection was present at the time of ED presentation or within 48 h from hospital admission.
- Patients over 18 years old.

The following exclusion criteria have been used: patients with a negative microbiological result (C1), colonized, not infected patients (C2), patients diagnosed with an infection after 3 days of hospitalization and those who presented in the ED with an infection but have been discharged for a maximum of 48 h from another hospital or are within 30 days postoperatively (90 days in case of implant) (C3), patients who come from chronic care or elderly care units (C4); 21 ED patients were excluded from the study based on these exclusion criteria (4-C1, 5-C2, 10-C3, 2-C4). Figure 1 presents the study flow diagram.

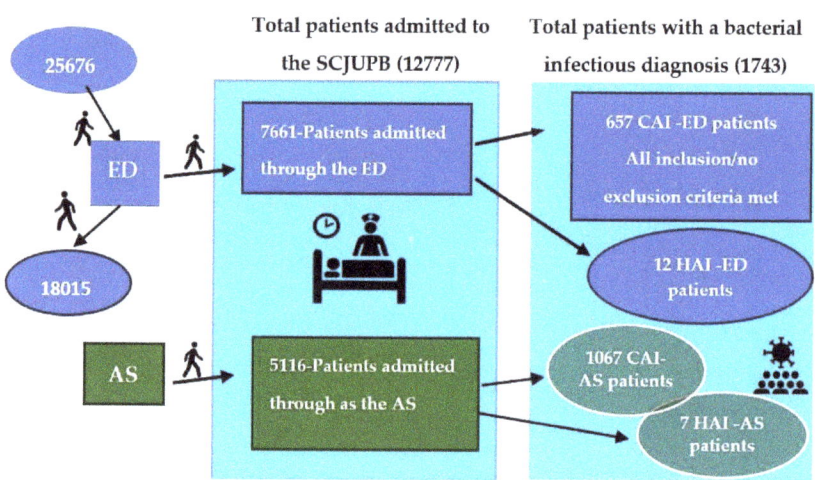

Figure 1. Study flow diagram. Legend: ED—emergency department, AS—admissions service, CAI—community-acquired infection, HAI—hospital-acquired infection.

The samples for microbiological diagnostics were collected from patients in the ED, but also from clinical wards where they were transferred to and only from the hospitalized patients, not from those discharged from the ED.

Samples were taken before antibiotic administration, and if this was not possible, empirical antibiotic therapy was initiated, followed by de-escalation, or changing the antibiotic depending on the antimicrobial susceptibility testing (AST) result. Regarding patients with sepsis, the blood culture was collected in the first hour after admission to the ED, just before the administration of the first dose of antibiotic. If this was not possible, BD BACTEC™ Plus Aerobic medium (Becton, Dickinson and Company, 7 Loveton Circle, Sparks, USA) was used, which contains resins for antibiotic neutralization.

Pathogen identification, AST, and minimum inhibitory concentration (MIC) were performed according to the protocols of the Microbiology Laboratory, using MALDI-TOF-Bruker and VITEK® 2 systems (Compact 60, BioMérieux, Marcy, l'Etoile, France). AST interpretation was performed according to CLSI standards [13].

For the clinically significant bacteria, depending on their acquired antibiotic resistance phenotypes, according to the CLSI standard, as well as the classifications of Magiorakos, Kadri, and other researchers, the following classifications have been used [13–18]:

- Methicillin-resistant *S. aureus* (MRSA): *S. aureus* with MIC ≥ 4 to oxacillin [14].
- Multidrug-resistant (MDR) bacteria: with resistance to at least one antibiotic from three or more classes of antibiotics active for a given species [15].
- Extensively drug-resistant bacteria (XDR): with resistance to at least one agent from all antimicrobial classes except one or two classes [15].
- Extended-spectrum beta-lactamase (ESBL) secreting Gram-negative bacilli (GNB): with resistance to all penicillins/cephalosporins [13,16].
- Carbapenem-resistant GNB (CR-GNB): enterobacteria with MIC ≥ 4 to imipenem, meropenem, and non-fermentative GNB with MIC ≥ 8 to imipenem, meropenem [13,17].
- Difficult-to-treat resistance (DTR): bacteria resistant to all first-line antibiotics, represented by: carbapenems (imipenem, meropenem, ertapenem/doripenem), extended-

spectrum cephalosporins (those relevant to the respective pathogens), fluoroquinolones (ciprofloxacin, levofloxacin, moxifloxacin) [18].

Statistical analysis of the data was performed using the EPI INFO version 7.2.50 (CDC, Atlanta, GA, USA). Numerical variables were defined by median and interquartile range (IQR) and category variables were defined by value, percentage, and CI 95%. The category-type variables were compared with the 2 × 2 contingency tables and the application of the hi^2 test (Fisher exact test). The tests were two-tailed and the threshold value was set at $p < 0.05$.

3. Results

During the period under study, a total of 25,676 patients were presented to the ED, out of which 7661 (29.83%) were admitted through the ED. The total number of patients admitted to the SCJUPB was 12,777, so patients admitted through the ED accounted for 59.96% of the total admissions.

Evaluation of the proportion of transfer wards of ED admissions showed that the most requested specialties were Surgery (SUR), Neurology (NEUR), and Gastroenterology (GE) (16.88%/14.25%/10.31%), followed by Vascular Surgery (VS), Cardiology (CD), and Urology (URO) (Table 1).

Table 1. The share of patients admitted through the ED on different wards of SCJUPBT.

ED Admissions by Ward of Total ED Admissions (%), January–June 2021					
Ward	No.	%	Ward	No.	%
Surgery (SUR)	1293	16.88	Orthopedics-Traumatology (OT)	629	8.21
Neurology (NEUR)	1092	14.25	Nephrology (NEF)	469	6.12
Gastroenterology (GE)	790	10.31	Neurosurgery (NSUR)	542	5.63
Vascular Surgery (VS)	717	9.36	Diabetes and Nutrition (DN)	338	4.41
Cardiology (CD)	652	8.51	Plastic and Reconstructive Surgery (PS)	311	4.06
Urology (URO)	623	8.13	Other	205	4.13
Total 7661 (100%)					

Regarding the share of ED admissions compared to total hospital admissions, this was almost 100% for Cardiology (CD) (99.54%), Vascular Surgery (VS) (99.54%), and Nephrology (NEF) (99.54%) and over 80% for Neurology (NEUR) (99.54%), Neurosurgery (NSUR) (99.54%), Gastroenterology (GE) (84.67%), and Diabetes and Nutrition (DN) (83.25%), respectively.

From the study group of 7661 ED inpatients, 657 (8.57%) were diagnosed with CAI, causing, or associated with inpatient illness, for which treatment was instituted according to microbiological diagnosis and AST. ED patients with an infectious diagnosis accounted for 37.69% of all patients with bacterial infections admitted during this period (FD, AS, CAI, and HAI) (Figure 1). Table 2 presents the demographic and comorbidity characteristics of the ED-CAI patients.

In terms of the distribution of ED-CAI admissions by ward, the data obtained showed that Gastroenterology (GE) was the most requested ward for ED admissions, hospitalizing more than $\frac{1}{4}$ of the total of this group of patients (26.79%). These patients were admitted with a diagnosis of GI infection—angiocolitis (26.13%), pancreatitis (15.34%), or for an acute infectious complication of an underlying chronic GI disease—liver neoplasm (20.45%), pancreatitis (15.34%). At a distance, registering half of the GE frequencies was Surgery (13.7%), followed by Nephrology (10.65%) (Figure 2).

Surgery admissions were indicated for diagnosis of abscess/phlegmon/gangrene/ plague (36.67%), peritonitis (21.12%), appendicitis (15.56%), and intestinal occlusions (7.78%), while on the Nephrology ward, patients were transferred for sepsis with renal origine (48.57%), chronic kidney disease (47.14%), acute kidney injury (34.28%), and acute pyelonephritis (18.57%).

Table 2. Demographic and comorbidity characteristics of the cohort (657 patients).

Variable	N = 657	95% CI
M (n(%))	355 (54.03)	50.21–57.81
F (n (%))	302 (45.97)	42.19–49.79
Average age (average (IQR))	62.38 (53–73)	/
Comorbid conditions		
Peripheral artery disease (n (%))	61 (9.28)	7.30–11.75
Hypertensive patients (n (%))	112 (17.04)	14.37–20.11
SARS-CoV2 (n (%))	106 (16.13)	13.52–19.14
Diabetes mellitus (n (%))	69 (10.5)	8.38–13.08
Coronary artery disease (n (%))	43 (6.54)	4.90–8.70
Ischemic stroke (n (%))	41 (6.24)	4.63–8.36
Kidney stones (n (%))	9 (1.37)	0.72–2.58
Chronic kidney disease (CKD) (n (%))	47 (7.15)	5.42–9.38
Acute kidney injury (AKI) (n (%))	39 (5.93)	4.37–8.01
Renal neoplasia (n (%))	7 (1.06)	0.52–2.18
Cirrhosis (n (%))	61 (9.28)	7.30–11.75
Biliary lithiasis (n (%))	50 (7.61)	5.82–9.89
GI tract neoplasia (n (%))	53 (8.06)	6.22–10.40

Legend: GI—gastrointestinal.

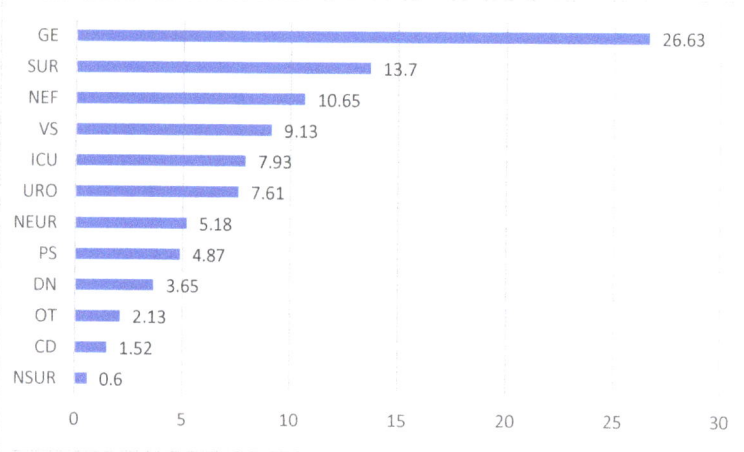

Figure 2. Breakdown by ward of CAI admitted through the ED (%). Legend: GE—Gastroenterology, SUR—Surgery, NEF—Nephrology, VS—Vascular Surgery, ICU—Intensive Care Unit, URO—Urology, NEUR—Neurology, PS—Plastic Surgery, DN—Diabetes and Nutrition, OT—Orthopedics-Traumatology, CD—Cardiology, NSUR—Neurosurgery.

A special group of ED inpatients was the group of burned patients (N = 28) and the patients with trauma of various etiologies (N = 67), road traffic accidents, accidents at work, or domestic accidents.

Out of the group of patients with burns, 54% (N = 15) were major burns, transferred to the Functional Burns Unit (FBU), while 46% (N = 13) were with limited injuries, admitted to the Plastic Surgery ward (PS). Burned patients accounted for 0.36% of all ED admissions. Burned patients with infected burn injuries (23) represented 3.5% of all ED-CAI patients being admitted to the PS (60%) and FBU (40%) wards.

In terms of age decade distribution, of the 657 ED-CAI patients, 80.42% (456 patients) were in the 50–80 age decade. The study showed that women's referral to ED services increases from age 50 onwards and peaks in the 70–79 age range. For men, referral increases from 40 years of age and peaks between 60 and 69 years of age.

Regarding the study of ED-CAI infections, from 657 ED-CAI patients, 767 clinical samples were collected for bacteriological diagnosis. The most numerous were urine cultures, wound drainage, and blood cultures (27.64%, 23.08%, 13.95%). Internal fluids together account for a significant percentage of 11.60% (Figure 3).

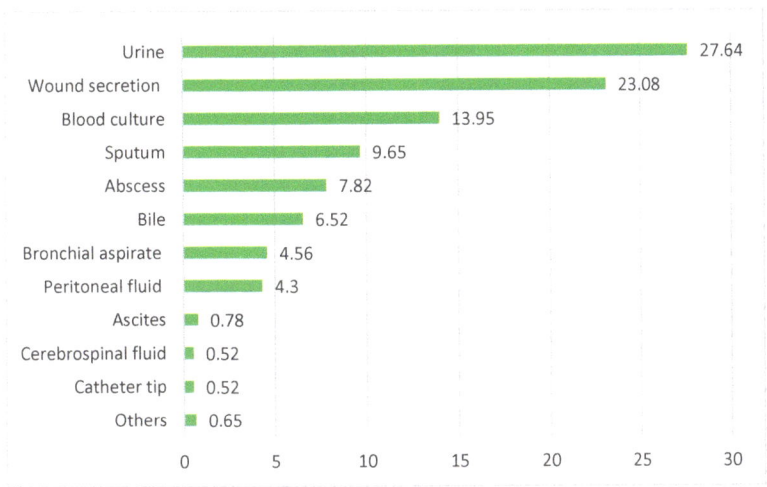

Figure 3. Clinical samples collected from ED-CAI patients (%).

Out of the 767 samples analyzed, 903 microbial isolates were identified, of which 48.95% were *Enterobacterales*, 10.08% non-fermentative GNB, 34.22% Gram-positive cocci (GPC), and 4.98% fungi. The bacterial species most represented were *E. coli*, accounting for approximately $\frac{1}{4}$ of the total strains isolated (24.25%), followed by *Klebsiella* spp. (13.73%) and *S. aureus* (10.63%) (Table 3).

Table 3. Proportion of microbial isolates identified from ED-CAI patients (% from 903 isolates).

903 Isolates	EC	KB	SA	EnC	CNS	STR	PSE	CAN	PRO	EnB	AcB	CIT	Other
Nr.	219	124	96	85	79	49	62	45	37	22	17	17	51
% from 903	24.25	13.73	10.63	9.41	8.75	5.43	6.87	4.98	4.1	2.44	1.88	1.88	5.65

Legend: EC—*E. coli*, KB—*Klebsiella* spp., SA—*S. aureus*, EnC—*Enterococcus* spp., CNS—coagulase-negative staphylococci, STR—*Streptococcus* spp., PSE—*Pseudomonas* spp., CAN—*Candida* spp., PRO—*Proteus* spp., EnB—*Enterobacter* spp., AbC—*Acinetobacter* spp., CIT—*Citrobacter* spp.

Tables 4 and 5 show the distribution of isolates in clinical samples and the distribution of AMR phenotypes.

Nearly 50% of the identified *E. coli* strains (47.03%) were from urine cultures, followed by wound drainage (12.32%) and internal fluids: bile fluid, peritoneal fluid, blood cultures (9.59%, 8.68%, 7.76%) (Table 4). In terms of AMR, 25% of *E. coli* strains showed resistance to trimethoprim/sulfamethoxazole (SXT) and 17.8% showed resistance to fluoroquinolones (FQ); 6.4% recorded ESBL phenotype and 9% fell into the MDR category (Table 5).

The second most common isolate in ED-CAI was *Klebsiella* spp. The highest number of *Klebsiella* isolates was in urine cultures (24.20%), followed by sputum (16.93%) and abscess cultures (10.48%) (Table 4). AMR was marked by the identification of ESBL (11.30%) and CR (7.28%) strains, respectively, SXT- and FQ-resistant strains (14.51% and 15.32%). As a result, 12.09% of strains were MDR type, 7.28% DTR type, and 2.50% were XDR strains (Table 5).

Table 4. Distribution of microbial isolates in clinical samples (%).

Bacterial Species (n)	Urine (%)	Wound Drainage (%)	Blood Culture (%)	Sputum (%)	Bronchial Aspirate (%)	Abscess (%)	Bile (%)	Peritoneal Fluid (%)
E. coli (219)	47.03	12.32	7.76	3.2	2.28	7.76	9.59	8.68
K. pneumoniae (124)	24.2	8.87	7.26	16.93	7.25	10.48	6.45	0
S. aureus (96)	6.25	53.12	9.37	10.42	10.42	6.25	0	0
Pseudomonas spp. (62)	12.9	40.32	6.45	12.9	6.45	1.61	12.9	3.22
Acinetobacter spp. (17)	0	58.83	5.88	5.88	11.7	0	5.88	11.76

Table 5. Classification of the most important GNB into resistance phenotypes (%).

Bacterial Species	DTR	MDR	XDR	ESBL	CR-GNB	R-AG	R-FQ	R-SXT	R-TE
E. coli (%)	0.5	9	0	6.4	0.45	1.8	17.8	25.2	1.8
Klebsiella spp. (%)	7.28	12.09	2.50	11.30	7.28	4.84	15.32	14.51	2.5
Pseudomonas spp. (%)	11.29	24.19	6.45	/	19.35	11.29	17.74	/	/
Acinetobacter spp. (%)	52.94	58.82	23.50	/	52.94	52.94	47.05	52.94	/

Klebsiella spp. were highlighted by the statistically significant higher frequency of the phenotypes: XDR ($p = 0.046$), DTR ($p < 0.001$), CRE ($p < 0.001$), and R-SXT ($p < 0.001$) vs. those of E. coli. ESBL isolates or strains with resistance to aminoglycosides, respectively, and resistance to fluoroquinolones, were identified in similar proportions ($p = 0.149/0.177/0.653$), as well as MDR strains ($p = 0.849$).

Non-fermentative GNB species had a low representation, with a frequency of 6.87% for Pseudomonas spp. and 1.88% for Acinetobacter spp., respectively (Table 3).

Pseudomonas spp. had the highest frequencies in cultures from wound drainage (40.32%), followed by cultures from bile fluids (12.9%) and urine cultures (12.90%) (Table 4); 19.35% were CR-resistant strains, 17.74% showed resistance to FQ, and 11.29% resistance to AG; 24.19% of strains were identified in the MDR and 11.29% in the DTR category, while the frequency of strains with extremely limited therapeutic options (XDR) was 6.45% (Table 5).

Acinetobacter spp. had the highest frequencies in cultures from wound drainage (58.83%). The remaining strains were present in bronchial aspirates and peritoneal fluid samples (Table 4). AMR studies reported high incidences of acquired resistance phenotypes of Acinetobacter spp. strains: over 50% CR and AG resistance phenotype. Accordingly, 52.94% of isolates fell into the DTR, 58.82% in the MDR category, and 23.15% were XDR strains (Table 5).

Among non-fermenters, Acinetobacter spp. isolates were statistically significant more resistant vs. those of Pseudomonas spp., both for the phenotypes: DTR ($p < 0.001$), MDR/ESBL ($p = 0.004$), CRE ($p = 0.011$), R-AG ($p < 0.001$), and R-FQ ($p = 0.022$). Only the XDR strains had similar percentages ($p = 0.060$).

Among the GPC, the highest frequency was recorded by Staphylococcus aureus (SA) strains. The majority of SA-positive cultures were taken from wounds (53.12%), followed by sputum and bronchial aspirates (10.42%, 10.42%) (Table 4). Phenotypic analysis showed that SA strains from CAI were resistant to antibiotics commonly used for the treatment of these infections. Thus 52% were beta-lactamase-producing strains, 32.3% were MRSA and 30.2% were identified with macrolide-lincosamide-streptogramin (MLSB) resistance phenotype, respectively. Consequently, the frequency of MDR strains was 37.5%. Penicillin resistance of S. aureus was significantly higher versus enterococci ($p < 0.001$) and macrolide resistance did not differ ($p = 1.00$).

4. Discussion

The present study was conducted during January–June 2021, namely, 181 days. The year 2021 was a pandemic year, located in the middle of the interval dominated by the SARS CoV-2 infection (February 2020–March 2022), in which hospital admissions were carried out according to well-established protocols, with limitations aimed at preventing intra-hospital transmission of the virus. The SCJUPBT-ED was requested by an average of 142 patients/day (25,676/181 days), of which, an average of 42 patients/day were admitted, out of an average total of 71 admissions/day/hospital, a flow that represented a percentage of approximately 60% ED admissions out of total admissions in the entire hospital.

The pathology of ED-CAI patients was split between surgical and medical specialties, but surgical pathology was noted to have a higher frequency of cases than medical pathology (53.64% versus 46.35%). This distribution is explained by the fact that the study covered the first 6 months of the second pandemic year 2021. In that year, the addressability of patients to tertiary medical units was strongly influenced by the restrictions imposed by the epidemiological situation, with the prioritization and admission of severe cases and medical/surgical emergencies. The hospitalization ward indirectly reflects the prevalent types of severe pathologies, which required hospitalization and immediate treatment, despite the pandemic context.

Most of the antibiotic treatments initiated in the ED for these patients are empirical. Antibiotic administration is profoundly influenced by patient demographic variables as well as diagnosis. High prescription rate use of antimicrobial treatments, regardless of these variables, however, has been observed in ED low-resource settings, highlighting the importance of surveillance in order to implement targeted intervention [19,20]. Moreover, in countries with a high consumption of antibiotics in Europe (such as Romania), an increase in antibiotic consumption is observed in winter and spring, thus causing a selective pressure and subsequently, an increase in multidrug resistance in community bacterial strains after a time delay of several months. These seasonal variations were also noticed by other researchers [21].

In our ED, antibiotics are administered only in cases of suspicion of sepsis, in the first hour after admission, immediately after having taken the samples intended for the microbiological examination, in accordance with the suspected source of sepsis. To medical practice, it is important that blood culture positivity is reduced by antimicrobial therapy, but remains high after a single dose of antibiotics, as shown in recent studies [22].

In this study, the majority of ED-CAI patients were over 50 years old, with approximately 55% falling within the 60–79 age range, consistent with findings from other studies [23,24]. ED-CAI patients over 80 years old were lower in number (15%) and they represented more than 2/3 of all admitted patients. The gender distribution of ED patients was not significant; however, the need for hospital medical care was significantly higher in men than in women for the age group 60–69 years ($p = 0.043$).

The strategy for dealing with the ED-CAI infectious patient depends on the framing of the disease—medical or surgical pathology. In the present study, ED-CAI patients with surgical pathology were 7.29% more common than those with medical diagnosis. It was noted that surgical patients (SUR+VS) accounted for about 23% of all infection admissions and renal patients (NEF+URO) achieved a significant frequency of 18.26%.

The problem of burned and trauma patients is a great challenge for the ED and transfer wards (BFU, respectively, ICU, OT, NSUR, PS), both in terms of medical treatment, length of stay, and cost of care. From the 28 burned patients admitted through the ED, 294 positive bacterial cultures were recorded throughout the admission, which means an average of 10.50 positive samples/patient and an average length of stay of 30 days, with a maximum of 156 days in isolation [25]. These figures show the importance of sampling for the diagnosis of microbial biofilms in these infections, as the biofilm is known to delay the healing even with optimal treatment instituted early [26,27].

The same issue of biofilm detection is posed for all types of wounds and catheter tip cultures, but also for respiratory tract cultures (sputum and bronchial aspirate). The most common bacterial species in wound biofilms (burn, ischemic, gangrenous) are *S. aureus* [28,29] and *P. aeruginosa* [30,31] with AMR to local and general treatments. *Pseudomonas* spp. are known to form biofilms in secretions of pulmonary patients, especially those with cystic fibrosis. Consequently, in these cases, genotypic investigation and biofilmography should be viewed as routine investigations for the institution of treatment.

The implementation of ASP-ED strategies for the management of CAI patients must take into consideration the peculiarities of ED functioning—rapid treatment decision-making in the context of time-constrained bacteriological investigation and access to rapid diagnostic tools. In this regard, Nauclér [32] has illustrated that rapid initiation of antibiotic treatment is crucial for patients with severe infections. He concluded that the literature supports prompt administration of effective antibiotics for septic shock and bacterial meningitis, but there is no clear evidence that delayed initiation of therapy is associated with a worse outcome for less severe infectious syndromes. For patients in whom bacterial infections are suspected, suspending antibiotic therapy until microbiological diagnostic results are available (e.g., up to 4–8 h) seems acceptable in most cases, except in the situation where septic shock or bacterial meningitis is suspected. This approach promotes the use of ecologically favorable antibiotics in the ED, reducing the risks of side effects and resistance selection.

To initiate an AB treatment in the ED, May [7] shows that the most important questions related to AMS to be answered at this stage are: "Is there a rationale for starting antimicrobial treatment for this diagnosis? Should I treat now? Or can I wait?" Currently, the answer to initiating antibiotic therapy in the ED is facilitated by the provision of rapid diagnostics through molecular techniques for the diagnosis of viral infections and the presence of biomarkers needed to differentiate bacterial from viral infections. Incorporating these findings into the clinical diagnostic process in the ED has the potential to significantly reduce unnecessary antibiotic use [10,33,34].

The use of procalcitonin as a biomarker has been considered when decision-making in chronic lung disease. There are studies that have shown a reduction in total antibiotic exposure (days of administration) and adverse effects based on values of this biomarker [35,36].

Multiplex PCR investigation on platforms such as rapid syndromic testing is another method that would allow rapid identification of pathogens and detection of resistance genes. Thus, Sun L. (2021) [37] showed in his study the overall sensitivity and specificity of Unyvero at detecting bacteria in lower respiratory tract infections was high (84.0% and 98.0%). The overall concordance between Unyvero and routine culture was 69/84 (82.1%). In addition, Unyvero showed good performance for antibiotic-resistant bacteria, except for *Pseudomonas aeruginosa*.

Similar agreements were published by Collins et al. [38], who compared the performance of the Unyvero LRT panel with routine bacterial culture methods on 175 bronchoalveolar lavage (BAL) samples and reported a sensitivity of 96.5% and a specificity of 99.6% among microbial targets. For antibiotic resistance markers in the LRT BAL lower respiratory tract panel, a positive predictive value (PPV) of 100% was reported. In another recent publication, Pickens et al. [39] reported a sensitivity of 85.7% and a specificity of 98.4% for 620 respiratory samples (395 bronchoscopic or none bronchoscopic BAL samples, 225 aspirates) using the Unyvero LRT panel.

Regarding GNB resistance genes, Klein [40] showed that the detection of a resistance gene does not necessarily link it to the host bacteria. However, for GNB, there were strong genotypic and phenotypic correlations of Unyvero results with the corresponding isolates. The reporting of resistance genes may provide a clue over the presence of an underlying resistant organism, which may have implications regarding infection prevention and control (e.g., if blaKPC, blaNDM, blaVIM, or blaOXA-48 is detected), even if the species with which the gene is associated is unknown.

Such an approach was adopted for some patients in the present study, so that multiplex PCR investigation on the Unyvero platform of an ED-CAI patient with polytrauma identified in blood culture the association of *A. baumannii* and *P. aeruginosa*, with the presence of NDM, OXA-24, SUL1, gyrA83 Pseu resistance genes, and of an ED-CAI patient transferred in GE, Unyvero investigation of a bronchial aspirate identified *A. baumannii* and *P. aeruginosa* and SUL1, gyrA83 Pseu resistance genes.

In the present study, the identification of germs responsible for ED-CAI infections has shown that the most frequently isolated strains were *E. coli* (24.25%), followed by *Klebsiella* species (13.73%) and *S. aureus* (10.63%). Benkő [41] showed in the ED study conducted in 2020 that she identified germs in the same hierarchy (*E. coli* (44.10%), *Klebsiella* spp. (13.40%), *S. aureus* (11.30%)), with the caveat that in this study, *E. coli* isolates had almost double the frequency, tending to account for half of the total number of strains.

Most ED-CAI patients with *E. coli* strains were admitted to GE wards (31.96%), kidney disease wards (NEF+URO, 21.46%), and SUR wards (18.26%). Isolates were identified in urine cultures and internal fluids (biliary, peritoneal, blood) and posed no AMR problems, with a small number being MDR, respectively, DTR strains. However, resistance to sulfonamides (R-S) and fluoroquinolones (R-FQ) was noted, which argues for the frequent use of these antibiotics in community infectious pathology [42] and draws attention to their use in the empiric therapy in ED.

Klebsiella spp. (13.73%) were isolated from urine cultures, RT cultures (sputum and bronchial aspirate), and wounds/abscesses of ED-CAI patients transferred to the GE, NEF+URO, SUR, and ICU wards (35.92%, 23.30%, 14.56%, and 11.65%). *Klebsiella* strains showed a higher percentage of MDR (12.9%), with acquired beta-lactam resistance phenotypes (ESBL and CR) and high frequencies of R-FQ, a fact also presented in other studies [10]. The difficult problem of establishing treatment regards the XDR strains (2.5%), with treatment options limited to, at most, two classes of antibiotics, which were identified in GE and SUR patients.

As for *S. aureus* strains, they were mostly identified in wound samples, respectively, RT samples of patients who were transferred to SUR, GE, NEF+URO, and ICU wards (48.14%, 14.81%, 11.12%, and 8.64%). The incidence of SA-MDR was high, (37.5%), explained by the frequency of MRSA and MLSB strains. A much lower rate of MRSA (only 0.4%) was identified in a study that set out to determine AMR in microorganisms causing community-onset bacteremia [43].

Non-fermentative GNBs were represented by *Pseudomonas* spp. and *Acinetobacter* spp., known to have high AMR behavior in hospital environments [44–46].

Pseudomonas spp. were reduced in number (6.87%), being mainly identified in wound drainage, RT samples (bronchial aspirates and sputum), and internal fluids (biliary and peritoneal). Approximately $\frac{1}{4}$ of these strains were MDR, with high frequencies of CR and FQ resistance phenotypes (almost 20% of them). Samples were from ED-CAI patients with transfer diagnoses for GE, SUR, and NEF+URO (30.07%, 30.18%, and 18.86%).

Acinetobacter spp. were present in low numbers, in samples from ED-CAI patients. The majority were identified in wound drainage of burned patients, patients with lower limb pathology (ischemia, gangrene), and infected traumatic injuries, 81.25% being transferred to surgical wards (VS, PS) and FBU. The problem raised by these isolates, however, is the high degree of AMR, with a frequency of almost $\frac{1}{4}$ of their number of XDR strains. The high resistance to carbapenems, the only effective beta-lactams on *Acinetobacter* species (52.94%), together with resistance to AG and FQ (52.94%, 47.05%) made infections caused by these strains extremely difficult to treat, due to the lack of effective therapy.

The current study brings more information about CAI patients hospitalized by the ED, a topic that is not often addressed in the literature, at least in our geographical area, where there is little data in this regard.

Moreover, because of the AMR studies published by our team and in accordance with the Stanford Antimicrobial Safety & Sustainability Program 2019 [47], the SCJUPBT Antibiotic Prophylaxis Guide has been updated.

Also, our recommendations regarding the purchase and installation of an Unyvero equipment in the ED, for the rapid molecular identification of MDR pathogens, as well as the screening of patients to identify colonization with these organisms in the ED, were discussed with the hospital management.

However, the current study has some limitations. It addresses infectious pathology hospitalized through a single ED, and a single hospital, which is a reason why its generalizability may be limited. The study was conducted in a particular pandemic period, burdened by restrictions imposed by the health system, but also by the decreasing addressability of the population. The descriptive design did not allow clear evidence of these differences. Also, as with any retrospective study, there are potential biases such as selection and information bias.

5. Conclusions

During the period under study, the proportion of ED admissions increased, with a significant percentage of patients with infectious diagnoses, mostly elderly, with associated pathologies, hospitalized mainly in surgical wards. It was found that the disease state and the need for hospital care in men was earlier than in women.

Of the identified pathogens, GNB were mostly predominant. *E. coli* was isolated most frequently, but with maintenance of susceptibility to the usual ABs, while non-fermenters were isolated less frequently, but with increased AMR rates. In the case of SA strains, we noted the significantly increased percentage of community-acquired MRSA strains.

The ongoing study of AMR in ED isolates, as well as the introduction of rapid microbiological diagnostic methods are imperative to timely identify MDR strains and improve therapeutic protocols. We also emphasize the need for ASP in the ED with the identification of interventions to improve patient outcomes and care and reduce the consequences of antimicrobial use in the hospital and community.

Author Contributions: Conceptualization, C.M. and M.L.; methodology, C.M. and S.I.M.; software, O.I.; validation, M.L., D.M. and S.I.M.; formal analysis, S.I.M.; investigation, A.V. and O.I.; resources, L.M.B. and O.I.; data curation, A.V.; writing—original draft preparation, S.I.M., R.J. and O.I.; writing—review and editing, D.M., A.V. and R.J.; supervision, M.L. and D.M.; project administration, S.I.M. and M.L. All authors have read and agreed to the published version of the manuscript.

Funding: This research received no external funding.

Institutional Review Board Statement: The study was conducted in accordance with the Declaration of Helsinki and approved by the Ethics Committee of "Pius Brînzeu" Emergency Clinical County Hospital Timisoara, Romania (No 306/16.06.2022).

Informed Consent Statement: Informed consent was obtained from all subjects involved in the study.

Data Availability Statement: Data are contained within the article.

Acknowledgments: A part of this study was presented in oral form at the Interdisciplinary Congress of Emergency Medicine, Cluj Napoca, Romania, in 2022.

Conflicts of Interest: The authors declare no conflicts of interest.

References

1. Han, J.H.; Kasahara, K.; Edelstein, P.H.; Bilker, W.B.; Lautenbach, E. Risk factors for infection or colonization with CTX-M extended-spectrum-β-lactamase-positive *Escherichia coli*. *Antimicrob. Agents Chemother.* **2012**, *56*, 5575–5580. [CrossRef] [PubMed]
2. Moran, G.J.; Krishnadasan, A.; Gorwitz, R.J.; Fosheim, G.E.; McDougal, L.K.; Carey, R.B.; Talan, D.A. Methicillin-resistant *S. aureus* infections among patients in the emergency department. *N. Engl. J. Med.* **2006**, *355*, 666–674. [CrossRef]
3. Kroening-Roche, J.C.; Soroudi, A.; Castillo, E.M.; Vilke, G.M. Antibiotic and bronchodilator prescribing for acute bronchitis in the emergency department. *J. Emerg. Med.* **2012**, *43*, 221–227. [CrossRef] [PubMed]
4. Gonzales, R.; Camargo, C.A.; MacKenzie, T.; Kersey, A.S.; Maselli, J.; Levin, S.K.; McCulloch, C.E.; Metlay, J.P. Antibiotic treatment of acute respiratory infections in acute care settings. *Acad. Emerg. Med.* **2006**, *13*, 288–294. [CrossRef] [PubMed]
5. Metlay, J.P.; Camargo, C.A.; MacKenzie, T.; McCulloch, C.; Maselli, J.; Levin, S.K.; Kersey, A.; Gonzales, R. Cluster-randomized trial to improve antibiotic use for adults with acute respiratory infections treated in emergency departments. *Ann. Emerg. Med.* **2007**, *50*, 221–230. [CrossRef] [PubMed]
6. May, L.; Cosgrove, S.; L'Archeveque, M.; Talan, D.A.; Payne, P.; Jordan, J.; Rothman, R.E. A call to action for antimicrobial stewardship in the emergency department: Approaches and strategies. *Ann. Emerg. Med.* **2013**, *62*, 69–77. [CrossRef] [PubMed]
7. May, L.; Martin-Quirós, A.; Ten Oever, J.; Hoogerwerf, J.; Schoffelen, T.; Schouten, J. Antimicrobial stewardship in the emergency department: Characteristics and evidence for effectiveness of interventions. *Clin. Microbiol. Infect.* **2021**, *27*, 204–209. [CrossRef]

8. Lawton, R.M.; Fridkin, S.K.; Gaynes, R.P.; McGowan, J.E. Practices to improve antimicrobial use at 47 US hospitals: The status of the 1997 SHEA/IDSA position paper recommendations. Society for Healthcare Epidemiology of America/Infectious Diseases Society of America. *Infect. Control Hosp. Epidemiol.* **2000**, *21*, 256–259. [CrossRef]
9. Policy statement on antimicrobial stewardship by the Society for Healthcare Epidemiology of America (SHEA), the Infectious Diseases Society of America (IDSA), and the Pediatric Infectious Diseases Society (PIDS). *Infect. Control Hosp. Epidemiol.* **2012**, *33*, 322–327. [CrossRef]
10. Bishop, B.M. Antimicrobial Stewardship in the Emergency Department: Challenges, Opportunities, and a Call to Action for Pharmacists. *J. Pharm. Pract.* **2016**, *29*, 556–563. [CrossRef]
11. Garner, J.S.; Jarvis, W.R.; Emori, T.G.; Horan, T.C.; Hughes, J.M. CDC definitions for nosocomial infections. *Am. J. Infect. Control.* **1988**, *16*, 128–140, Erratum in *Am. J. Infect. Control* **1988**, *16*, 177. [CrossRef] [PubMed]
12. Dabar, G.; Harmouche, C.; Salameh, P.; Jaber, B.L.; Jamaleddine, G.; Waked, M.; Yazbeck, P. Community- and healthcare-associated infections in critically ill patients: A multicenter cohort study. *Int. J. Infect. Dis.* **2015**, *37*, 80–85. [CrossRef] [PubMed]
13. CLSI. *Performance Standards for Antimicrobial Susceptibility Testing*, M100, 31st ed.; Clinical and Laboratory Standards Institute: Wayne, PA, USA, 2021. Available online: https://clsi.org/media/z2uhcbmv/m100ed31_sample.pdf (accessed on 12 November 2023).
14. Turner, N.A.; Sharma-Kuinkel, B.K.; Maskarinec, S.A.; Eichenberger, E.M.; Shah, P.P.; Carugati, M.; Holland, T.L.; Fowler, V.G., Jr. Methicillin-resistant Staphylococcus aureus: An overview of basic and clinical research. *Nat. Rev. Microbiol.* **2019**, *17*, 203–218. [CrossRef] [PubMed]
15. Magiorakos, A.-P.; Srinivasan, A.; Carey, R.B.; Carmeli, Y.; Falagas, M.E.; Giske, C.G.; Harbarth, S.; Hindler, J.F.; Kahlmeter, G.; Olsson-Liljequist, B.; et al. Multidrug-resistant, extensively drug-resistant and pandrug-resistant bacteria: An international expert proposal for interim standard definitions for acquired resistance. *Clin. Microbiol. Infect.* **2012**, *18*, 268–281. [CrossRef] [PubMed]
16. Pitout, J.D.D.; Laupland, K.B. Extended-spectrum beta-lactamase-producing Enterobacteriaceae: An emerging public-health concern. *Lancet Infect. Dis.* **2008**, *8*, 159–166. [CrossRef]
17. Nordmann, P.; Naas, T.; Poirel, L. Global spread of Carbapenemase-producing Enterobacteriaceae. *Emerg. Infect. Dis.* **2011**, *17*, 1791–1798. [CrossRef] [PubMed]
18. Kadri, S.S.; Adjemian, J.; Lai, Y.L.; Spaulding, A.B.; Ricotta, E.; Prevots, D.R.; Palmore, T.N.; Rhee, C.; Klompas, M.; Dekker, J.P.; et al. Difficult-to-Treat Resistance in Gram-negative Bacteremia at 173 US Hospitals: Retrospective Cohort Analysis of Prevalence, Predictors, and Outcome of Resistance to All First-line Agents. *Clin. Infect. Dis.* **2018**, *67*, 1803–1814. [CrossRef]
19. Yi, S.; Ramachandran, A.; Epps, L.; Mayah, A.; Burkholder, T.W.; Jaung, M.S.; Haider, A.; Whesseh, P.; Shakpeh, J.; Enriquez, K.; et al. Emergency department antimicrobial use in a low-resource setting: Results from a retrospective observational study at a referral hospital in Liberia. *BMJ Open* **2022**, *12*, e056709. [CrossRef]
20. Shankar, P.R. Medicines use in primary care in developing and transitional countries: Fact book summarizing results from studies reported between 1990 and 2006. *Bull. World Health Organ.* **2009**, *87*, 804–805. [CrossRef]
21. Martínez, P.; Rosmalen, J.; Bustillos Huilca, R.; Natsch, S.; Mouton, J.; Verbon, A. Trends, seasonality and the association between outpatient antibiotic use and antimicrobial resistance among urinary bacteria in the Netherlands. *J. Antimicrob. Chemother.* **2020**, *75*, 2314–2325. [CrossRef]
22. Zornitzki, L.; Anuk, L.; Frydman, S.; Morag-Koren, N.; Zahler, D.; Freund, O.; Biran, R.; Liron, Y.; Tau, L.; Tchebiner, J.Z.; et al. Rate and predictors of blood culture positivity after antibiotic administration: A prospective single-center study. *Infection* **2023**. [CrossRef] [PubMed]
23. Hong, S.-I.; Kim, J.-S.; Kim, Y.-J.; Seo, D.-W.; Kang, H.; Kim, S.J.; Han, K.S.; Lee, S.W.; Kim, W.Y. Characteristics of Patients Who Visited Emergency Department: A Nationwide Population-Based Study in South Korea (2016–2018). *Int. J. Environ. Res. Public Health* **2022**, *19*, 8578. [CrossRef] [PubMed]
24. Lee, J.H.; Park, G.J.; Kim, S.C.; Kim, H.; Lee, S.W. Characteristics of frequent adult emergency department users: A Korean tertiary hospital observational study. *Medicine* **2020**, *99*, e20123. [CrossRef] [PubMed]
25. Licker, M.; Musuroi, C.; Muntean, D.; Crainiceanu, Z. Updates in the management of multidrug-resistant bacterial infections in burn patients. In Proceedings of the 16th National Conference on Microbiology and Epidemiology, Bucharest, Romania, 9–11 November 2023. Available online: https://www.srm.ro/media/2023/11/volum-rezumate-cnme-1.pdf (accessed on 12 November 2023).
26. Percival, S.L.; McCarty, S.M.; Lipsky, B. Biofilms and Wounds: An Overview of the Evidence. *Adv. Wound Care* **2015**, *4*, 373–381. [CrossRef]
27. Schultz, G.; Bjarnsholt, T.; James, G.A.; Leaper, D.J.; McBain, A.J.; Malone, M.; Stoodley, P.; Swanson, T.; Tachi, M.; Wolcott, R.D.; et al. Consensus guidelines for the identification and treatment of biofilms in chronic nonhealing wounds. *Wound Repair Regen.* **2017**, *25*, 744–757. [CrossRef]
28. Di Lodovico, S.; Bacchetti, T.; D'ercole, S.; Covone, S.; Petrini, M.; Di Giulio, M.; Di Fermo, P.; Diban, F.; Ferretti, G.; Cellini, L. Complex Chronic Wound Biofilms Are Inhibited in vitro by the Natural Extract of Capparis spinose. *Front. Microbiol.* **2022**, *13*, 832919. [CrossRef]
29. Roy, S.; Santra, S.; Das, A.; Dixith, S.; Sinha, M.; Ghatak, S.; Ghosh, N.; Banerjee, P.; Khanna, S.; Mathew-Steiner, S.; et al. Staphylococcus aureus Biofilm Infection Compromises Wound Healing by Causing Deficiencies in Granulation Tissue Collagen. *Ann. Surg.* **2020**, *271*, 1174–1185. [CrossRef]
30. Moreau-Marquis, S.; Stanton, B.A.; O'Toole, G.A. Pseudomonas aeruginosa biofilm formation in the cystic fibrosis airway. *Pulm. Pharmacol. Ther.* **2008**, *21*, 595–599. [CrossRef]

31. Jennings, L.K.; Dreifus, J.E.; Reichhardt, C.; Storek, K.M.; Secor, P.R.; Wozniak, D.J.; Hisert, K.B.; Parsek, M.R. Pseudomonas aeruginosa aggregates in cystic fibrosis sputum produce exopolysaccharides that likely impede current therapies. *Cell Rep.* **2021**, *34*, 108782. [CrossRef]
32. Nauclér, P.; Huttner, A.; van Werkhoven, C.; Singer, M.; Tattevin, P.; Einav, S.; Tängdén, T. Impact of time to antibiotic therapy on clinical outcome in patients with bacterial infections in the emergency department: Implications for antimicrobial stewardship. *Clin. Microbiol. Infect.* **2021**, *27*, 175–181. [CrossRef]
33. Pulia, M.; Redwood, R.; May, L. Antimicrobial Stewardship in the Emergency Department. *Emerg. Med. Clin. N. Am.* **2018**, *36*, 853–872. [CrossRef] [PubMed]
34. Barlam, T.F.; Cosgrove, S.E.; Abbo, L.M.; MacDougall, C.; Schuetz, A.N.; Septimus, E.J.; Srinivasan, A.; Dellit, T.H.; Falck-Ytter, Y.T.; Fishman, N.O.; et al. Implementing an Antibiotic Stewardship Program: Guidelines by the Infectious Diseases Society of America and the Society for Healthcare Epidemiology of America. *Clin. Infect. Dis.* **2016**, *62*, e51–e77. [CrossRef] [PubMed]
35. Mathioudakis, A.G.; Chatzimavridou-Grigoriadou, V.; Corlateanu, A.; Vestbo, J. Procalcitonin to guide antibiotic administration in COPD exacerbations: A meta-analysis. *Eur. Respir. Rev.* **2017**, *26*, 160073. [CrossRef] [PubMed]
36. Schuetz, P.; Wirz, Y.; Sager, R.; Christ-Crain, M.; Stolz, D.; Tamm, M.; Bouadma, L.; Luyt, C.E.; Wolff, M.; Chastre, J.; et al. Procalcitonin to initiate or discontinue antibiotics in acute respiratory tract infections. *Cochrane Database Syst. Rev.* **2017**, *10*, CD007498. [CrossRef] [PubMed]
37. Sun, L.; Li, L.; Du, S.; Liu, Y.; Cao, B. An evaluation of the Unyvero pneumonia system for rapid detection of microorganisms and resistance markers of lower respiratory infections-a multicenter prospective study on ICU patients. *Eur. J. Clin. Microbiol. Infect. Dis.* **2021**, *40*, 2113–2121. [CrossRef] [PubMed]
38. Collins, M.E.; Popowitch, E.B.; Miller, M.B. Evaluation of a Novel Multiplex PCR Panel Compared to Quantitative Bacterial Culture for Diagnosis of Lower Respiratory Tract Infections. *J. Clin. Microbiol.* **2020**, *58*, 02013-19. [CrossRef]
39. Pickens, C.; Wunderink, R.G.; Qi, C.; Mopuru, H.; Donnelly, H.; Powell, K.; Sims, M.D. A multiplex polymerase chain reaction assay for antibiotic stewardship in suspected pneumonia. *Diagn. Microbiol. Infect. Dis.* **2020**, *98*, 115179. [CrossRef]
40. Klein, M.; Bacher, J.; Barth, S.; Atrzadeh, F.; Siebenhaller, K.; Ferreira, I.; Beisken, S.; Posch, A.E.; Carroll, K.C.; Wunderink, R.G.; et al. Multicenter Evaluation of the Unyvero Platform for Testing Bronchoalveolar Lavage Fluid. *J. Clin. Microbiol.* **2021**, *59*, e02497-20. [CrossRef]
41. Benkő, R.; Gajdács, M.; Matuz, M.; Bodó, G.; Lázár, A.; Hajdú, E.; Papfalvi, E.; Hannauer, P.; Erdélyi, P.; Pető, Z. Prevalence and Antibiotic Resistance of ESKAPE Pathogens Isolated in the Emergency Department of a Tertiary Care Teaching Hospital in Hungary: A 5-Year Retrospective Survey. *Antibiot* **2020**, *9*, 624. [CrossRef]
42. Grignon, O.; EDBAC Study Group; Montassier, E.; Corvec, S.; Lepelletier, D.; Hardouin, J.-B.; Caillon, J.; Batard, E. Escherichia coli antibiotic resistance in emergency departments. Do local resistance rates matter? *Eur. J. Clin. Microbiol. Infect. Dis.* **2015**, *34*, 571–577. [CrossRef]
43. Rothe, K.; Wantia, N.; Spinner, C.D.; Schneider, J.; Lahmer, T.; Waschulzik, B.; Schmid, R.M.; Busch, D.H.; Katchanov, J. Antimicrobial resistance of bacteraemia in the emergency department of a German university hospital (2013–2018): Potential carbapenem-sparing empiric treatment options in light of the new EUCAST recommendations. *BMC Infect. Dis.* **2019**, *19*, 1091. [CrossRef] [PubMed]
44. El-Sokkary, R.; Uysal, S.; Erdem, H.; Kullar, R.; Pekok, A.U.; Amer, F.; Grgić, S.; Carevic, B.; El-Kholy, A.; Liskova, A.; et al. Profiles of multidrug-resistant organisms among patients with bacteremia in intensive care units: An International ID-IRI survey. *Eur. J. Clin. Microbiol. Infect. Dis.* **2021**, *40*, 2323–2334. [CrossRef] [PubMed]
45. Baditoiu, L.; Axente, C.; Lungeanu, D.; Muntean, D.; Horhat, F.; Moldovan, R.; Hogea, E.; Bedreag, O.; Sandesc, D.; Licker, M. Intensive care antibiotic consumption and resistance patterns: A cross-correlation analysis. *Ann. Clin. Microbiol. Antimicrob.* **2017**, *16*, 71. [CrossRef] [PubMed]
46. Axente, C.; Licker, M.; Moldovan, R.; Hogea, E.; Muntean, D.; Horhat, F.; Bedreag, O.; Sandesc, D.; Papurica, M.; Dugaesescu, D.; et al. Antimicrobial consumption, costs and resistance patterns: A two year prospective study in a Romanian intensive care unit. *BMC Infect. Dis.* **2017**, *17*, 358. [CrossRef]
47. Stanford Health Care. The SHC Antimicrobial Guidebook. Available online: https://med.stanford.edu/bugsanddrugs/guidebook.html (accessed on 12 November 2023).

Disclaimer/Publisher's Note: The statements, opinions and data contained in all publications are solely those of the individual author(s) and contributor(s) and not of MDPI and/or the editor(s). MDPI and/or the editor(s) disclaim responsibility for any injury to people or property resulting from any ideas, methods, instructions or products referred to in the content.

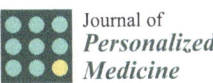

Article

Rate of Complications after Hip Fractures Caused by Prolonged Time-to-Surgery Depends on the Patient's Individual Type of Fracture and Its Treatment

Alina Daginnus [1,2], Jan Schmitt [1,3], Jan Adriaan Graw [4], Christian Soost [5] and Rene Burchard [1,2,3,*]

1. Faculty of Medicine, University of Marburg, 35037 Marburg, Germany
2. Department of Orthopaedics and Traumatology, University Hospital of Giessen and Marburg, 35043 Marburg, Germany
3. Department of Orthopaedics and Trauma Surgery, Lahn-Dill-Kliniken, 35683 Dillenburg, Germany
4. Department of Anesthesiology and Intensive Care Medicine, Ulm University Hospital, 89070 Ulm, Germany
5. Institute for Empirics & Statistics, FOM University of Applied Sciences, 45141 Essen, Germany
* Correspondence: burcharr@staff.uni-marburg.de; Tel.: +49-2771-396-4485; Fax: +49-2771-396-4487

Citation: Daginnus, A.; Schmitt, J.; Graw, J.A.; Soost, C.; Burchard, R. Rate of Complications after Hip Fractures Caused by Prolonged Time-to-Surgery Depends on the Patient's Individual Type of Fracture and Its Treatment. *J. Pers. Med.* **2023**, *13*, 1470. https://doi.org/10.3390/jpm13101470

Academic Editor: Ovidiu Alexandru Mederle

Received: 12 September 2023
Revised: 3 October 2023
Accepted: 6 October 2023
Published: 8 October 2023

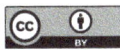

Copyright: © 2023 by the authors. Licensee MDPI, Basel, Switzerland. This article is an open access article distributed under the terms and conditions of the Creative Commons Attribution (CC BY) license (https://creativecommons.org/licenses/by/4.0/).

Abstract: Introduction: Hip fractures are common injuries in the elderly and are usually treated with timely surgery. While severe postoperative complications are reported for up to 10% of patients, many studies identified predictive factors for the occurrence of complications postoperatively. A controversially discussed factor is "time-to-surgery". The aim of the study was to examine if time-to-surgery was associated with the occurrence of complications and if the complication rate differed between the patient individual fracture types of intracapsular on the one hand and extracapsular hip fractures on the other hand. We hypothesized that time-to-surgery had less impact on complications in intracapsular hip fractures compared to extracapsular ones, and therefore, guidelines should pay attention to the patient individual case scenario. Materials and Methods: All patients who were admitted to the Department of Trauma and Orthopaedic Surgery of an academic teaching hospital for hip fracture surgery ($n = 650$) over a five-year period were included in the study. After the application of the exclusion criteria, such as periprosthetic or pathologic fractures, cases needed immediate surgical treatment, and after outlier adjustment, 629 cases remained in the study. Hip fractures were classified into intracapsular fractures (treated by hip arthroplasty) and extracapsular fractures (treated by intramedullary nailing osteosynthesis). The occurrence of severe complications in patients treated within 24 h was compared with patients treated later than 24 h after injury. For statistical evaluation, a multivariate logistic regression analysis was performed to investigate the impact of time-to-surgery interval on the occurrence of complications. Results: Patients with an extracapsular fracture, which was treated with intramedullary nailing (44.5%), rarely suffered a serious complication when surgery was performed within 24 h after injury. However, when the interval of the time-to-surgery was longer than 24 h, the complication rate increased significantly (8.63% vs. 25.0%, $p = 0.002$). In contrast to this finding in patients with intracapsular fractures (55.5%), which were treated with cemented arthroplasty, complication rates did not depend on the 24 h interval (26.17% vs. 20.83%, $p = 0.567$). Conclusions: The occurrence of complications after surgical treatment of hip fractures is associated with the time interval between injury and surgery. A 24 h time interval between injury and surgical procedure seems to play a major role only in extracapsular fractures treated with osteosynthesis but not in intracapsular fractures treated with arthroplasty. Therefore, guidelines should take notice of the patient individual case scenario and, in particular, the individual hip fracture type.

Keywords: hip fracture; time to surgery; complications; intracapsular hip fracture; extracapsular hip fracture

1. Introduction

Hip fractures are one of the most common bone injuries of the musculoskeletal system in the elderly, and the incidence per year rises with age [1,2]. Across Europe, incidences are

0.5–1.6% per year [3,4]. For example, in Germany, annual incidences for those over 65 years of age range from 0.6 to 0.9% [5–7]. In industrialized countries, there is an expected yearly increase in the incidence of hip fractures of 3–5%, and therefore, a doubling of cases can be anticipated by 2040 [8,9]. Hip fractures predominantly occur in women, with men having only half the estimated risk [10]. For people in the age group above 65 years, hip fractures are the most common cause of admission and hospitalization to an orthopedic or trauma department. The prognosis after these injuries is unfavorable since a worldwide 1-year mortality rate of 22% is calculated based on a review article including 229,851 patients [11]. Hip fractures are a worldwide major public health burden with high costs for health systems and social care through hospital stays and subsequent rehabilitation or home care. Costs for fractures close to the hip add up to two to four billion EUR per year [1,12–14].

Hip fractures are usually treated with surgery depending on the fracture type, and a timely operation of these serious injuries results in good outcomes and fewer complication rates [15]. Potential complications such as wound infections or embolisms can lead to dependency, immobility, impaired quality of life, and death. [7,16]. For instance, Seong and colleagues and Klestil and colleagues described a one-year mortality rate of 14–36% after surgery [2,17]. These results are in line with data described in a review by Downey and colleagues [11]. Furthermore, there is a significant rate of postoperative complications in both, systemic complications such as myocardial infarction, deep vein thrombosis, pulmonary embolism, and urinary tract infection and surgical complications such as wound infections, expanded hematomas, and any other serious condition with the need for revision surgery [1,2]. In addition to others, Palma and colleagues described a rate for severe complications ranging from loss of mobility or loss of independence up to death between 8 and 28% [18–20].

Many studies revealed predictive factors for the occurrence of perioperative complications after hip fracture, such as gender, age, comorbidities, systemic anticoagulation, and the general physical status at the time of the injury [1,11,17,19,21–32]. The most controversial factor recognized and examined in multiple studies on the therapy of hip fractures is the "time-to-surgery" interval [19,33,34]. While some studies found an increased complication rate for surgical procedures performed after 24 h, other study groups found disadvantages for a too-early operation or detected no significant association between the time-to-surgery interval and complication rates [19,21–26,35]. Some guidelines, such as the "German guideline for the treatment of femoral fracture close to the hip joint", recommend surgery for these fractures without differentiating the fracture type patient individual within 24 h after injury [27]. Others recommend treatment within 48 h after hospital admission [36,37]. However, there is no consensus about the optimal time window for treatment in international literature.

However, none of the aforementioned studies to date examined fracture type or type of surgical procedure in terms of the optimal time to surgery. Due to the completely different pathoanatomical conditions of the various fracture types, the distinction between intra- and extracapsular fractures should be of particular interest [38]. Analyzing Swedish registry data, Mattisson and colleagues recommended surgery within 36 h for extracapsular fractures due to the more problematic results [39]. However, they could not give any recommendations for intracapsular fractures. In addition, the common surgical approach to address these two different fracture types differs too: while intracapsular fractures are usually treated with arthroplasty, extracapsular fractures are mainly treated with osteosynthesis, e.g., with intramedullary nailing [40].

Therefore, the aim of this study was to investigate whether the occurrence of complications after treatment of hip fractures differs according to the patient individual type of fractures and the specific treatment procedures.

2. Materials and Methods

2.1. Ethical Approval

The ethics committee of the State Medical Chamber of Westfalia-Lippe approved the present study according to the ethical standards (number of ethical approval: 2015-497-f-S). Written informed consent of included patients was waived by the ethics committee because of the retrospective nature of the presented study. All methods were performed in accordance with the relevant guidelines and regulations as stated in the Helsinki Declarations.

2.2. Study Design

This single-center retrospective observational study includes a reanalyzed subset of data from a patient population from a previous study examining the gender-specific circumstances of required transfusion in the setting of hip fractures [41]. All patients admitted to the Department of Trauma and Orthopaedic Surgery of a 595-bed-academic teaching hospital of the University of Marburg for hip fracture surgery ($n = 650$) in the years 2010 to 2014 were included in the study. The following exclusion criteria were stated: periprosthetic fracture, fractures that had to be treated directly by osteosynthesis such as intracapsular fractures of young and healthy patients (age < 65), pathologic fractures such as metastasis, postoperative conditions that forbid an immediate full weight-bearing, and fractures including the pelvic bone. After application of the exclusion criteria and after outlier adjustment, 629 cases remained in the study collective. According to the major study target, all hip fractures were classified into intracapsular fractures (treated by hip arthroplasty) and extracapsular fractures (treated by intramedullary nailing).

2.3. Surgical Technique and Postoperative Care

All surgical procedures in both study groups were performed under general anesthesia. Neither during osteosynthesis of extracapsular fractures nor during arthroplasty of intracapsular fractures, tranexamic acid was used. Disinfection administration and perioperative care, such as warming, pain and physiotherapy, and patient blood management, were performed according to the national guidelines and the recommendations of the World Health Organization (WHO).

2.3.1. Intracapsular Fractures

Since urgent cases of intracapsular hip fractures, just as younger patients needed immediate osteosyntheses with, for example, cannulated screws, were excluded, all intracapsular fractures of the presented study collective were treated by hip arthroplasty. The surgical procedure was performed under single-shot antibiotic prophylaxis 30–45 min prior to surgery, applying 2 g of Cefazoline intravenous. A muscle-protecting anterolateral approach using the so-called Watson-Jones interval was performed, and after resection of the fractured femoral neck by a saw cut, the femoral head was removed, too. Femoral bone was prepared for the implantation of a cemented straight stem. In all cases, the Excia T Standard stem was implanted (Aesculap AG, Tuttlingen, Germany). After cementing a bipolar steel head according to the patient, the individual diameter of the removed bony head was applied (Bipolar Head, Aesculap AG, Tuttlingen, Germany). After the insertion of two suction drains into the subfascial and subcutaneous tissue, the wound was closed and draped. Postoperative treatment included immediate gait training with full weight-bearing on crutches beginning from day 1 after surgery. Prophylaxis of embolic complications was performed by standardized anticoagulation by low molecular weight heparin.

2.3.2. Extracapsular Fractures

Extracapsular fractures were treated by intramedullary nailing osteosynthesis. The surgical procedure was performed under single-shot antibiotic prophylaxis 30–45 min prior to surgery applying 2 g of Cefazoline intravenous. First fracture reduction was established using a classic reduction table. Therefore, the injured leg was fixed and repositioned under X-ray control in anterior posterior view and in lateral view. To fix the reposition, an intramedullary nail was inserted (Targon PFT, Aesculap AG, Tuttlingen, Germany). This proximal femur nail has a gliding femoral neck screw and an additional anti-rotation pin above the neck screw. Distally the nail was fixed with one bicortical screw. Wound closure included a multilayer closing and a sterile draping after the application of one subfascial suction drain. Postoperative treatment included immediate gait training with full weight-bearing on crutches beginning from day 1 after surgery. Prophylaxis of embolic complications was performed by standardized anticoagulation by low molecular weight heparin.

2.4. Data Collection

Cases were identified by ICD (International Statistical Classification of Diseases and Related Health Problems) codes (S72.00-08 and S72.10-11) using the hospital patient data management system (MCC Meierhofer®, Meierhofer AG, Munich, Germany). The following variables were extracted from the electronic patient data files: demographic patient data such as age, sex, date of accident, time to surgery interval, length of surgery (incision to end of suture), patient individual type of fracture, surgical treatment such as arthroplasty or osteosynthesis, medication profile, overall length of hospital stay, admittance to intensive care unit, cumulated costs of the hospital stay, patients' residential status (living at home or living in a nursing home), and common laboratory values (hemoglobin concentration, International Normalized Ratio (INR), blood glucose, electrolytes such as natrium, kalium, calcium, and kidney retention parameters). Presence of a comorbidity was considered if the following previous illnesses were identified: dementia, symptomatic heart failure, previous ischemic stroke, gait disorder, living in a nursing home before hospitalization, and the presence of polypharmacy, which was defined as 4 or more medications taken.

2.5. Study Outcome Parameters

Occurrence of severe perioperative complications was defined as primary outcome parameter. The need for revision surgery and the occurrence of any deep wound infection were considered severe surgical complications. In addition, occurrence of severe systemic perioperative complications was defined as secondary outcome parameter, including death, thromboembolic events, perioperative pneumonia, and urinary tract infection. Thromboembolic events were defined as pulmonary embolism, deep vein thromboembolism, ischemic stroke, and myocardial infarction.

2.6. Statistical Analysis

The statistical analysis of the data was conducted using the R software package, version 4.0.4, developed by the R Foundation for Statistical Computing in Vienna, Austria. Categorical data and bivariate relationships were assessed using two statistical tests: Pearson's Chi-Square test of independence and the two-sample proportion test. For the bivariate analysis, results are presented in terms of absolute numbers and frequencies (%) or means unless otherwise specified. In addition, the standard errors are also reported. To delve deeper into the relationships between variables and control for potential confounding factors, multivariate analysis was employed, specifically logistic regression. This method enables us to identify the influence of multiple factors simultaneously and allows us to control for potential influence factors and obtain a more accurate understanding of the factors affecting the outcome, reducing the risk of selection bias in our study. Standard errors presented in parentheses alongside the regression results were included. A significance level of $p < 0.05$ was set as the threshold for statistical significance.

3. Results

Table 1 shows the characteristics of the 629 patients undergoing surgical hip fracture treatment. There were 449 (71.38%) female and 180 (28.62%) male patients (3:1 female to male ratio). The mean age of all patients was 79.29 years (range 20–102). In addition, a mean length of stay in the hospital of 14.44 days (sd 6.92 days, range 1–79 days) was recognized.

Table 1. Patient characteristics ($n = 629$).

Age, mean (sd)	79.29 years (11.94 years)
Range	20–102 years
Gender, n (%)	
female	449 (71.38%)
male	180 (28.62%)
Comorbidities, n (%)	
dementia	138 (21.94%)
symptomatic heart failure	241 (38.31%)
stroke	88 (14.00%)
gait disorder	145 (23.05%)
Place of residence, n (%)	
live at home	507 (80.60%)
live in a nursing home	98 (15.58%)
unknown	24 (3.82%)
Medication, n (%)	
none	90 (14.31%)
1–3	145 (23.05%)
4–6	133 (21.14%)
>7	351 (55.80%)
INR, n (%)	
≤1.5	566 (91.14%)
>1.5	55 (8.86%)

Based on the fracture type, two groups were compared: patients with intracapsular hip fractures (44.52%) and patients with extracapsular fractures (55.48%). Patients with an extracapsular fracture rarely suffered a serious complication if the surgical treatment was performed within the 24 h interval, but when the 24 h window was exceeded, complications increased significantly in this group (27 (8.63%) vs. (9 (25.0%), $p = 0.002$). In the group of intracapsular fractures, the complication frequency did not differ between a surgical treatment within 24 h on the one hand and a treatment minimum 24 h after the injury on the other hand (67 (26.17%) vs. 5 (20.83%), $p = 0.567$).

To reduce the probability of a possible selection bias, multivariate analysis was performed using logistic regression and stepwise integration of patient characteristics of age, sex, place of residence, comorbidities, and hospital length of stay. The results in Table 2 show a significant increase in the probability of complications for the extracapsular fracture type and duration to surgery greater than 24 h compared to the intracapsular fracture type for models 1–3 ($p < 0.05$). The addition of the control variables leads only to marginal changes in the regression coefficients but not to a change in the significant interaction. This allows us to show that the effect is not biased by the sociodemographic characteristics of the study participants. The significant interaction effect of the most comprehensive model 3 (probability to suffer from a complication regarding the time to surgery (within 24 h vs. >24 h)) is shown in Figure 1, allowing a more intuitive interpretation of the findings.

In addition, logistic regression analysis (most comprehensive model 3) provides results for the influence of the control variables and reveals that the probability of occurrence of complications increased with increasing age ($b = 0.040$, OR = 1.041, $p < 0.05$). The probability of occurrence of complications also increased if dementia ($b = 0.999$, OR = 2.714, $p < 0.01$) or heart failure ($b = 1.260$, OR = 3.525, $p < 0.001$) was present.

Table 2. Logistic regression model in which predictors of complication occurrence are added stepwise in models 1, 2, and 3.

	Complication		
	(1)	(2)	(3)
Intracapsular fracture	0.063	−0.025	0.067
	(0.314)	(0.317)	(0.330)
Time to surgery > 24 h	1.262 **	1.200 **	1.093 *
	(0.434)	(0.448)	(0.476)
Age		0.057 ***	0.040 *
		(0.017)	(0.019)
Male		−0.142	−0.329
		(0.338)	(0.360)
Residence: live at home			0.429
			(0.436)
Residence: live in a nursing home			0.275
			(0.418)
Residence: unknown			1.146
			(0.646)
Dementia			0.999 **
			(0.323)
Symptomatic heart failure			1.260 ***
			(0.319)
Stroke			0.093
			(0.434)
Gait disorder			−0.026
			(0.371)
Length of stay			0.029
			(0.017)
Intracapsular fracture * Time to surgery > 24 h	−1.559 *	−1.453 *	−1.596 *
	(0.679)	(0.691)	(0.716)
Constant	−2.360 ***	−6.932 ***	−7.259 ***
	(0.201)	(1.439)	(1.708)
Observations	629	629	629
Log Likelihood	−193.936	−185.973	−169.866
Akaike Inf. Crit.	395.872	383.946	367.731

Notes: * Significant at the 5 percent level. ** Significant at the 1 percent level. *** Significant at the 0.1 percent level.

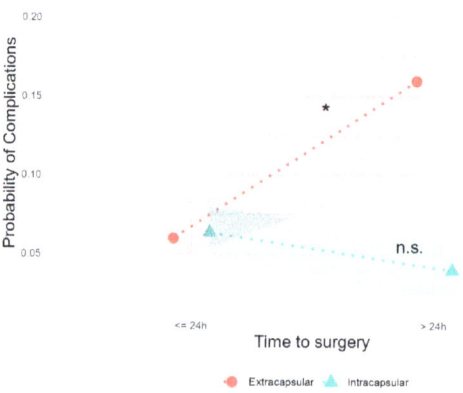

Figure 1. Comparison of the complication rates between the extra- and intracapsular groups. A significant increase in the complication probability can only be seen in the extracapsular group instead of the intracapsular group (* = $p < 0.05$, n.s. = not significant).

4. Discussion

This retrospective study demonstrates that patients with an extracapsular hip fracture rarely suffered a serious perioperative complication when surgery was performed within 24 h after injury. However, when the interval of the time-to-surgery was >24 h, the complication rate increased significantly. In patients with intracapsular fractures, complication rates did not differ between patients treated within 24 h and patients with surgery performed >24 h after injury.

Due to the demographic development of humankind and medical progress, geriatric medicine is one of the challenges of modern medicine [8]. Hip fractures are among the most common traumas of the elderly, and because these people are usually pre-diseased, a higher risk for the occurrence of perioperative complications is present [16]. The study collective was comparable to other studies, including epidemiologic parameters such as age, gender distribution, BMI, blood values, and presence of comorbidities [2,7,11,15–17]. Furthermore, the general complication rate (9.54% of all cases) was comparable to the complication rates reported from similar study cohorts [18–20].

4.1. The Time to Surgery Interval in Hip Fractures

The optimal time for surgery associated with the lowest risk of complications after hip fracture surgery has been the subject of numerous studies in the literature. While some authors found advantages for surgery within 24 h, others could not confirm these results [1,17,19,21–26,28–32,35,42–44]. These heterogeneous results thus leave room for interpretation also for national guidelines. Taken together, most of the studies recommend surgery as soon as possible for all types of hip fractures without considering individual fracture types. In the German guidelines, for example, treatment within 24 h is recommended as mandatory [27]. In contrast, U.S. and U.K. guidelines recommend surgical treatment of hip fractures within 48 h of admission [36,37]. The American Academy of Orthopaedic Surgeons (AAOS) recommends surgery within 48 h and claims moderate evidence [17]. The discrepancy between recommendations can be explained by the heterogeneity of studies and the lack of a clearly definable cutoff for the safest time between admission and the start of surgery.

4.2. Impact of Patient Individual Hip Fracture Type

In all the studies mentioned, the type of fracture has not been considered differentiated in the analysis of the results [1,17,19,21–26,28–32,35,42–44]. Reasons for the assumed influence of the fracture type on the complication rate are mainly to be found in the anatomy of the hip joint or the proximal femur [40]. Intracapsular fractures usually have low primary blood loss because of the confinement by the capsule itself [38]. Extracapsular fractures, on the other hand, may have much more extensive bleeding into the soft tissues of the entire femur [38]. Therefore, Harper and colleagues describe a "hidden blood loss" of extracapsular fractures compared to intracapsular fractures [38]. These findings are well explained by the anatomy of the proximal femoral region. Intracapsular fractures usually have very limited blood loss until the time of surgery because the rough and tight capsule limits the blood loss to only a few milliliters. In contrast, blood loss in extracapsular fractures differs substantially due to the absence of the limiting capsule. Bleeding from the medullary cavity of the largest human bone is limited only by the capacity of the soft tissue space. Therefore, significant blood loss up to hemorrhagic shock is known from traumatic extracapsular fractures of the femur [45]. Stacey's research group was also able to show significant differences in preoperative blood loss related to the patient individual fracture type in hip fractures [46]. In intracapsular hip fractures, hemoglobin levels dropped about an average of 1.1 g/dL. On the other hand, extracapsular fractures showed much more extensive blood loss with an average loss in hemoglobin concentration of 1.7 g/dL. The differences in blood loss were also evident in immediate postoperative blood count measurement as a consequence of the already higher preoperative blood loss. Thus, patients with intracapsular fractures left the operation theatre with an average hemoglobin value of 10.1 g/dL, while those with extracapsular fractures had a value of only 8.8 g/dL [46]. Further examination of the pathophysiological processes in the context of increased blood loss, especially in mono-injury of the large tubular bones, reveals a significantly increased inflammatory response with potential consequences for several organ systems in various animal models in pigs and mice [47,48]. A significantly increased expression of Interleukin-6-related genes, as well as the infiltration of polymorphonuclear (PMN) leukocytes into the tissue, could be detected [47]. In particular, the lungs and liver were affected. Furthermore, increased age was found to be a predictive factor for exacerbating liver inflammation and, for this reason, also an additional disorder of coagulation [48].

Due to the lack of limitation of the peri-trochanteric bone regions by a rough capsule, extracapsular hip fractures are associated with significantly increased soft tissue damage, especially in the skeletal muscles resulting from trauma by the sharp-edged fragments of the dislocated bone parts. Such soft tissue damage leads to both an increased inflammatory response and increased blood loss. In this context, Pierce and Pittet described a vicious circle of soft tissue damage and inflammatory response [49]. The soft tissue damage and the subsequent response result in damage to the endothelium with a corresponding change in permeability and subsequent soft tissue edema. This edema further leads to worsened tissue perfusion and oxygenation. This, in turn, increases the soft tissue damage and closes the vicious circle [50]. Infiltration of tissue, particularly muscle, by inflammation-mediating cells and mediators peaks between 12 and 24 h after trauma [50]. These pathophysiological correlations further suggest that early therapy might be useful in extracapsular hip fractures with concomitant soft tissue trauma.

In summary, extracapsular hip fractures offer a higher risk profile regarding a prolonged time to surgery due to their anatomical and pathophysiological circumstances. These are not found to the same extent in intracapsular fractures, and therefore, the reduction and stabilization of extracapsular fractures might be of increased priority.

In addition, intracapsular fractures have a correspondingly lower influence on the entire body because of the usually better preoperative physical condition of the patients [51]. Hershkovitz and Rutenberg recently reported that the patient populations with extracapsular and intracapsular hip fractures differed in physical condition, with patients with intracapsular fractures having a better physical condition on average [52]. The patient cohort with intracapsular fractures had a slightly higher proportion of male gender, a higher level of education, and more frequent access to home care than those with extracapsular fractures. This is also reflected in the fact that postoperative recovery is faster in intracapsular fractures and is more often associated with a favorable outcome [51,52]. The results found in this study support the differentiated view and suggest that individual consideration of the patient-specific fracture type is useful in hip fractures.

Based on the high frequency of hip fractures in the elderly and, therefore, the high relevance of this disease for healthcare systems particularly in the Western world, guidelines support maintaining the quality of treatment at a consistently high level [27,36]. Nevertheless, as this study supports, patient-specific aspects might also be considered in the decision-making process [40]. Besides the medical quality of treatment, appropriated resource allocation is a growing factor for each healthcare system with an impact on healthcare economics [12,14]. The high costs of holding hip fractures coupled with a growing shortage of specialists challenges many hospitals in the timely treatment of hip fractures [53]. In particular, the treatment of intracapsular fractures of the elderly by means of arthroplasty is in focus here [40]. The fact that these latter cases are now less prone to delayed surgery could be a finding of great interest with a corresponding health policy impact.

4.3. Limitations

Although the work presented is based on a large patient population, this study is limited by the retrospective and single-center study design. While the surgeons performing the operations remained constant during the study period, intracapsular fractures of younger patients requiring acute care (<6 h) by primary osteosynthesis were excluded.

In summary, the results currently available in the international literature on the question of the best possible surgical timing in patients with hip fractures do not provide clear evidence for a 24 h rule. The lack of data on differentiation for different patient individual fracture types and the influence of fracture type on the occurrence of complications after hip fracture has not been adequately studied. The present study provides new additional insights that could facilitate the approach in orthopedic and trauma surgery departments through a patient-specific treatment approach to hip fracture surgery and a more differentiated application of the guideline recommendations.

5. Conclusions

Occurrence of a severe complication after surgical treatment of hip fractures is associated with the time interval between injury and surgery. A 24 h time interval to surgery seems to play a role only in extracapsular fractures treated with osteosynthesis but not in intracapsular fractures treated with arthroplasty. Therefore, recommendations of current national and international guidelines on hip fracture surgery should be reevaluated with respect to the patient individual hip fracture type.

Author Contributions: All authors contributed to the study conception and design. Material preparation, data collection, and analysis were performed by A.D., J.S., J.A.G., C.S. and R.B. The first draft of the manuscript was written by A.D. and R.B. and all authors commented on previous versions of the manuscript. All authors have read and agreed to the published version of the manuscript.

Funding: This research received no external funding.

Institutional Review Board Statement: The ethics committee of the State Medical Chamber of Westfalia-Lippe approved the present study (number of ethics approval: 2015-497-f-S).

Informed Consent Statement: Written informed consent was waived by the ethics committee of the State Medical Chamber of Westfalia-Lippe.

Data Availability Statement: The datasets used and/or analyzed during the current study are available from the corresponding author upon reasonable request.

Conflicts of Interest: The authors declare no conflict of interest.

References

1. Saul, D.; Riekenberg, J.; Ammon, J.C.; Hoffmann, D.B.; Sehmisch, S. Hip Fractures: Therapy, Timing, and Complication Spectrum. *Orthop. Surg.* **2019**, *11*, 994–1002. [PubMed]
2. Klestil, T.; Röder, C.; Stotter, C.; Winkler, B.; Nehrer, S.; Lutz, M.; Klerings, I.; Wagner, G.; Gartlehner, G.; Nussbaumer-Streit, B. Impact of timing of surgery in elderly hip fracture patients: A systematic review and meta-analysis. *Sci. Rep.* **2018**, *8*, 13933. [PubMed]
3. Abrahamsen, B., Vestergaard, P. Declining incidence of hip fractures and the extent of use of anti-osteoporotic therapy in Denmark 1997–2006. *Osteoporos. Int.* **2010**, *21*, 373–380. [PubMed]
4. Leal, J.; The REFReSH Study Group; Gray, A.M.; Prieto-Alhambra, D.; Arden, N.K.; Cooper, C.; Javaid, M.K.; Judge, A. Impact of hip fracture on hospital care costs: A population-based study. *Osteoporos. Int.* **2016**, *27*, 549–558. [CrossRef] [PubMed]
5. Stöckle, U.; Lucke, M.; Haas, N.P. Zertifizierte medizinische Fortbildung: Der Oberschenkelhalsbruch. *Dtsch Arztebl Int.* **2005**, *102*, A3426.
6. Minne, H.W.; Pfeifer, M.; Wittenberg, R.; Würtz, R. Schenkelhalsfrakturen in Deutschland: Prävention, Therapie, Inzidenz und sozioökonomische Bedeutung. *Dtsch Arztebl Int.* **2001**, *98*, 1751–1756.
7. Hoffmann, F.; Glaeske, G. Inzidenz proximaler Femurfrakturen in Deutschland. *Pers. Anal. Einer Versich.* **2006**, *68*, 161–164. [CrossRef]
8. Hoenig, H.; Rubenstein, L.V.; Sloane, R.; Horner, R.; Kahn, K. What is the role of timing in the surgical and rehabilitative care of community-dwelling older persons with acute hip fracture? *Arch. Intern. Med.* **1997**, *157*, 513–520. [CrossRef]
9. Muhm, M.; Walendowski, M.; Danko, T.; Weiss, C.; Ruffing, T.; Winkler, H. Einflussfaktoren auf den stationären Verlauf von Patienten mit hüftgelenknahen Femurfrakturen. *Z. Gerontol. Geriatr.* **2014**, *48*, 339–345.
10. Kanis, J.A.; Odén, A.; McCloskey, E.V.; Johansson, H.; Wahl, D.A.; Cooper, C. A systematic review of hip fracture incidence and probability of fracture worldwide. *Osteoporos. Int.* **2012**, *23*, 2239–2256. [CrossRef]

11. Downey, C.; Kelly, M.; Quinlan, J.F. Changing trends in the mortality rate at 1-year post hip fracture—A systematic review. *World J. Orthop.* **2019**, *10*, 166–175.
12. Boufous, S.; Finch, C.; Close, J.; Day, L.; Lord, S. Hospital admissions following presentations to emergency departments for a fracture in older people. *Inj. Prev.* **2007**, *13*, 211–214. [PubMed]
13. Muhm, M.; Walendowski, M.; Danko, T.; Weiss, C.; Ruffing, T.; Winkler, H. Verweildauer von Patienten mit hüftgelenknahen Femurfrakturen. *Der Unfallchirurg* **2014**, *119*, 560–569.
14. Parker, M.; Johansen, A. Hip fracture. *BMJ* **2006**, *333*, 27–30. [CrossRef]
15. Moja, L.; Piatti, A.; Pecoraro, V.; Ricci, C.; Virgili, G.; Salanti, G.; Germagnoli, L.; Liberati, A.; Banfi, G. Timing matters in hip fracture surgery: Patients operated within 48 hours have better outcomes. A meta-analysis and meta-regression of over 190,000 patients. *PLoS ONE* **2012**, *7*, e46175.
16. Tan, L.; Wong, S.; Kwek, E. Inpatient cost for hip fracture patients managed with an orthogeriatric care model in Singapore. *Singap. Med. J.* **2017**, *58*, 139–144. [CrossRef]
17. Seong, Y.J.; Shin, W.C.; Moon, N.H.; Suh, K.T. Timing of Hip-fracture Surgery in Elderly Patients: Literature Review and Recommendations. *Hip Pelvis* **2020**, *32*, 11–16.
18. de Palma, L.; Torcianti, M.; Meco, L.; Catalani, A.; Marinelli, M. Operative delay and mortality in elderly patients with hip fracture: An observational study. *Eur. J. Orthop. Surg. Traumatol.* **2014**, *24*, 783–788.
19. Orosz, G.M.; Magaziner, J.; Hannan, E.L.; Morrison, R.S.; Koval, K.; Gilbert, M.; McLaughlin, M.; Halm, E.A.; Wang, J.J.; Litke, A.; et al. Association of timing of surgery for hip fracture and patient outcomes. *JAMA* **2004**, *291*, 1738–1743. [CrossRef]
20. Gdalevich, M.; Cohen, D.; Yosef, D.; Tauber, C. Morbidity and mortality after hip fracture: The impact of operative delay. *Arch. Orthop. Trauma Surg.* **2004**, *124*, 334–340.
21. Nyholm, A.M.; Gromov, K.; Palm, H.; Brix, M.; Kallemose, T.; Troelsen, A.; Danish Fracture Database Collaborators. Time to Surgery Is Associated with Thirty-Day and Ninety-Day Mortality after Proximal Femoral Fracture: A Retrospective Observational Study on Prospectively Collected Data from the Danish Fracture Database Collaborators. *J. Bone Joint Surg. Am.* **2015**, *97*, 1333–1339.
22. Ryan, D.J.; Yoshihara, H.; Yoneoka, D.; Egol, K.A.; Zuckerman, J.D. Delay in Hip Fracture Surgery: An Analysis of Patient-Specific and Hospital-Specific Risk Factors. *J. Orthop. Trauma* **2015**, *29*, 343–348. [CrossRef] [PubMed]
23. Craik, J.; Geleit, R.; Hiddema, J.; Bray, E.; Hampton, R.; Railton, G.; Ward, D.; Windley, J. The effect of time to surgery on outcomes and complication rates following total hip arthroplasty for fractured neck of femur. *Ann. R. Coll. Surg. Engl.* **2019**, *101*, 342–345. [PubMed]
24. Grimes, J.P.; Gregory, P.M.; Noveck, H.; Butler, M.S.; Carson, J.L. The effects of time-to-surgery on mortality and morbidity in patients following hip fracture. *Am. J. Med.* **2002**, *112*, 702–709.
25. Ii, A.T.; Jarvis, S.; Orlando, A.; Nwafo, N.; Madayag, R.; Roberts, Z.; Corrigan, C.; Carrick, M.; Bourg, P.; Smith, W.; et al. A three-year retrospective multi-center study on time to surgery and mortality for isolated geriatric hip fractures. *J. Clin. Orthop. Trauma* **2020**, *11*, S56–S61.
26. Bergeron, E.; Lavoie, A.; Moore, L.; Bamvita, J.M.; Ratte, S.; Gravel, C.; Clas, D. Is the delay to surgery for isolated hip fracture predictive of outcome in efficient systems? *J. Trauma* **2006**, *60*, 753–757. [CrossRef]
27. Neumann, C.J.; Schulze-Raestrup, U.; Müller-Mai, C.M.; Smektala, R. Entwicklung der stationären Versorgungsqualität operativ behandelter Patienten mit einer proximalen Femurfraktur in Nordrhein-Westfalen. *Die Unfallchirurgie* **2022**, *125*, 634–646. [PubMed]
28. Verbeek, D.O.F.; Ponsen, K.J.; Goslings, J.C.; Heetveld, M.J. Effect of surgical delay on outcome in hip fracture patients: A retrospective multivariate analysis of 192 patients. *Int. Orthop.* **2008**, *32*, 13–18.
29. Simunovic, N.; Devereaux, P.J.; Sprague, S.; Guyatt, G.H.; Schemitsch, E.; DeBeer, J.; Bhandari, M. Effect of early surgery after hip fracture on mortality and complications: Systematic review and meta-analysis. *CMAJ* **2010**, *182*, 1609–1616. [CrossRef]
30. Al-Ani, A.N.; Samuelsson, B.; Tidermark, J.; Norling, Å.; Ekström, W.; Cederholm, T.; Hedström, M. Early operation on patients with a hip fracture improved the ability to return to independent living. A prospective study of 850 patients. *J. Bone Joint Surg. Am.* **2008**, *90*, 1436–1442. [CrossRef]
31. Muhm, M.; Arend, G.; Ruffing, T.; Winkler, H. Mortality and quality of life after proximal femur fracture-effect of time until surgery and reasons for delay. *Eur. J. Trauma Emerg. Surg.* **2013**, *39*, 267–275. [PubMed]
32. Ma, R.-S.; Gu, G.-S.; Wang, C.-X.; Zhu, N.; Zhang, X.-Z. Relationship between surgical time and postoperative complications in senile patients with hip fractures. *Chin. J. Traumatol.* **2010**, *13*, 167–172.
33. Vidal, E.I.D.O.; Moreira-Filho, D.C.; Coeli, C.M.; Camargo Jr, K.R.; Fukushima, F.B.; Blais, R. Hip fracture in the elderly: Does counting time from fracture to surgery or from hospital admission to surgery matter when studying in-hospital mortality? *Osteoporos. Int.* **2009**, *20*, 723–729. [PubMed]
34. Parker, M.J.; Pryor, G.A. The timing of surgery for proximal femoral fractures. *J. Bone Joint Surg. Br.* **1992**, *74*, 203–205. [CrossRef] [PubMed]
35. Smektala, R.; Endres, H.G.; Dasch, B.; Maier, C.; Trampisch, H.J.; Bonnaire, F.; Pientka, L. The effect of time-to-surgery on outcome in elderly patients with proximal femoral fractures. *BMC Musculoskelet. Disord.* **2008**, *9*, 171. [CrossRef] [PubMed]
36. National Clinical Guideline Centre. National Clinical Guideline Centre. National Institute for Health and Clinical Excellence: Guidance. In *The Management of Hip Fracture in Adults*; Royal College of Physicians: London, UK, 2011.

37. Roberts, K.C.; Brox, W.T.; Jevsevar, D.S.; Sevarino, K. Management of hip fractures in the elderly. *J. Am. Acad. Orthop. Surg.* **2015**, *23*, 131–137. [CrossRef] [PubMed]
38. Harper, K.D.; Navo, P.; Ramsey, F.; Jallow, S.; Rehman, S. "Hidden" Preoperative Blood Loss with Extracapsular Versus Intracapsular Hip Fractures: What Is the Difference? *Geriatr. Orthop. Surg. Rehabil.* **2017**, *8*, 202–207. [CrossRef]
39. Mattisson, L.; Bojan, A.; Enocson, A. Epidemiology, treatment and mortality of trochanteric and subtrochanteric hip fractures: Data from the Swedish fracture register. *BMC Musculoskelet. Disord.* **2018**, *19*, 369.
40. Kim, D.C.; Honeycutt, M.W.; Riehl, J.T. Hip fractures: Current review of treatment and management. *Curr. Orthop. Pract.* **2019**, *30*, 385–394.
41. Soost, C.; Daginnus, A.; Burchard, R.; Schmitt, J.; Graw, J. Gender differences in blood transfusion strategy for patients with hip fractures—A retrospective analysis. *Int. J. Med. Sci.* **2020**, *17*, 620–625.
42. Pincus, D.; Ravi, B.; Wasserstein, D.; Huang, A.; Paterson, J.M.; Nathens, A.B.; Kreder, H.J.; Jenkinson, R.J.; Wodchis, W.P. Association Between Wait Time and 30-Day Mortality in Adults Undergoing Hip Fracture Surgery. *JAMA* **2017**, *318*, 1994–2003. [CrossRef] [PubMed]
43. Vidán, M.T.; Sánchez, E.; Gracia, Y.; Maranón, E.; Vaquero, J.; Serra, J.A. Causes and effects of surgical delay in patients with hip fracture: A cohort study. *Ann. Intern. Med.* **2011**, *155*, 226–233. [CrossRef] [PubMed]
44. Leer-Salvesen, S.; Engesæter, L.B.; Dybvik, E.; Furnes, O.; Kristensen, T.B.; Gjertsen, J.E. Does time from fracture to surgery affect mortality and intraoperative medical complications for hip fracture patients? An observational study of 73,557 patients reported to the Norwegian Hip Fracture Register. *Bone Joint J.* **2019**, *101*, 1129–1137. [CrossRef] [PubMed]
45. Mitchnik, I.Y.; Talmy, T.; Radomislensky, I.; Chechik, Y.; Shlaifer, A.; Almog, O.; Gendler, S. Femur fractures and hemorrhagic shock: Implications for point of injury treatment. *Injury* **2022**, *53*, 3416–3422. [PubMed]
46. Stacey, J.; Bush, C.; DiPasquale, T. The hidden blood loss in proximal femur fractures is sizeable and significant. *J. Clin. Orthop. Trauma* **2021**, *16*, 239–243. [CrossRef] [PubMed]
47. Störmann, P.; Wagner, N.; Köhler, K.; Auner, B.; Simon, T.-P.; Pfeifer, R.; Horst, K.; Pape, H.-C.; Hildebrand, F.; Wutzler, S.; et al. Monotrauma is associated with enhanced remote inflammatory response and organ damage, while polytrauma intensifies both in porcine trauma model. *Eur. J. Trauma Emerg. Surg.* **2020**, *46*, 31–42. [CrossRef]
48. Meng, F.; Zhou, Y.; Wagner, A.; Bülow, J.M.; Köhler, K.; Neunaber, C.; Bundkirchen, K.; Relja, B. Impact of age on liver damage, inflammation, and molecular signaling pathways in response to femoral fracture and hemorrhage. *Front. Immunol.* **2023**, *14*, 1239145. [CrossRef]
49. Pierce, A.; Pittet, J.F. Inflammatory response to trauma: Implications for coagulation and resuscitation. *Curr. Opin. Anaesthesiol.* **2014**, *27*, 246–252.
50. Muire, P.J.; Mangum, L.H.; Wenke, J.C. Time Course of Immune Response and Immunomodulation During Normal and Delayed Healing of Musculoskeletal Wounds. *Front. Immunol.* **2020**, *11*, 1056.
51. Fox, K.M.; Magaziner, J.; Hebel, J.R.; Kenzora, J.E.; Kashnei, T.M. Intertrochanteric versus femoral neck hip fractures: Differential characteristics, treatment, and sequelae. *J. Gerontol. A Biol. Sci. Med. Sci.* **1999**, *54*, M635–M640. [CrossRef]
52. Hershkovitz, A.; Frenkel Rutenberg, T. Are extracapsular and intracapsular hip-fracture patients two distinct rehabilitation subpopulations? *Disabil. Rehabil.* **2022**, *44*, 4761–4766. [CrossRef] [PubMed]
53. Fluck, B.; Yeong, K.; Lisk, R.; Robin, J.; Fluck, D.; Fry, C.H.; Han, T.S. Identification of preoperative factors and postoperative outcomes in relation to delays in surgery for hip fractures. *Clin. Med.* **2022**, *22*, 313–319. [CrossRef] [PubMed]

Disclaimer/Publisher's Note: The statements, opinions and data contained in all publications are solely those of the individual author(s) and contributor(s) and not of MDPI and/or the editor(s). MDPI and/or the editor(s) disclaim responsibility for any injury to people or property resulting from any ideas, methods, instructions or products referred to in the content.

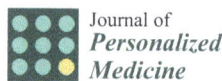

Review

Point-of-Care Lung Ultrasound in the Intensive Care Unit—The Dark Side of Radiology: Where Do We Stand?

Marco Di Serafino [1,*,†], Giuseppina Dell'Aversano Orabona [1,†], Martina Caruso [1], Costanza Camillo [1], Daniela Viscardi [2], Francesca Iacobellis [1], Roberto Ronza [1], Vittorio Sabatino [1], Luigi Barbuto [1], Gaspare Oliva [1] and Luigia Romano [1]

1. Department of General and Emergency Radiology, "Antonio Cardarelli" Hospital, 80131 Naples, Italy; giuseppina.dellaversanoorabona@aocardarelli.it (G.D.O.); martina.caruso@aocardarelli.it (M.C.); costanza.camillo@aocardarelli.it (C.C.); francesca.iacobellis@aocardarelli.it (F.I.); roberto.ronza@aocardarelli.it (R.R.); vittorio.sabatino@aocardarelli.it (V.S.); luigi.barbuto@aocardarelli.it (L.B.); gaspare.oliva@aocardarelli.it (G.O.); luigia.romano@aocardarelli.it (L.R.)
2. Department of Intensive Care and Resuscitation, "Antonio Cardarelli" Hospital, 80131 Naples, Italy; daniela.viscardi@aocardarelli.it
* Correspondence: marco.diserafino@aocardarelli.it
† These authors contributed equally to this work.

Abstract: Patients in intensive care units (ICUs) are critically ill and require constant monitoring of clinical conditions. Due to the severity of the underlying disease and the need to monitor devices, imaging plays a crucial role in critically ill patients' care. Given the clinical complexity of these patients, who typically need respiratory assistance as well as continuous monitoring of vital functions and equipment, computed tomography (CT) can be regarded as the diagnostic gold standard, although it is not a bedside diagnostic technique. Despite its limitations, portable chest X-ray (CXR) is still today an essential diagnostic tool used in the ICU. Being a widely accessible imaging technique, which can be performed at the patient's bedside and at a low healthcare cost, it provides additional diagnostic support to the patient's clinical management. In recent years, the use of point-of-care lung ultrasound (LUS) in ICUs for procedure guidance, diagnosis, and screening has proliferated, and it is usually performed at the patient's bedside. This review illustrates the role of point-of-care LUS in ICUs from a purely radiological point of view as an advanced method in ICU CXR reports to improve the interpretation and monitoring of lung CXR findings.

Keywords: intensive care unit; chest X-ray; lung ultrasound; point-of-care ultrasound

1. Introduction

The anterior–posterior supine chest X-ray (CXR) is a routine investigation performed in intensive care units (ICUs). Being a widely accessible imaging technique, which can be performed at the patient's bedside and at a low healthcare cost, it provides additional diagnostic support to the clinical examination of patients who usually require respiratory assistance and constant monitoring of vital functions and devices [1]. However, its limitations in terms of technical and diagnostic performance are equally well known when compared to both a standard CXR and the better performing and more panoramic chest computed tomography (CT) scan, with image quality often resulting in a frustrating experience for both the clinician, who has to manage a critical patient, and the radiologist, who has to provide the best diagnostics guidance [2]. The technical limitations of the image produced are mitigated by the widespread availability of sufficiently powered X-ray tubes, image digitization, and a rigorous execution technique. Nevertheless, interpretative shortcomings in the cardiopulmonary findings obtained remain, which are unavoidable and inherent in the method [1–4]. If on the one hand the chest CT scan can be considered the diagnostic gold standard in view of the critical state of these patients, it is quite understandable that, since they are critical patients, they cannot be easily transported to the diagnostic radiology departments in order to undergo a chest CT scan [5–7].

In addition, the frequency of diagnostic procedures required for these patients, often with daily monitoring of the chest, is to date still a widely controversial issue, and anterior–posterior supine CXR performed at the patient's bedside is still the best solution [8–10].

The well-established role of bedside lung ultrasound (LUS) performed by the resuscitation team itself represents a crucial turning point in the diagnosis and management of the critically ill patient as well as a guide to the interventional procedures to be performed at the patient's bedside, such as pleural drainage or the insertion and monitoring of devices (Figure 1) [11–13].

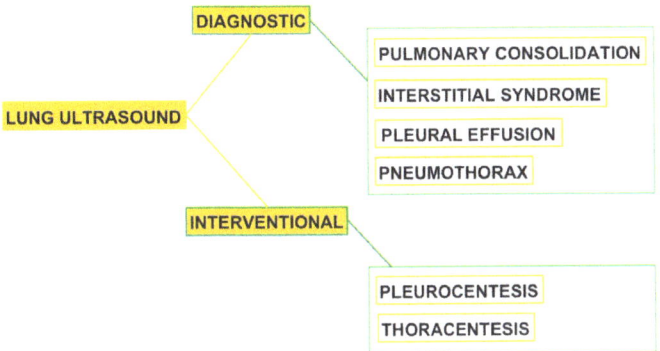

Figure 1. Utility of LUS in the ICU. Modified from [11].

LUS is thus widely accepted in several codified clinical management protocols, as summarized in Table 1 [5,14,15].

Table 1. Validated clinical management LUS protocols.

Validated Clinical Management LUS Protocol	Purpose
BLUE protocol (Bedside Lung Ultrasonography in Emergency)	Emergency protocol for immediate diagnosis of acute respiratory failure.
FALLS protocol (Fluid Administration Limited by Lung Sonography)	Emergency protocol designed to sequentially rule out differential diagnoses such as cardiogenic and hypovolemic shock, allowing an early diagnosis of septic shock.
CAUSE protocol (Cardiac Arrest Ultrasound Exam)	Emergency protocol in cardiac arrest management. It has the potential to reduce the time required to determine the etiology of a cardiac arrest and thus decrease the time between arrest and appropriate therapy.

Furthermore, the specificity and sensitivity of LUS when compared with anterior–posterior supine CXR are encouraging enough to make it an attractive and often alternative choice to CXR (Table 2) [4,5,16].

All this is also amplified in view of the method's proximity to resuscitation areas, its high clinical value, and the absence of the use of ionizing radiation, albeit settling for a partial view, limited to artifactual deductions of the subpleural lung parenchyma, which is highly subjective with the risks of operator dependence [4]. The integration of these methods, i.e., CXR and LUS, could be an incisive turning point, especially in complex clinical settings such as ICUs, where management decisions must be made rapidly and coordinated among the various specialists [17,18].

In this imaging review, we provide some food for thought by drawing on our organizational expertise in interpreting CXR findings and lowering the number of serial CXR checks through the use of LUS as a clinical radiology point of care. This is conducted solely to supplement the CXR findings, monitor those that are readily accessible to the investigation itself, and reduce the produced radiant dose. Finally, but just as importantly, we focus more on the CXR reading through a more insightful echo-mediated clinical interpretation (Figure 2).

Table 2. Lung ultrasound and chest X-ray sensitivity and specificity in many lung diseases. Modified from [5].

Pulmonary Acute Disease	CXR	LUS
Pulmonary Consolidation	Sensitivity of plain chest radiography in detection of pulmonary consolidation has been reported as 38% to 76%.	Sensitivity and specificity of LUS for detection of pulmonary consolidation have been reported as 86–97% and 89–94%, respectively.
Interstitial Syndrome (Cardiogenic pulmonary edema, ARDS)	CXR showed a sensitivity of 36%, specificity of 90%, PPV of 29% and NPV of 92% while these results combined with clinical examination findings became 50%, 84%, 28% and 93% respectively.	US abnormalities may precede those of radiography and can be diagnostic, with a sensitivity and specificity of 97% and 95%, respectively.
Pleural Effusion	Supine chest radiography may reveal abnormality when the amount of fluid reaches 175–525 mL, which is higher than that for upright chest radiography.	US may detect 5–20 mL of pleural fluid with an overall sensitivity of 89–100% and specificity of 96–100%.
Pneumothorax	Portable chest radiography has a sensitivity of 19.8–31.8% and specificity of 99.3–100%.	The overall sensitivity and specificity of US in the detection of pneumothorax are 78.6–100% and 96.5–100%.

Table 3 shows the main pleural–parenchymal complications observed in ICUs that are the subject of this imaging review [19].

Table 3. ICU pleural–parenchymal and device complications grouped by CXR general findings with literature references reporting LUS-validated findings.

ICU Pulmonary Acute Disease	CXR General Findings	LUS-Validated Findings
Pulmonary Consolidation (Atelectasis/Pneumonia/Contusion)	Areas of decreased transparency	Yes [11,13–15,19–22]
Interstitial Syndrome (Cardiogenic pulmonary edema, ARDS)		Yes [13–15,22–24]
Pleural Effusion		Yes [11,13,14,20,25,26]
Pneumothorax	Areas of increased transparency	Yes [11,13,20,27]
Device Complication	Displacement	Empirical

They are divided into three specific paragraphs where the use of LUS, as a methodological advance in the bedside CXR reports in ICUs, is crucial for diagnosing and monitoring areas of decreased transparency around the chest found on X-rays (atelectasis, pneumonia, pleural effusion, pulmonary edema, acute respiratory distress syndrome (ARDS), and pulmonary contusions), in pneumothorax and device monitoring.

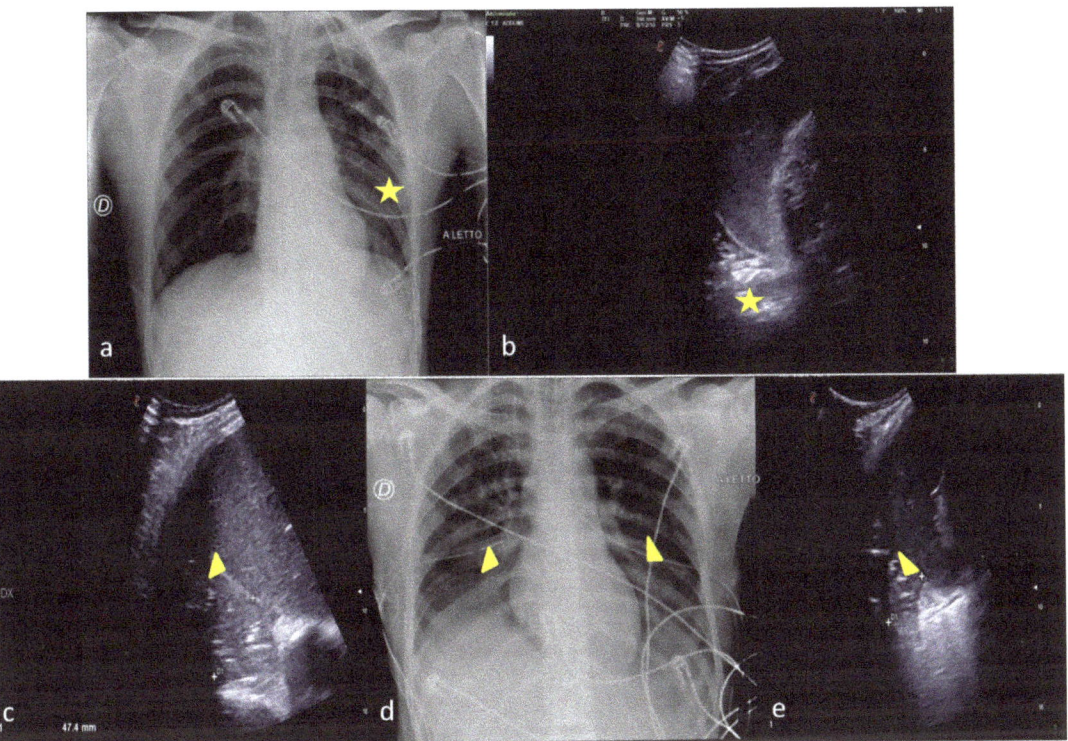

Figure 2. Two examples of CXR and LUS diagnostic integration. Bedside CXR (**a**,**d**) and LUS diagnostic integration (**b**,**c**,**e**). In the first case (top line) the CXR showed small, blurred opacities in the left inferior pulmonary field (**a**, star); LUS of the left basis confirmed the consolidative area with hyperechogenic spots as signs of an air bronchogram (**b**, star). In the second case (below line), the CXR showed small, blurred opacities in the inferior pulmonary field bilaterally (**d**, arrowhead); LUS confirmed areas of lung consolidation with an air bronchogram in the lower right and left pulmonary fields without pleural effusion (**c**,**e**, arrowhead).

2. Characterizing and Monitoring Areas of Decreased Transparency on the CXR

LUS allows us to read the CXR by identifying and better characterizing areas of decreased transparency found on X-rays and also defining their solid or liquid nature and assisting drainage procedures (Figures 3 and 4) [28–32].

However, the initial CXR is still an essential diagnostic tool to obtain an overview of pleural–parenchymal—but not necessarily subpleural—findings and cardio-mediastinal findings, just like an "open window to the chest". It is then supplemented by a targeted LUS investigation where these findings are available to the investigation itself, in order to make the diagnosis and undertake a correct evolutionary/resolutive monitoring in line with the clinical course of the patient being treated [17,18]. Furthermore, the potential role of contrast-enhanced ultrasound (CEUS) cannot be excluded [33–35]. CEUS could be a valuable diagnostic tool in differentiating peripheral areas of parenchymal-enhancing consolidation, such as pneumonic foci, atelectasis, or tumors from peripheral areas of non-enhancing parenchymal infarction [33–35]. However, dynamic CEUS parameters cannot effectively differentiate between benign and malignant peripheral pulmonary lesions due to an overlap of CEUS timings and patterns [36]. On the other hand, CEUS plays an additional role in diagnosing pleuritis or empyema and in guiding their drainage or the biopsy of solid lesions [33–35]. Figure 5 illustrates an example of CEUS diagnostic utility for LUS.

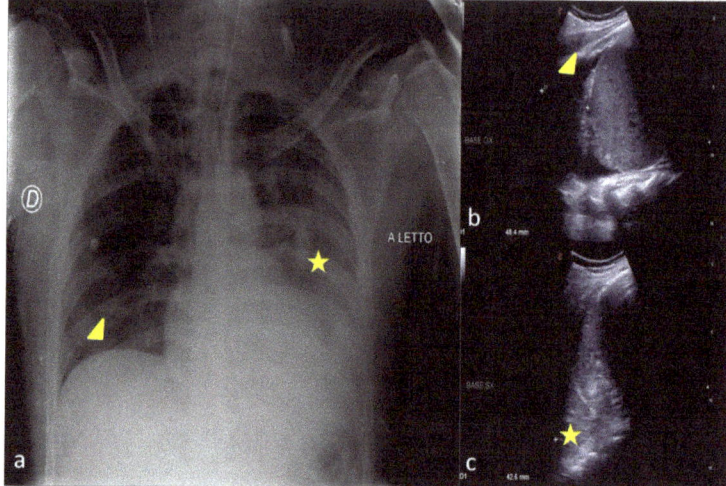

Figure 3. A 30-year-old male patient admitted to the ICU for motor vehicle crash polytrauma resulting in multiple costal fractures and coma status. Bedside CXR (**a**) and LUS (**b**,**c**). (**a**) The CXR showed a blurred opacity in the left inferior pulmonary field (star); the basal field of the right lung appeared normally expanded (arrowhead). (**c**,**d**) LUS diagnostic integration performed on the same day showed a fluid collection in the basal region of the right lung indicating the presence of a small pleural effusion (**b**, arrowhead) that was not clearly demonstrable in the bedside CXR and also an inhomogeneous hypo-echogenicity indicating a parenchymal consolidation in the basal region of the left lung without fluid collection (**c**, star).

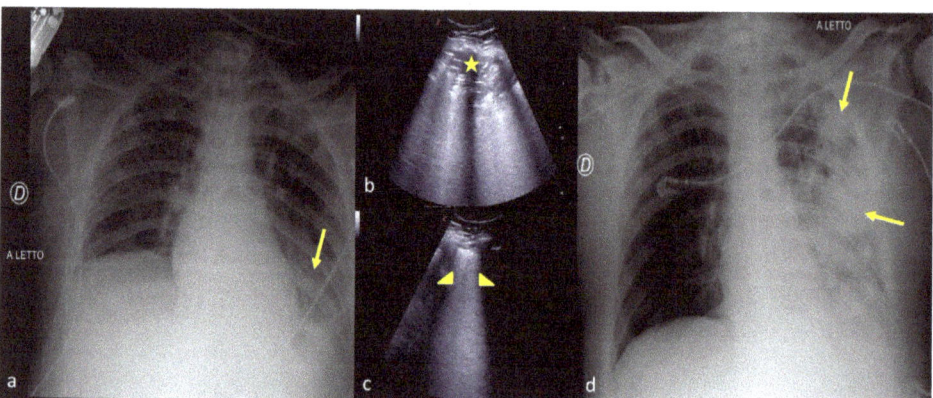

Figure 4. A 27-year-old male patient admitted to the ICU for high-grade gunshot trauma with abdominal involvement and a clinically worsened condition after intubation. Bedside CXR (**a**,**d**) and LUS (**b**,**c**). (**a**) The admission CXR showed a good expansion of the lungs with just a subtle and blurred opacity in the left inferior field (arrow). (**b**,**c**) LUS follow-up was performed after 2 days with evidence of hypoechogenic consolidative change in the left parenchyma (**b**, star) and a compact disposition of the B-lines as a sign of interstitial involvement (**c**, arrowhead) suggestive of phlogistic parenchymal complication. (**d**) The CXR confirmed the LUS findings showing some ovular opacity with a confluence trend occupying the left superior, middle, and inferior pulmonary fields (**d**, arrows).

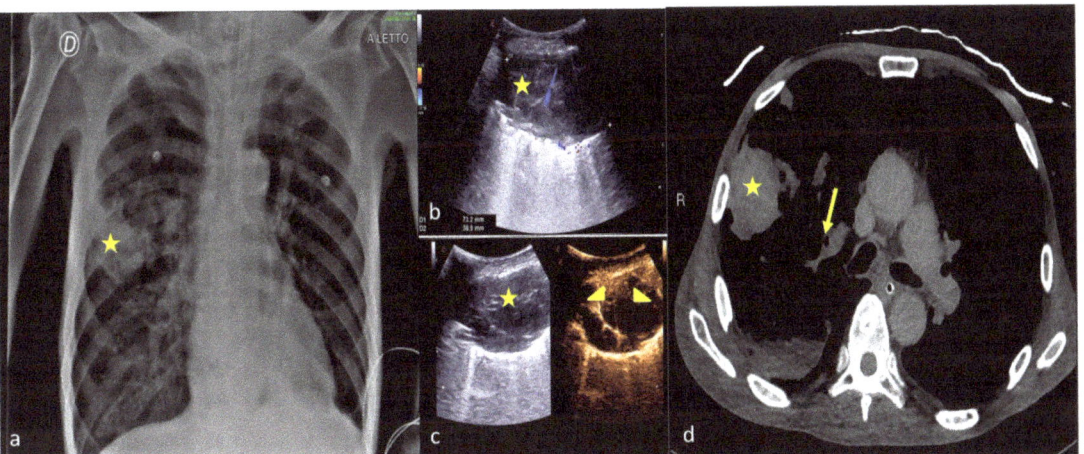

Figure 5. A 70-year-old male patient admitted to the ICU with acute respiratory failure from chronic obstructive pulmonary disease. Bedside CXR (**a**) LUS (**b**), CEUS (**c**), and CT scan (**d**). (**a**) The bedside CXR showed an area of pseudo-nodular consolidation (star) in the medium right pulmonary field. (**b**) LUS confirmed the parenchymal consolidation (star) that appears as a large heterogeneous hypoechoic area in the subpleural lung parenchyma. (**c**) CEUS examination with the administration of a sonographic contrast agent (Sonovue®, Bracco, Milan IT) showed no significative contrast enhancement in the pulmonary consolidation area (**c**, star) during the different phases of the study (**c**, arrowhead) concerning bronchial consolidation with the segmentary obstructive atelectatic area. (**d**) The CT scan highlighted areas of segmental parenchymal consolidation (**d**, star) caused by mucoid obstruction (**d**, arrow).

2.1. Atelectasis

The term atelectasis refers to the collapse of groups of alveoli resulting in a concurrent decrease in intrapulmonary airflow sustained by a dysfunction of the diaphragm, causing respiratory impairment, as in post-operative adhesions [37]. The main physiologic causes of atelectasis are compression of lung tissue, absorption of alveolar air, and impairment of surfactant function [37–39].

Compression atelectasis occurs when the transmural pressure is reduced to a level that allows the alveolus to collapse. The supine position, positive-pressure ventilation, and muscle paralysis, when applied in ICUs, cause a cephalad shift of the diaphragm, which normally permits differential pressures in the abdomen and chest, resulting in a concurrent decrease in intrapulmonary airflow. In an anesthetized patient a cephalad diaphragm displacement, differential regional diaphragmatic changes, a shift of thoracic central vascular blood into the abdomen, and an increase in regional pleural pressure result in negative transpulmonary pressure and compressive atelectasis [37–39].

Resorption atelectasis or gas atelectasis stems from the resorption of gas from alveoli when communication between the alveoli and the trachea is obstructed. The obstruction leads to a non-ventilation of the distal airways; the gas residing in that region is completely absorbed by pulmonary blood flowing through that area. Aspirated foreign bodies, food and gastric contents, malpositioned endotracheal tubes, and mucous plugs favor the appearance of resorption atelectasis in ICUs [37–39]. Resorption atelectasis can also be seen in acute bronchitis and pneumonia from the obstruction of small bronchi and bronchioles by inflammatory exudate and tumors (bronchogenic carcinoma, bronchial carcinoid, metastastates, lymphoma) [37–39].

A number of conditions impair muco-ciliary clearance: thoracic and abdominal pain, thoracic and abdominal surgery or trauma, central venous system depression, respiratory depressant medication, anticholinergic medication, general anesthesia, endotracheal intubation, ventilation with dry gases, inspiring oxygen in higher concentrations. Impairment of muco-ciliary transport causes the pooling of retained secretions in the smaller airways, and it favors the appearance of atelectasis. In the post-operative patient and in patients recovering in the ICU many factors are combined [40].

Development of atelectasis is associated with the development of several pathophysiologic effects, including decreased compliance, impairment of oxygenation, increased pulmonary vascular resistance, and development of lung injury. Atelectasis produces alveolar hypoxia and pulmonary vasoconstriction to prevent ventilation–perfusion mismatching and to minimize arterial hypoxia [37–40]. Atelectasis itself is often asymptomatic unless hypoxemia or pneumonia develops. Symptoms of hypoxemia tend to be related to acuity and extent of atelectasis. Dyspnea or even respiratory failure can develop with rapid, extensive atelectasis [37–40].

The main CXR sign is a lobar or sub-lobar parenchymal thickening often evident at the lower lobes with partial or total disappearance of the profile of the hemidiaphragms or cardiac silhouette and also with the mediastinum that is shifted toward the collapsed lung area [41,42].

On LUS, the common finding is the sign of tissue, the so-called pulmonary "hepatization", suggesting collapsed parenchyma with air bronchograms frequently static or unaffected by respiratory dynamics as they are trapped in the area of consolidation; the bronchi are often in a parallel arrangement, unlike the typical tree-like arrangement of the pneumonia consolidation, in line with a reduction in lung volume [5,21,29,30,38,43]. Furthermore, in the collapsed parenchymal area the "lung sliding" is usually absent while the "lung pulse" appears more represented, which is a sign of the perception of the impact of cardiac activity on the collapsed lung [44].

Figure 6 is an example of CXR and LUS diagnostic integration in detecting atelectasis.

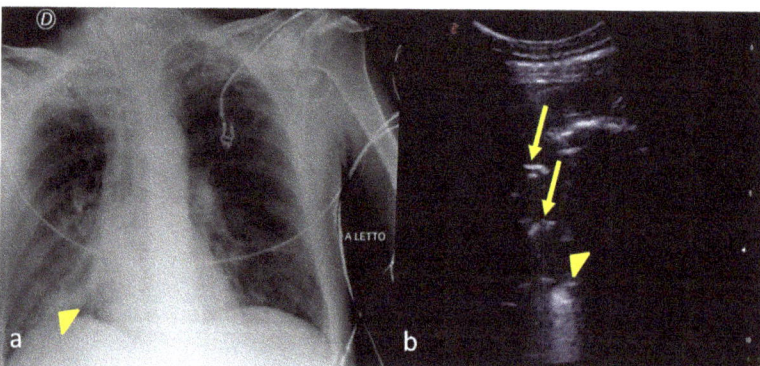

Figure 6. A 48-year-old male patient admitted to the ICU for post-traumatic subarachnoid hemorrhage and acute respiratory failure. Bedside CXR (**a**) and LUS (**b**). (**a**) The CXR showed an inhomogeneous opacity in the right inferior pulmonary field (arrowhead). (**b**) LUS confirmed a parenchymal consolidation area at the basis of the right lung (**b**, arrowhead) showing some hyperechogenic spots as signs of a static bronchogram (**b**, arrows) related to the diagnostic hypothesis of an atelectatic area.

2.2. Pneumonia

Pneumonia ranks among the more common nosocomial infections [45–47]. The mechanisms of contamination may depend on the aspiration of active flora in the oropharynx, inhalation of aerosols containing pathogenic microorganisms, or more rarely, hematogenous spread to the lungs [45–47].

In ICUs, hospital-acquired pneumonia (HAP) and ventilator-associated pneumonia (VAP) occur more frequently. HAP is a new pneumonia (a lower respiratory tract infection verified by the presence of a new pulmonary infiltrate on imaging) that develops more than

48 h after admission in non-intubated patients. VAP, the most common and fatal nosocomial infection in critical care, is a new pneumonia that develops after 48 h of endotracheal intubation. Importantly, by the time of VAP onset, patients may have already been extubated [45–47]. Aspiration is an important contributor to the pathogenesis of HAP and VAP. Further, proton-pump inhibitors and histamine-2 receptor blockers, by suppressing acid production, can allow nosocomial pathogens to colonize the oropharynx and endotracheal tube and be aspirated [45–47]. Owing to their low sensitivity and specificity, history and physical examination are considered suboptimal to confirm or exclude the diagnosis.

Guidelines recommend that a new pulmonary infiltrate at the CXR should be present to classify a hospitalized patient as having the diagnosis of pneumonia. Oxygen saturation (SpO_2) and arterial gas analysis can provide important information about severity. In an attempt to determine whether a typical pathogen is the etiology of pneumonia, all patients should have a sputum specimen for Gram stain and culture as well as two sets of blood cultures obtained before the institution of antimicrobial therapy. Fluid samples from the pleural space and bronchoscopy represent invasive tests that are also useful in pneumonia diagnosis [45–47].

The CXR shows the presence and extent of the condition, any concurrent cavities, and the appearance of parapneumonic effusions or abscesses [41,42].

On LUS examination, areas of subpleural consolidation with a hypoechogenic echostructure, irregular margins, and of various shapes and sizes with a tendency to confluence can be found, often associated with the detection of dynamic air bronchograms or hyperechogenic punctiform foci representing air in the bronchi that moves in line with the respiratory excursion. Furthermore, if a significant peripheral abscess cavitation develops, it appears on the LUS as a colliquated central lacuna with debris and gas or with a pseudo-solid appearance related to suppuration development [5,21,29,30,43].

Figure 4, Figure 7, and Figure 8 show some examples of CXR and LUS diagnostic integration in detecting pneumonia.

2.3. Pleural Effusion

A pleural effusion is defined as an excess of pleural fluid within the pleural space. It represents a disturbance of equilibrium between production and resorption. Normally, a small amount of pleural liquid (5–10 mL, 0.1 mL/kg per hemithorax in healthy adults) exists within the pleural space [48]. The volume of the pleural fluid is determined by the balance of the hydrostatic and oncotic pressure differences that are present between the systemic and pulmonary circulation and the pleural space. Both the visceral and the parietal pleura play an important role in fluid homeostasis in the pleural space; especially, the parietal side of the pleura accounts for most of the production of pleural fluid and for most of its resorption [48–50]. Excess fluid accumulation in the pleural space can be caused by both benign and life-threatening conditions. A transudate occurs when systemic factors influencing the formation and absorption of pleural fluid (hydrostatic and oncotic pressures) are altered so that fluid accumulates. The reason to make this differentiation is that the existence of a transudative pleural effusion indicates that systemic factors such as heart failure or cirrhosis are responsible for the effusion, with the existence of examples such as congestive heart failure, cirrhosis, nephrotic syndrome, urinothorax, hypoalbuminemia, and cerebrospinal fluid leak [48–50].

An exudative effusion indicates that local factors are responsible for the effusion. Malignant disease (carcinoma of any origin, but especially lung and breast; lymphoma; mesothelioma); infections (parapneumonic effusion; tuberculous pleurisy; fungal, parasitic or viral infections); autoimmune inflammatory diseases (systemic lupus erythematosus and other connective tissue diseases; rheumatoid arthritis); pulmonary embolism; intra-abdominal processes (pancreatitis; subphrenic/hepatic abscess); drugs (amiodarone, methotrexate, nitrofurantoin and others); traumatic hemothorax; cardiac bypass surgery; post-cardiac injury syndrome; and post-radiation therapy could cause exudative effusion [48–50].

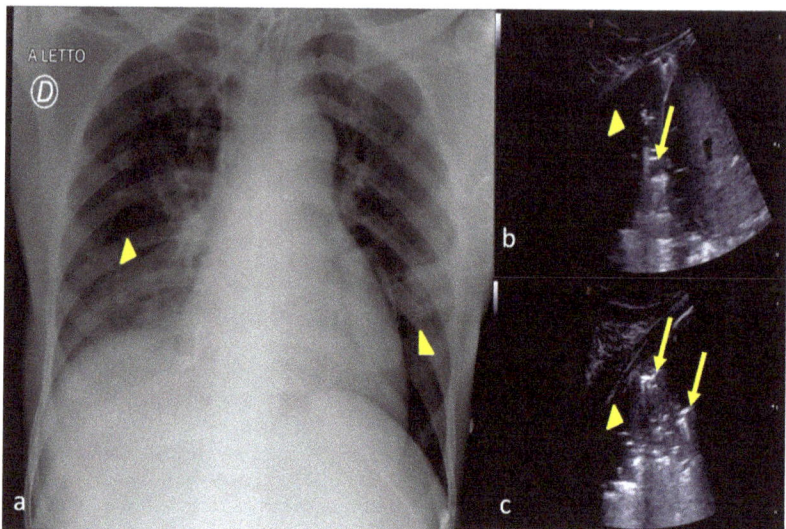

Figure 7. A 36-year-old female patient admitted to the ICU for a comatose state related to cerebral hemorrhage with fever and dyspnea after endotracheal intubation. Bedside CXR (**a**) and LUS (**b**,**c**). (**a**) The CXR showed faint areas of decreased parenchymal transparency in the right and left inferior pulmonary field (**a**, arrowheads); (**b**). LUS confirmed the consolidative areas at the lung basis (**b**,**c**, arrowheads) with hyperechogenic spots as signs of an air bronchogram (**b**,**c**, arrows) that moved in line with the respiratory excursion. The clinical scenario and imaging findings were suggestive of phlogistic bronchopneumonia.

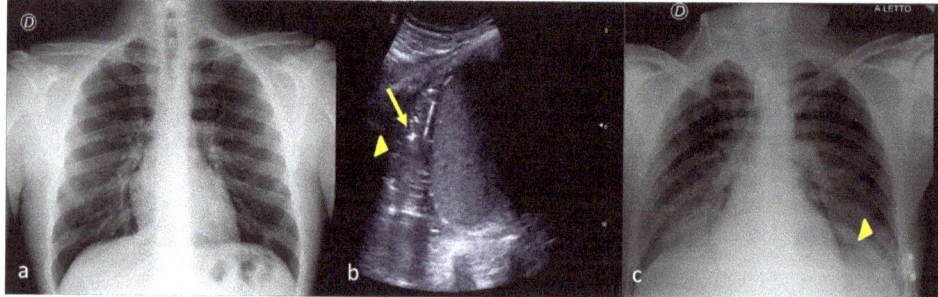

Figure 8. A 26-year-old male patient admitted to the ICU for a comatose state related to high-energy trauma due to a car accident. Bedside CXR (**a**,**c**) and LUS (**b**). (**a**) The CXR on the day of admission into the ICU showed normal lung expansion with no evidence of parenchymal change. (**b**) LSU was performed after 24 h endotracheal intubation with the onset of a respiratory worsening and showed an inhomogeneous area of mixed hypoechogenic change at the basis of the left lung (**b**, arrowhead) with some hyperechogenic spots suggestive of consolidation with an air bronchogram (**b**, arrow). (**c**) The CXR confirmed the LUS findings showing an area of reduced diaphony in the basal left field that was considered the manifestation of parenchymal consolidation (**c**, arrowhead). The clinical scenario and imaging findings were suggestive of phlogistic bronchopneumonia.

Clinical assessment to determine the appropriate investigation and management is essential. Although symptoms specific to the underlying cause may be present, pleural effusions usually present with nonspecific symptoms such as dyspnea, cough, and pleuritic pain. Such symptoms, if present, reflect an inflammatory response of the pleura, a restriction of pulmonary mechanics, or a disturbance of gas exchange; the severity of these symptoms depends on effusion size and the patient's cardiopulmonary reserve [48–50]. The most common symptom of pleural effusion is dyspnea. The severity of dyspnea is only loosely correlated with the size of the effusion, and it could require patient endotracheal intubation and hospitalization in the ICU.

Detection of a pleural effusion by examination is determined by its size. A pleural effusion of less than 300 mL is likely to be clinically undetectable, whereas a large effusion (>1500 mL) may cause significant hemithorax asymmetry. Chest examination typically reveals dullness to percussion, the absence of fremitus, and diminished breath sounds or their absence. Distended neck veins, an S3 gallop, or peripheral edema suggests congestive heart failure, and a right ventricular heave or thrombophlebitis suggests pulmonary embolus [48–50].

Moderate effusion often goes undetected by CXR, especially by supine CXR, which can document abnormalities when the amount of pleural effusion reaches 175–525 mL; therefore, only when the amount of fluid increases, the hemithorax becomes hazy, the pulmonary vessels become less recognizable, and the profile of the hemidiaphragm fades and becomes unrecognizable [28,41,42].

According to this evidence, the LUS plays an important role in the identification and quantification of small pleural effusions not detectable by CXR. Simple transudate fluid collections are evident on LUS as anechogenic spaces between the pleural layers; debris that moves on respiratory movement may also be present. A more compact septated collection with a tendency to sacculate may indicate a pleural empyema [5,26,29,30].

LUS may also be a guiding imaging tool both for diagnostic pleural drainage, rather than for therapeutic pleural drainage or thoracentesis, and for follow-up procedures such as iatrogenic pneumothorax occurrences [26,50].

Figures 9 and 10 show examples of CXR and LUS diagnostic integration in detecting pleural effusion.

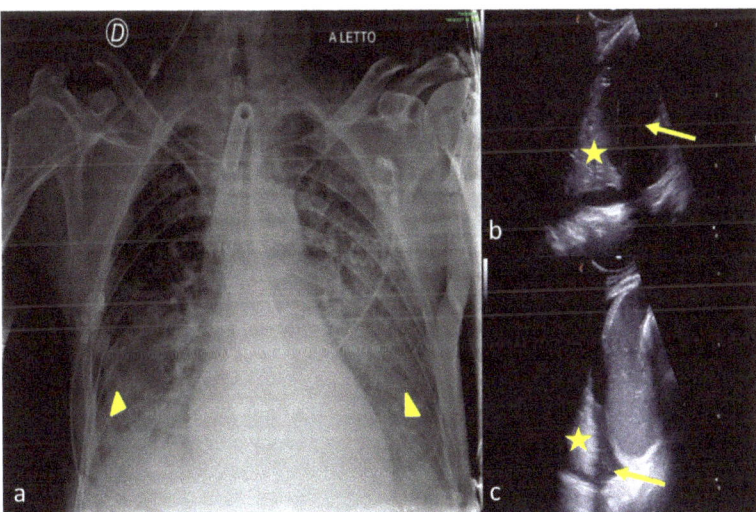

Figure 9. A 67-year-old male patient referred to the ICU after major trauma by a fall from a height. Bedside CXR (**a**) and LUS (**b**,**c**). (**a**) The CXR showed bilateral pulmonary opacities associated with pleural effusion (**a**, arrowheads). (**b**,**c**) Bilateral minimal pleural fluid was also confirmed by LUS (**b**,**c**, arrows) both on the right (**b**) and on the left (**c**) sides; lung consolidation was also visible (**b**,**c**, asterisks).

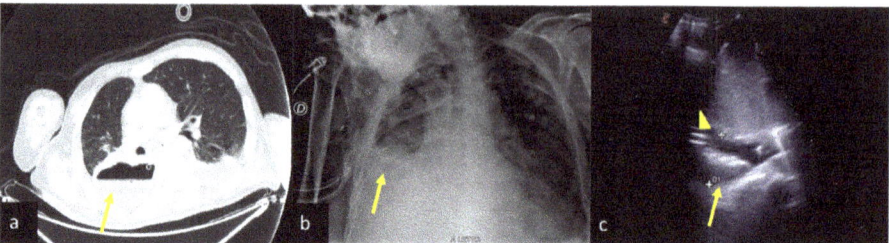

Figure 10. A 54-year-old male patient in respiratory failure. CT scan (**a**), CXR (**b**), and LUS (**c**). (**a**) The axial CT scan of the chest showed a parenchymal consolidation area with the air–fluid level in the basal segments of the right inferior pulmonary lobe suggestive of a pleural empyema (**a**, arrow). (**b**) The subsequent CXR control revealed a basal right-side decreased parenchymal transparency consistent with a persistent amount of the empyematous effusion (**b**, arrow). (**c**) LUS follow-up showed a better quantification of the residual fluid amount, with an inhomogeneous content of echogenic substance in suspension (**c**, arrow) and also confirmed the correct position of the surgical drainage tube (**c**, arrowhead).

2.4. Cardiogenic Pulmonary Edema

Pulmonary edema is defined as increased fluid in the interstitial and/or alveolar spaces of the lung parenchyma. Acute cardiogenic and/or volume overload edema usually have increased pulmonary venous pressure because of elevations in left atrial and left ventricle end-diastolic pressure [51,52].

The most frequent cause of congestive heart failure is myocardial infarction, although heart failure has many causes, including hypertension, myocarditis, acute onset cardiomyopathy, left ventricle dysfunction or failure, papillary muscle dysfunction, ventricular septal rupture, acute severe aortic insufficiency, acute severe mitral regurgitation, arrhythmias, myocardial contusion/post-cardiac arrest stunning, cardiac tamponade, toxic and metabolic, beta block or calcium channel antagonist overdose, and pheochromocytoma [51,52].

Clinical presentation is characterized by shortness of breath at rest and worsens with exertion, tachypnea, tachycardia, and relative hypoxemia. The lung exam reveals crackles or gasps. Jugular venous pressure may be normal or increased. The S3 gallop on the electrocardiographic exam is relatively specific for cardiogenic edema. A focused exam for cardiac murmurs consistent with valvular stenosis, regurgitation, or signs of right heart failure is of high importance [51,52].

On the CXR, when the edema is still confined to the interstitium, it occurs as a thickening of the associated spaces, especially in the declivities of the lungs where the hydrostatic pressure is higher, so that a thickening of the interlobular septa or so-called Kerley lines, thickening of the walls of the bronchi, shading of the vessel profile, and thickening of the subpleural interstitium can be detected [41,42]. As the edema worsens, vascular and bilateral cotton wool opacities with no aero-bronchogram appear [41,42]. Usually, the heart is enlarged and pleural effusion coexists [41,42].

Multiple B-lines tending to confluence (so-called white lung) are evident on LUS depending on the severity of the condition and are associated with pleural effusion, inferior vena cava ectasia, and heart failure [5,14,15,29,30].

Figure 11 shows an example of CXR and LUS diagnostic integration in detecting cardiogenic pulmonary edema.

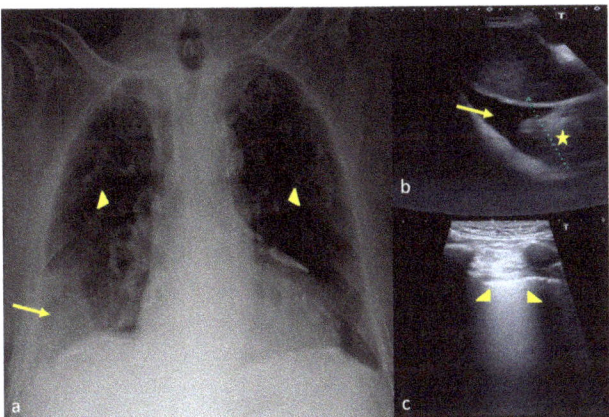

Figure 11. A 79-year-old male patient suspected of having pulmonary edema. CXR (**a**) and LUS (**b**,**c**). (**a**) On the CXR opacity of the middle and inferior field was detected bilaterally (**a**, arrowheads) with right lung basis consolidation (**a**, arrow). (**b**,**c**) LUS integration showed on the right lung basis (**b**) a pleural anechoic effusion (**b**, arrow) associated with a consolidative area (**b**, star); the evaluation of the right and left lungs (**c**) showed a compact appearance of the B-lines on the explorable lung areas in the intercostal space (**c**, arrowheads). In this case LUS allowed us to better clarify the nature of the CXR lung opacities.

2.5. Acute Respiratory Distress Syndrome

ARDS is a syndrome of acute respiratory failure caused by non-cardiogenic pulmonary edema representing the most severe stage of acute lung damage due to alveolar–capillary endothelial damage with leakage of fluid from the intravascular to the extravascular compartment [53]. ARDS accounts for 10% of ICU admissions, representing more than 3 million patients with ARDS annually [53,54]. ARDS progresses through several phases (exudative, proliferative, and fibrotic) after a direct pulmonary or indirect extrapulmonary insult, and it is classified as low, moderate, and severe according to Berlin criteria [53,54].

ARDS initially manifests as dyspnea, tachypnea, and hypoxemia, then quickly evolves into respiratory failure. Identification of a specific cause for ARDS remains a crucial therapeutic goal to improve outcomes associated with ARDS. There is still no effective pharmacotherapy for this syndrome, and the treatment remains primarily supportive and includes mechanical ventilation, fluid management strategy, prophylaxis for stress ulcers and venous thromboembolism, nutritional support, and treatment of the underlying injury [53,54].

The CXR shows the presence of more or less homogeneously distributed patches at an already advanced stage in both lungs with less gravitational tendency and less confluence as well as evidence of an internal air bronchogram [41,42]. It may regress, evolve into fibrosis, or in adverse cases show a mosaic evolution with temporal changes in opacities [41,42].

On a LUS, multiple B-lines with irregular distribution alternate with areas of hypoechogenic subpleural consolidation with concurrent air bronchograms [29,30]. The pleural line is also frequently irregular [29–31]. Furthermore, the possibility of highlighting healthy lung areas allows for orientation in the differential diagnosis of hydrostatic pulmonary edema [29–31].

Figure 12 shows an example of CXR and LUS diagnostic integration in detecting and monitoring ARDS.

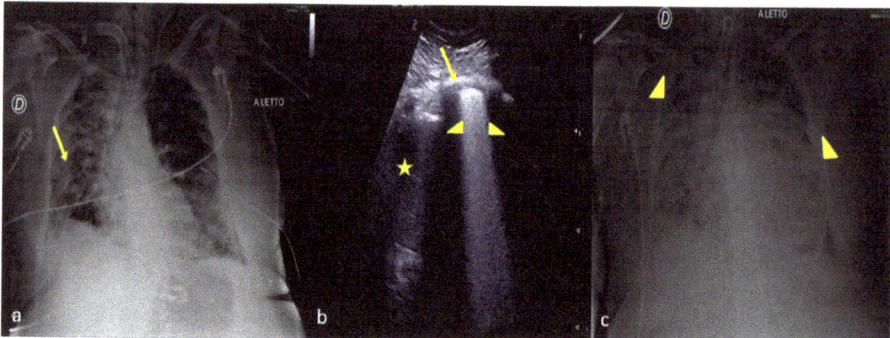

Figure 12. A 57-year-old female patient with acute respiratory failure during interstitial pneumonia not related to SARS-CoV2 infection. Bedside CXR (**a**,**c**) and LUS (**b**). (**a**) The CXR revealed on the right side multiple small opacities with signs of interstitial thickening suggestive of an interstitial and alveolar infective process (**a**, arrow). (**b**) The LUS examination performed after 5 days showed in the middle right pulmonary field and on the left side a compact appearance of B-lines (**b**, arrowheads) associated with some areas of parenchymal consolidation (**b**, star) with an irregular pleural line (**b**, arrow) that was suggestive of ARDS complication, according to the clinical worsening refractory to therapies. (**c**) The CXR confirmed massive involvement of the interstitial compartment and bilateral consolidation of the parenchyma with an internal air bronchogram suggestive of ARDS according to the clinical scenario (**c**, arrowheads).

2.6. Pulmonary Contusion

A pulmonary contusion is an entity defined as an alveolar hemorrhage caused by an injury to the alveolar capillaries and pulmonary parenchymal destruction after blunt chest trauma. It is a common finding after mechanisms of injury that impart substantial kinetic energy to the thorax, and often the rate of pulmonary contusion is linearly associated with the severity of injury to the bony thorax. Lung tissue injury occurs when the chest wall bends inward following the trauma [22,55]. The possible mechanisms are based on inertial effects, mainly on different tissue densities, light alveolar tissue, and heavy hilar structures. Rib fractures and their degree of displacement, as well as flail chest and penetrating mechanisms, contribute to the severity of the underlying lung injury [22,55].

Parenchymal lung injury leads to pathophysiologic changes, the severity of which depends on the extent of injury. The number of affected lobes has been reported to determine the outcome. The physiologic consequences of alveolar hemorrhage and pulmonary parenchymal destruction typically manifest themselves within 24–48 h of injury and usually resolve within approximately 7–14 days, but delayed deterioration may occur [22,55].

Clinical manifestations include increased work at breathing, respiratory distress with hypoxemia and hypercarbia. Patients may present with a rapid respiratory rate, rhonchi or wheezes, or even hemoptysis. Bleeding into uninvolved lung segments may cause bronchospasm and may compromise alveolar function [22,55].

On the CXR, pulmonary contusions appear as diffuse or patchy parenchymal opacities. However, CXRs have a low sensitivity in detecting foci of contusion, in view of the possible coexistence of hemothorax or pneumothorax [41,42].

In view of the fact that the areas of contusion are predominantly subpleural in extension and at the site of impact, LUS may document and monitor obvious foci of contusion as hypoechogenic areas with poorly defined margins often coexisting with multiple confluent B-lines [22,29,30].

Figure 13 shows an example of CXR and LUS diagnostic integration in detecting pulmonary contusion.

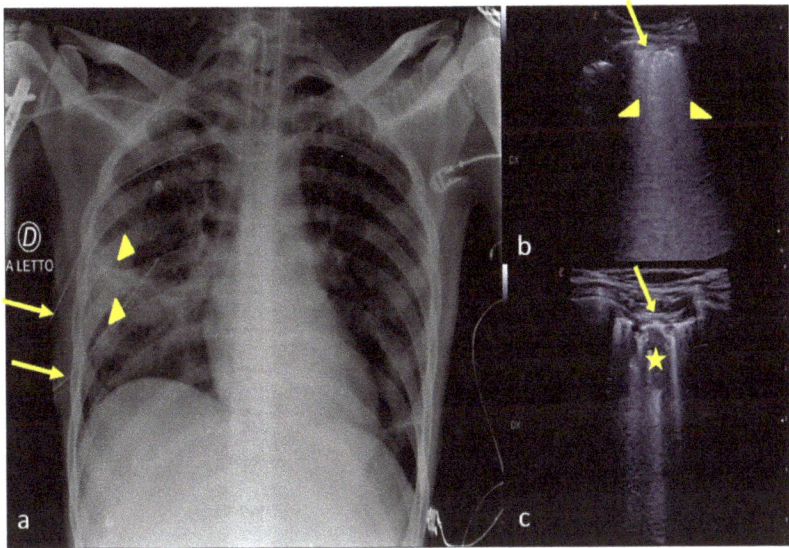

Figure 13. A 33-year-old male patient referred to the ICU after major trauma by defenestration. Bedside CXR (**a**) and LUS (**b**,**c**). (**a**) The CXR revealed on the right side the presence of two thoracic tube drainages (**a**, arrows) after pneumothorax (not shown) with middle and lower right lung zones indicating several confluent opacities (**a**, arrowheads). (**b**,**c**) LUS revealed on the same side the presence of a thick pleural line (**b**,**c**, arrow) with multiple B-line artifacts (**b**, arrowheads) and hypoechoic alveolar consolidation (**c**, star) corresponding to lung contusion.

3. Confirming or Excluding Pneumothorax and Monitoring its Evolution

Pneumothorax is defined as the presence of air in the pleural space. It indicates the loss of visceral or parietal pleural membrane integrity, thereby allowing air from the environment or respiratory tract to accumulate in the pleural space. Although intrapleural pressures are negative throughout most of the respiratory cycle, air does not enter into the pleural space [27,56]. Iatrogenic pneumothorax is one of the main iatrogenic complications in ICU patients, and its occurrence increases the duration of ICU and hospital stays.

Iatrogenic pneumothorax occurs chiefly as a complication of barotrauma related to mechanical ventilation or as a post-procedural event (transthoracic needle biopsy, subclavian vein catheterization, thoracentesis, transbronchial, lung biopsy, pleural biopsy) [27,56]. The development of lung-protective strategies for ventilation and of new material, techniques, and recommendations for inserting central vein catheters (CVCs) makes iatrogenic pneumothorax largely preventable in routine practice. Nevertheless, its occurrence is closely related to the underlying disease, such as in patients with adult ARDS [27,56]. Other causes of pneumothorax such as spontaneous or traumatic-acquired may represent an additional portion of patients admitted to the ICU who need diagnosis and monitoring [27,56].

Symptoms of a pneumothorax can include chest pain, shortness of breath, cough, and increases in heart rate or breathing.

Different treatments are used depending on the size of the air volume in the pleural space and the amount of pressure it puts on the lung [27,56]. Small and asymptomatic iatrogenic pneumothoraxes often do not need any treatment and resolve spontaneously. Parenchymal lung damage can effectively heal, and the intrapleural air will be resorbed over time. In larger or symptomatic pneumothoraxes, simple manual aspiration or placement of a small catheter or chest tube attached to a Heimlich valve usually is successful. Tension pneumothorax presents as a life-threatening emergency that requires prompt recognition and treatment. When tension pneumothorax develops, urgent thoracic decompression is recommended [27,56]. For this reason, it is understandable how an early diagnosis can lead to the best therapeutic direction.

On the CXR, radiolucent air and the absence of juxtaposed lung markings between a compressed lobe or lung and the parietal pleura are indicative of pneumothorax. Tracheal deviation and mediastinal shift occur in a large tensive pneumothorax [41,42]. However, for the aforementioned diagnostic CXR limitations that are also due to the supine patient's position, the risk of incurring an occult small pneumothorax is not negligible where the failure to recognize it is important, especially if the patient must undergo ventilation [27,56]. In such contexts, LUS offers an important contribution to the diagnosis and in the same way to monitoring.

On LUS, the most specific finding is the lung point, i.e., the boundary between the airy lung and pneumothorax visible as a change in physiological pleural sliding; the presence of air will also generate overlapping A-lines and the complete absence of B-lines [27,29,30].

Figure 14 shows an example of CXR and LUS diagnostic integration in detecting pneumothorax.

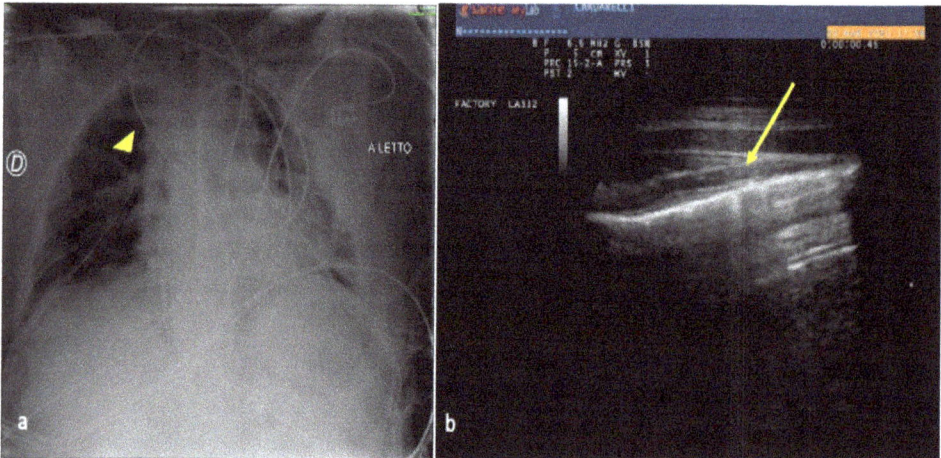

Figure 14. A 50-year-old male patient referred to the ICU after major trauma. Bedside CXR (**a**) and LUS (**b**). (**a**) The CXR showed the surgical drainage tube (arrowhead), with poor confidence on the entity of the residual pneumothorax. (**b**) LUS showed the presence of "lungs points" (arrow) confirming the residual pneumothorax that was not clearly demonstrable on the CXR.

4. Checking and Monitoring the Devices

Medical devices, including ventilators, infusion pumps, breathing and feeding support, and others, improve patient care and outcomes in the ICU. Despite the staff's ability to manage them, using them properly and checking their correct position reduces the development of adverse events associated with them [57]. The correct positioning of the various life-sustaining devices in the ICU represents a further diagnostic challenge in the correct reading of the CXR (Figure 15) [41].

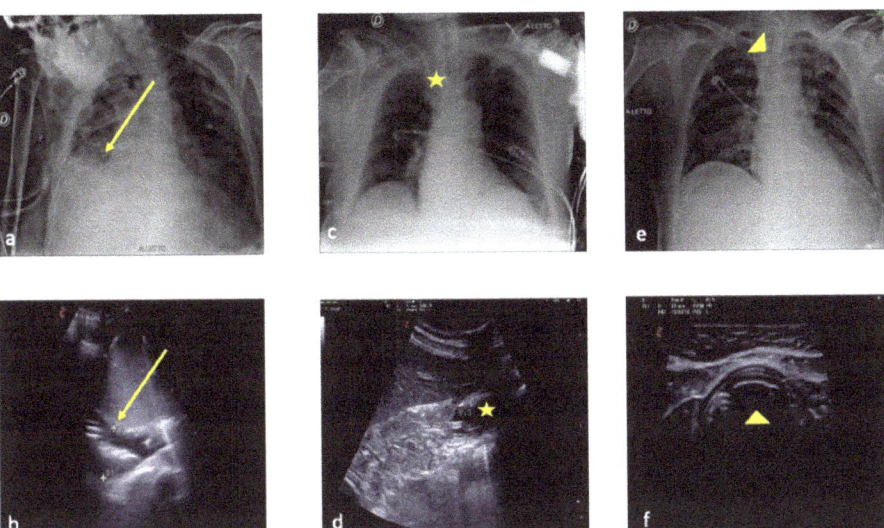

Figure 15. Comparison between plain chest radiography and LUS in three different critical patients in the intensive care unit. (**a,b**) CXR and LUS surgical drainage tube evaluation (the same patient as in Figure 10) (**a,b**, arrow). (**c,d**) CXR and LUS nasogastric tube evaluation (**c,d**, star). (**e,f**) CXR and LUS endotracheal tube evaluation (**e,f**, arrowhead).

In addition to the well-known operative use of LUS in positioning CVCs and tracheostomy procedures, LUS is an integrative diagnostic tool with CXR for monitoring thrombosis or pneumothorax complications related to CVCs and nasogastric tube displacements (Figure 16) [58–60].

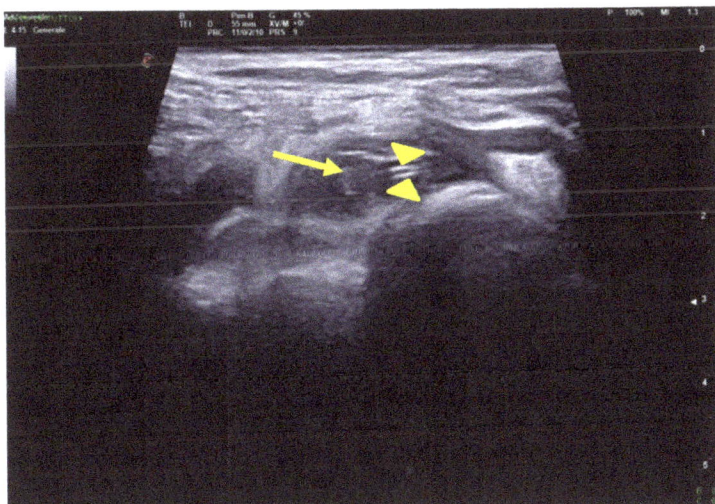

Figure 16. CVC thrombosis. Right supraclavicular ultrasound exploration highlights the presence of an isocogenic, non-compressible area attributable to thrombosis in the lumen of the subclavian vein (arrow); it also allows visualization of the course of the catheter, visible as a hyperechoic tubular structure (arrowheads).

5. Conclusions

LUS is a well-established diagnostic tool inextricably linked to the clinical environment and frequently used in ICUs. Despite their reduced diagnostic sensitivity in the anteroposterior supine projection, CXRs nevertheless remain an indispensable 'open window' to the chest that also provide information on parenchymal changes far from the pleura as well as on the cardio-mediastinum.

From a purely radiological point of view, in addition to a well-codified organization, the use of point-of-care LUS as an advanced method in ICU CXR reports can be an essential tool for diagnosing and monitoring areas of decreased transparency around the chest found on CXRs, such as atelectasis, pneumonia, pleural effusion, pulmonary edema, ARDS, and pulmonary contusions, as well as in diagnosing and monitoring pneumothorax and also when checking the positioning of the devices or the complications associated with them.

Author Contributions: Conceptualization, M.D.S., G.D.O. and M.C.; methodology, M.D.S., G.D.O., M.C. and D.V.; validation, L.R.; resources, M.D.S., G.D.O., M.C., D.V. and F.I.; data curation, M.D.S., G.D.O., M.C., C.C., R.R., V.S., L.B. and G.O.; writing—original draft preparation, M.D.S., G.D.O., M.C. and D.V.; writing—review and editing, M.D.S., G.D.O., M.C., C.C. and F.I.; supervision, L.R. All authors have read and agreed to the published version of the manuscript.

Funding: This research received no external funding.

Institutional Review Board Statement: Ethical review and approval were waived due to the nature of the manuscript.

Informed Consent Statement: Patient consent was waived due to the nature of the manuscript.

Data Availability Statement: Not applicable.

Acknowledgments: In this section, you can acknowledge any support given which is not covered by the author contribution or funding sections. This may include administrative and technical support, or donations in kind (e.g., materials used for experiments). Thanks to Nazareno Capasso for data collection.

Conflicts of Interest: The authors declare no conflict of interest.

References

1. Expert Panel on Thoracic Imaging; Laroia, A.T.; Donnelly, E.F.; Henry, T.S.; Berry, M.F.; Boiselle, P.M.; Colletti, P.M.; Kuzniewski, C.T.; Maldonado, F.; Olsen, K.M.; et al. ACR Appropriateness Criteria® Intensive Care Unit Patients. *J. Am. Coll. Radiol.* **2021**, *18*, S62–S72. [CrossRef] [PubMed]
2. Swensen, S.J.; Peters, S.G.; LeROY, A.J.; Gay, P.C.; Sykes, M.W.; Trastek, V.F. Radiology in the Intensive-Care Unit. *Mayo Clin. Proc.* **1991**, *66*, 396–410. [CrossRef]
3. Fabre, C.; Proisy, M.; Chapuis, C.; Jouneau, S.; Lentz, P.-A.; Meunier, C.; Mahé, G.; Lederlin, M. Radiology residents' skill level in chest x-ray reading. *Diagn. Interv. Imaging* **2018**, *99*, 361–370. [CrossRef]
4. Trotman-Dickenson, B. Radiology in the Intensive Care Unit (Part I). *J. Intensiv. Care Med.* **2003**, *18*, 198–210. [CrossRef]
5. Di Serafino, M.; Notaro, M.; Rea, G.; Iacobellis, F.; Paoli, V.D.; Acampora, C.; Ianniello, S.; Brunese, L.; Romano, L.; Vallone, G. The lung ultrasound: Facts or artifacts? In the era of COVID-19 outbreak. *La Radiol. medica* **2020**, *125*, 738–753. [CrossRef] [PubMed]
6. Quarato, C.M.I.; Mirijello, A.; Lacedonia, D.; Russo, R.; Maggi, M.M.; Rea, G.; Simeone, A.; Borelli, C.; Feragalli, B.; Scioscia, G.; et al. Low Sensitivity of Admission Lung US Compared to Chest CT for Diagnosis of Lung Involvement in a Cohort of 82 Patients with COVID-19 Pneumonia. *Medicina* **2021**, *57*, 236. [CrossRef]
7. Trotman-Dickenson, B. Radiology in the Intensive Care Unit (Part 2). *J. Intensiv. Care Med.* **2003**, *18*, 239–252. [CrossRef]
8. Al Shahrani, A.; Al-Surimi, K. Daily routine versus on-demand chest radiograph policy and practice in adult ICU patients-clinicians' perspective. *BMC Med. Imaging* **2018**, *18*, 4. [CrossRef]
9. Keveson, B.; Clouser, R.D.; Hamlin, M.P.; Stevens, P.; Stinnett-Donnelly, J.M.; Allen, G.B. Adding value to daily chest X-rays in the ICU through education, restricted daily orders and indication-based prompting. *BMJ Open Qual.* **2017**, *6*, e000072. [CrossRef] [PubMed]
10. Ganapathy, A.; Adhikari, N.K.; Spiegelman, J.; Scales, D.C. Routine chest x-rays in intensive care units: A systematic review and meta-analysis. *Crit. Care* **2012**, *16*, R68. [CrossRef]
11. Deshpande, R.; Akhtar, S.; Haddadin, A.S. Utility of ultrasound in the ICU. *Curr. Opin. Anaesthesiol.* **2014**, *27*, 123–132. [CrossRef]

12. Gil-Rodríguez, J.; de Rojas, J.P.; Aranda-Laserna, P.; Benavente-Fernández, A.; Martos-Ruiz, M.; Peregrina-Rivas, J.-A.; Guirao-Arrabal, E. Ultrasound findings of lung ultrasonography in COVID-19: A systematic review. *Eur. J. Radiol.* **2022**, *148*, 110156. [CrossRef]
13. Smit, J.M.; Haaksma, M.E.; Winkler, M.H.; Heldeweg, M.L.A.; Arts, L.; Lust, E.J.; Elbers, P.W.G.; Meijboom, L.J.; Girbes, A.R.J.; Heunks, L.M.A.; et al. Lung ultrasound in a tertiary intensive care unit population: A diagnostic accuracy study. *Crit. Care* **2021**, *25*, 339. [CrossRef]
14. Lichtenstein, D.A. BLUE-Protocol and FALLS-Protocol: Two applications of lung ultrasound in the critically ill. *Chest* **2015**, *147*, 1659–1670. [CrossRef] [PubMed]
15. Bekgoz, B.; Kilicaslan, I.; Bildik, F.; Keles, A.; Demircan, A.; Hakoglu, O.; Coskun, G.; Demir, H.A. BLUE protocol ultrasonography in Emergency Department patients presenting with acute dyspnea. *Am. J. Emerg. Med.* **2019**, *37*, 2020–2027. [CrossRef]
16. Rea, G.; Sperandeo, M.; Di Serafino, M.; Vallone, G.; Tomà, P. Neonatal and pediatric thoracic ultrasonography. *J. Ultrasound* **2019**, *22*, 121–130. [CrossRef] [PubMed]
17. Sperandeo, M.; Rea, G.; Filabozzi, P.; Carnevale, V. Lung Ultrasound and Chest X-Rays: Together to Improve the Diagnosis. *Respiration* **2017**, *93*, 226–227. [CrossRef]
18. Di Serafino, M.; Vallone, G. The role of point of care ultrasound in radiology department: Update and prospective. A statement of Italian college ultrasound. *La Radiol. Medica* **2020**, *126*, 636–641. [CrossRef] [PubMed]
19. Das Villgran, V.; Lyons, C.; Nasrullah, A.; Abalos, C.C.; Bihler, E.D.; Alhajhusain, A. Acute Respiratory Failure. *Crit. Care Nurs. Q.* **2022**, *45*, 233–247. [CrossRef]
20. Lichtenstein, D. Lung ultrasound in the critically ill. *Curr. Opin. Crit. Care* **2014**, *20*, 315–322. [CrossRef] [PubMed]
21. Haaksma, M.E.; Smit, J.M.; Heldeweg, M.L.A.; Nooitgedacht, J.S.B.; de Grooth, H.J.; Jonkman, A.H.M.; Girbes, A.R.J.; Heunks, L.; Tuinman, P.R. Extended Lung Ultrasound to Differentiate Between Pneumonia and Atelectasis in Critically Ill Patients: A Diagnostic Accuracy Study. *Crit. Care Med.* **2021**, *50*, 750–759. [CrossRef] [PubMed]
22. Dicker, S.A. Lung Ultrasound for Pulmonary Contusions. *Vet. Clin. North Am. Small Anim. Pract.* **2021**, *51*, 1141–1151. [CrossRef] [PubMed]
23. Assaad, S.; Kratzert, W.B.; Shelley, B.; Friedman, M.B.; Perrino, A. Assessment of Pulmonary Edema: Principles and Practice. *J. Cardiothorac. Vasc. Anesthesia* **2018**, *32*, 901–914. [CrossRef] [PubMed]
24. Wang, Y.; Shen, Z.; Lu, X.; Zhen, Y.; Li, H. Sensitivity and specificity of ultrasound for the diagnosis of acute pulmonary edema: A systematic review and meta-analysis. *Med. Ultrason.* **2018**, *1*, 32–36. [CrossRef]
25. Shao, R.-J.; Du, M.-J.; Xie, J.-T. Use of lung ultrasound for the diagnosis and treatment of pleural effusion. *Eur. Rev. Med. Pharmacol. Sci.* **2022**, *26*, 8771–8776. [CrossRef]
26. Brogi, E.; Gargani, L.; Bignami, E.; Barbariol, F.; Marra, A.; Forfori, F.; Vetrugno, L. Thoracic ultrasound for pleural effusion in the intensive care unit: A narrative review from diagnosis to treatment. *Crit. Care* **2017**, *21*, 325. [CrossRef]
27. Thachuthara-George, J. Pneumothorax in patients with respiratory failure in ICU. *J. Thorac. Dis.* **2021**, *13*, 5195–5204. [CrossRef]
28. Kitazono, M.T.; Lau, C.T.; Parada, A.N.; Renjen, P.; Miller, W.T. Differentiation of Pleural Effusions From Parenchymal Opacities: Accuracy of Bedside Chest Radiography. *Am. J. Roentgenol.* **2010**, *194*, 407–412. [CrossRef]
29. Wongwaisayawan, S.; Suwannanon, R.; Sawatmongkorngul, S.; Kaewlai, R. Emergency Thoracic US: The Essentials. *Radiographics* **2016**, *36*, 640–659. [CrossRef]
30. Breitkopf, R.; Treml, B.; Rajsic, S. Lung Sonography in Critical Care Medicine. *Diagnostics* **2022**, *12*, 1405. [CrossRef]
31. Mojoli, F.; Bouhemad, B.; Mongodi, S.; Lichtenstein, D. Lung Ultrasound for Critically Ill Patients. *Am. J. Respir. Crit. Care Med.* **2019**, *199*, 701–714, Erratum in: *Am. J. Respir. Crit. Care Med.* **2020**, *201*, 1015; Erratum in: *Am. J. Respir. Crit. Care Med.* **2020**, *201*, 1454. [CrossRef]
32. Mayo, P.H.; Copetti, R.; Feller-Kopman, D.; Mathis, G.; Maury, E.; Mongodi, S.; Mojoli, F.; Volpicelli, G.; Zanobetti, M. Thoracic ultrasonography: A narrative review. *Intensiv. Care Med* **2019**, *45*, 1200–1211. [CrossRef]
33. Sidhu, P.S.; Cantisani, V.; Dietrich, C.F.; Gilja, O.H.; Saftoiu, A.; Bartels, E.; Bertolotto, M.; Calliada, F.; Clevert, D.-A.; Cosgrove, D.; et al. The EFSUMB Guidelines and Recommendations for the Clinical Practice of Contrast-Enhanced Ultrasound (CEUS) in Non-Hepatic Applications: Update 2017 (Long Version). *Ultraschall der Med. Eur. J. Ultrasound* **2018**, *39*, e2–e44. [CrossRef]
34. Quarato, C.M.I.; Sperandeo, M. Letter to the Editor Regarding the Article: "Vascularization of Primary, Peripheral Lung Carcinoma in CEUS—A Retrospective Study (n = 89 Patients)" by Findeisen H et al. *Ultraschall der Med. Eur. J. Ultrasound* **2020**, *42*, 321–322. [CrossRef] [PubMed]
35. Quarato, C.M.; Cipriani, C.; Dimitri, L.; Lacedonia, D.; Graziano, P.; Copetti, M.; De Cosmo, S.; Simeone, A.; Scioscia, G.; Barbaro, M.F.; et al. Assessing value of contrast-enhanced ultrasound vs. conventional transthoracic ultrasound in improving diagnostic yield of percutaneous needle biopsy of peripheral lung lesions. *Eur. Rev. Med. Pharmacol. Sci.* **2021**, *25*, 5781–5789. [CrossRef]
36. Quarato, C.M.I.; Feragalli, B.; Lacedonia, D.; Rea, G.; Scioscia, G.; Maiello, E.; Di Micco, C.; Borelli, C.; Mirijello, A.; Graziano, P.; et al. Contrast-Enhanced Ultrasound in Distinguishing between Malignant and Benign Peripheral Pulmonary Consolidations: The Debated Utility of the Contrast Enhancement Arrival Time. *Diagnostics* **2023**, *13*, 666. [CrossRef]
37. Toy, D.; Siegel, M.D.; Rubinowitz, A.N. Imaging in the Intensive Care Unit. *Semin. Respir. Crit. Care Med.* **2022**, *43*, 899–923. [CrossRef] [PubMed]
38. Adler, A.C.; von Ungern-Sternberg, B.S.; Matava, C.T. Lung ultrasound and atelectasis—The devil is in the details. *Pediatr. Anesthesia* **2021**, *31*, 1269–1270. [CrossRef]

39. Peroni, D.; Boner, A. Atelectasis: Mechanisms, diagnosis and management. *Paediatr. Respir. Rev.* **2000**, *1*, 274–278. [CrossRef] [PubMed]
40. Duggan, M.; Kavanagh, B.P.; Warltier, D.C. Pulmonary Atelectasis: A pathogenic perioperative entity. *Anesthesiology* **2005**, *102*, 838–854. [CrossRef]
41. Maffessanti, M.; Berlot, G.; Bortolotto, P. Chest roentgenology in the intensive care unit: An overview. *Eur. Radiol.* **1998**, *8*, 69–78. [CrossRef]
42. Rubinowitz, A.N.; Siegel, M.D.; Tocino, I. Thoracic Imaging in the ICU. *Crit. Care Clin.* **2007**, *23*, 539–573. [CrossRef]
43. Lichtenstein, D.; Mezière, G.; Seitz, J. The The dynamic air bronchogram. A lung ultrasound sign of alveolar consolidation ruling out atelectasis. *Chest* **2009**, *135*, 1421–1425. [CrossRef]
44. Lichtenstein, D.A.; Lascols, N.; Prin, S.; Mezière, G. The "lung pulse": An early ultrasound sign of complete atelectasis. *Intensiv. Care Med.* **2003**, *29*, 2187–2192. [CrossRef]
45. Lanks, C.W.; Musani, A.I.; Hsia, D.W. Community-acquired Pneumonia and Hospital-acquired Pneumonia. *Med. Clin. N. Am.* **2019**, *103*, 487–501. [CrossRef] [PubMed]
46. Woodhead, M.; Welch, C.A.; Harrison, D.A.; Bellingan, G.; Ayres, J.G. Community-acquired pneumonia on the intensive care unit: Secondary analysis of 17,869 cases in the ICNARC Case Mix Programme Database. *Crit. Care* **2006**, *10* (Suppl. S2), S1. [CrossRef] [PubMed]
47. Papazian, L.; Klompas, M.; Luyt, C.-E. Ventilator-associated pneumonia in adults: A narrative review. *Intensiv. Care Med.* **2020**, *46*, 888–906. [CrossRef]
48. Walker, S.P.; Morley, A.J.; Stadon, L.; De Fonseka, D.; Arnold, D.T.; Medford, A.R.; Maskell, N.A. Nonmalignant Pleural Effusions: A Prospective Study of 356 Consecutive Unselected Patients. *Chest* **2017**, *151*, 1099–1105. [CrossRef] [PubMed]
49. Saguil, A.; Wyrick, K.; Hallgren, J. Diagnostic approach to pleural effusion. *Am. Fam. Physician.* **2014**, *90*, 99–104.
50. Aboudara, M.; Maldonado, F. Update in the Management of Pleural Effusions. *Med. Clin. N. Am.* **2019**, *103*, 475–485. [CrossRef]
51. Alwi, I. Diagnosis and management of cardiogenic pulmonary edema. *Acta Med. Indones.* **2010**, *42*, 176–184.
52. Aissaoui, N.; Hamzaoui, O.; Price, S. Ten questions ICU specialists should address when managing cardiogenic acute pulmonary oedema. *Intensiv. Care Med.* **2022**, *48*, 482–485. [CrossRef] [PubMed]
53. Meyer, N.J.; Gattinoni, L.; Calfee, C.S. Acute respiratory distress syndrome. *Lancet* **2021**, *398*, 622–637. [CrossRef] [PubMed]
54. Fan, E.; Brodie, D.; Slutsky, A.S. Acute Respiratory Distress Syndrome: Advances in Diagnosis and Treatment. *JAMA* **2018**, *319*, 698–710. [CrossRef]
55. Rendeki, S.; Molnár, T.F. Pulmonary contusion. *J. Thorac. Dis.* **2019**, *11* (Suppl. S2), S141–S151. [CrossRef]
56. Shah, K.; Tran, J.; Schmidt, L. Traumatic pneumothorax: Updates in diagnosis and management in the emergency department. *Emerg. Med. Pract.* **2022**, *25* (Suppl. S1), 1–28.
57. Alsohime, F.; Temsah, M.-H.; Al-Eyadhy, A.; Ghulman, S.; Mosleh, H.; Alsohime, O. Technical Aspects of Intensive Care Unit Management: A Single-Center Experience at a Tertiary Academic Hospital. *J. Multidiscip. Health.* **2021**, *14*, 869–875. [CrossRef]
58. Plata, P.; Gaszyński, T. Ultrasound-guided percutaneous tracheostomy. *Anaesthesiol. Intensiv. Ther.* **2019**, *51*, 126–132. [CrossRef] [PubMed]
59. Saugel, B.; Scheeren, T.W.L.; Teboul, J.-L. Ultrasound-guided central venous catheter placement: A structured review and recommendations for clinical practice. *Crit. Care* **2017**, *21*, 225. [CrossRef]
60. Tsujimoto, H.; Tsujimoto, Y.; Nakata, Y.; Akazawa, M.; Kataoka, Y. Ultrasonography for confirmation of gastric tube placement. *Cochrane Database Syst. Rev.* **2017**, *2017*, CD012083. [CrossRef]

Disclaimer/Publisher's Note: The statements, opinions and data contained in all publications are solely those of the individual author(s) and contributor(s) and not of MDPI and/or the editor(s). MDPI and/or the editor(s) disclaim responsibility for any injury to people or property resulting from any ideas, methods, instructions or products referred to in the content.

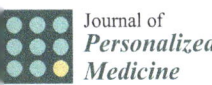

Case Report

The Arterial Axis Lesions in Proximal Humeral Fractures—Case Report and Literature Review

Cosmin Ioan Faur [1,2,3], Razvan Nitu [2,4,*], Simona-Alina Abu-Awwad [2,4], Cristina Tudoran [2,5,6] and Ahmed Abu-Awwad [1,2,3]

1. Department XV—Discipline of Orthopedics—Traumatology, "Victor Babes" University of Medicine and Pharmacy, Eftimie Murgu Square, No. 2, 300041 Timisoara, Romania; faur17@gmail.com (C.I.F.); ahm.abuawwad@umft.ro (A.A.-A.)
2. "Pius Brinzeu" Emergency Clinical County Hospital, Bld Liviu Rebreanu, No. 156, 300723 Timisoara, Romania; alina.abuawwad@umft.ro (S.-A.A.-A.); cristina13.tudoran@gmail.com (C.T.)
3. Research Center University Professor Doctor Teodor Șora, Victor Babes University of Medicine and Pharmacy, Eftimie Murgu Square, No. 2, 300041 Timisoara, Romania
4. Department XII—Discipline of Obstetrics and Gynecology, Victor Babes University of Medicine and Pharmacy, Eftimie Murgu Square, No. 2, 300041 Timisoara, Romania
5. Department VII, Internal Medicine II, Discipline of Cardiology, University of Medicine and Pharmacy "Victor Babes" Timisoara, E. Murgu Square, Nr. 2, 300041 Timisoara, Romania
6. Center of Molecular Research in Nephrology and Vascular Disease, Faculty of the University of Medicine and Pharmacy "Victor Babes" Timisoara, E. Murgu Square, Nr. 2, 300041 Timisoara, Romania
* Correspondence: nitu.dumitru@umft.ro

Abstract: Background: This comprehensive review delves into the nuanced domain of arterial axis lesions associated with proximal humeral fractures, elucidating the intricate interplay between fracture patterns and vascular compromise. Proximal humeral fractures, a common orthopedic occurrence, often present challenges beyond the skeletal realm, necessitating a profound understanding of the vascular implications. Methods: The study synthesizes the existing literature, presenting a collective analysis of documented cases and their respective clinical outcomes. The spectrum of arterial axis lesions, from subtle vascular compromise to overt ischemic events, is systematically examined, highlighting the varied clinical manifestations encountered in proximal humeral fractures. Diagnostic modalities, including advanced imaging techniques such as angiography and Doppler ultrasound, are scrutinized for their efficacy in identifying arterial axis lesions promptly. The review emphasizes the critical role of early and accurate diagnosis in mitigating the potential sequelae associated with vascular compromise, thereby underscoring the importance of a vigilant clinical approach. Results: Therapeutic strategies, ranging from conservative management to surgical interventions, are critically evaluated in the context of existing evidence. The evolving landscape of endovascular interventions and their applicability in addressing arterial axis lesions specific to proximal humeral fractures is explored, providing valuable insights for clinicians navigating the therapeutic decision-making process. Furthermore, the review addresses gaps in current knowledge and proposes avenues for future research, emphasizing the need for tailored, evidence-based guidelines in the management of arterial axis lesions in proximal humeral fractures. By consolidating current understanding and pointing towards areas warranting further exploration, this review contributes to the ongoing discourse surrounding the intricacies of vascular complications in orthopedic trauma. Conclusions: this comprehensive review provides a synthesized overview of arterial axis lesions in proximal humeral fractures, offering a valuable resource for clinicians, researchers, and educators alike. The findings underscore the multifaceted nature of these lesions and advocate for a holistic, patient-centered approach to their management.

Keywords: arterial axis lesions; proximal humeral fractures; vascular complications; diagnostic challenges; therapeutic strategies

Citation: Faur, C.I.; Nitu, R.; Abu-Awwad, S.-A.; Tudoran, C.; Abu-Awwad, A. The Arterial Axis Lesions in Proximal Humeral Fractures—Case Report and Literature Review. *J. Pers. Med.* **2023**, *13*, 1712. https://doi.org/10.3390/jpm13121712

Academic Editor: Ovidiu Alexandru Mederle

Received: 25 November 2023
Revised: 6 December 2023
Accepted: 12 December 2023
Published: 14 December 2023

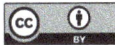

Copyright: © 2023 by the authors. Licensee MDPI, Basel, Switzerland. This article is an open access article distributed under the terms and conditions of the Creative Commons Attribution (CC BY) license (https://creativecommons.org/licenses/by/4.0/).

1. Introduction

Proximal humeral fractures, comprising approximately 5% of all fractures, present a unique set of challenges in clinical orthopedics due to their intricate anatomy and susceptibility to complications beyond the immediate skeletal injury [1,2].

The close proximity of the shoulder to significant neurovascular structures, particularly the axillary artery, makes it prone to arterial axis lesions. An in-depth comprehension of this phenomenon is imperative for effective clinical management. Proximal humeral fractures are associated with a spectrum of arterial axis lesions, ranging from transient perfusion deficits to critical ischemic events. The vulnerability of the axillary artery due to its anatomical proximity to the proximal humerus underscores the importance of recognizing and understanding these vascular complications. It is crucial to acknowledge the diverse clinical manifestations resulting from arterial axis compromise, as subtle perfusion deficits may be obscured by more evident fracture-related signs, potentially leading to delayed diagnosis and management. Diagnostic precision is paramount in addressing arterial axis lesions in the context of proximal humeral fractures. Advanced imaging modalities, such as angiography and Doppler ultrasound, play a pivotal role in delineating the extent and nature of vascular compromise [3,4].

These techniques not only aid in accurate diagnosis but also contribute to the formulation of targeted therapeutic strategies. However, navigating the nuances of diagnostic challenges, including differentiating arterial axis lesions from other complications and assessing the optimal timing for imaging, underscores the complexity of managing these cases. Therapeutically, the management of arterial axis lesions in proximal humeral fractures demands a tailored approach.

Conservative strategies, including close monitoring and anticoagulation, may be appropriate for less severe cases, while surgical interventions, such as vascular repair or revascularization, become imperative in the face of critical ischemia. Emerging endovascular techniques offer additional avenues for intervention, providing minimally invasive alternatives in select cases [3–6]. This article consolidates existing knowledge and identifies areas for future exploration. Research could enhance diagnostic and therapeutic algorithms, investigating long-term outcomes of varied management strategies. Aiming to deepen understanding of arterial axis lesions in proximal humeral fractures, this work seeks to contribute to evidence-based guidelines, optimizing patient care in orthopedic trauma.

2. Case Report

The study cohort comprised individuals presenting with proximal humeral fractures and concomitant arterial axis lesions at the Pius Brinzeu County Clinical Emergency Hospital between 2014 and 2022. Informed consent was obtained from each participant, and ethical approval was obtained from the Pius Brinzeu Ethics Committee.

A retrospective analysis of clinical and paraclinical data examines five cases of axillary arterial injuries secondary to proximal humeral fractures. The study spans a period of 9 years (2014–2022), describing axillary arterial pathology arising from proximal humeral fractures (PHFs). Through a literature review, the study provides insights for early diagnosis and effective treatment of these less common injuries.

Patients were monitored both preoperatively and postoperatively. However, given the rarity of this pathology, a comprehensive evaluation of incidence and prevalence was challenging. Instead, the study offers a detailed presentation of clinical cases, modes of presentation, and the instituted diagnostic and treatment modalities.

The research aims to contribute to the understanding of axillary arterial injuries associated with proximal humeral fractures, emphasizing the importance of early diagnosis and efficient management based on the findings from both the clinical cases and the literature review.

2.1. Clinical Data Collection

Detailed clinical histories, including the mechanism of injury, comorbidities, and presenting symptoms, were systematically recorded. Physical examinations, with specific attention to vascular status, were conducted for all participants. Relevant demographic data, such as age and gender, were documented.

Pain and functional impairment in the shoulder, with the hand displaying a "swan neck" appearance; paresthesia on the dorsal aspect of the left hand in the territory of the radial nerve; ecchymosis in the affected limb; absence of pulse at the radial artery.

2.2. Imaging Studies

Diagnostic imaging studies played a pivotal role in characterizing both the proximal humeral fractures and associated arterial axis lesions. Plain radiographs, computed tomography (CT) scans (Figure 1), and magnetic resonance imaging (MRI) were employed to delineate fracture patterns and identify potential vascular compromise. Angiography was utilized for a more comprehensive assessment of arterial integrity and blood flow.

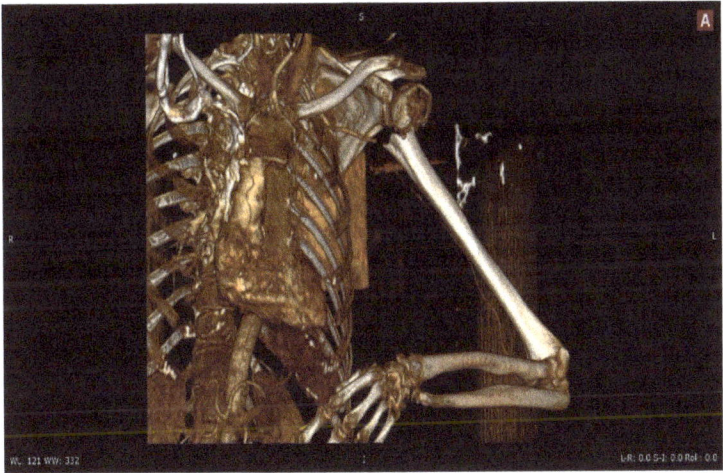

Figure 1. Angio CT left shoulder.

2.3. Diagnostic Criteria

Arterial axis lesions were defined based on angiographic findings, including arterial dissection, occlusion, or pseudoaneurysm formation. Vascular compromise was categorized according to severity, ranging from minor perfusion deficits to critical ischemic events.

2.4. Treatment Modalities

The therapeutic approach was determined through a multidisciplinary consensus involving orthopedic surgeons, vascular surgeons, and interventional radiologists. Treatment options included conservative management with close monitoring, anticoagulation, or surgical interventions such as vascular repair or revascularization. Endovascular techniques were considered when deemed appropriate.

2.5. Follow-Up

Patients were followed longitudinally to assess treatment outcomes and complications. Post-treatment imaging studies, including angiography when indicated, were conducted to evaluate vascular integrity. Functional outcomes, pain levels, and any recurrent symptoms were systematically documented.

2.6. Statistical Analysis

Descriptive statistics were employed to summarize demographic and clinical characteristics. Continuous variables were presented as means with standard deviations or as medians with interquartile ranges, while categorical variables were expressed as frequencies and percentages. The analysis aimed to provide a comprehensive overview of the patient cohort and highlight any trends or patterns in the presentation and management of arterial axis lesions in proximal humeral fractures.

2.7. Ethical Considerations

This study adhered to the principles outlined in the Declaration of Helsinki and was conducted in accordance with ethical standards for research involving human subjects. Patient confidentiality and privacy were rigorously maintained throughout the study period.

Case I.: 62y, female; X-ray; pain in the left shoulder, with the hand displaying a "swan neck" appearance; paresthesia on the dorsal aspect of the left hand in the territory of the radial nerve. (Figure 2).

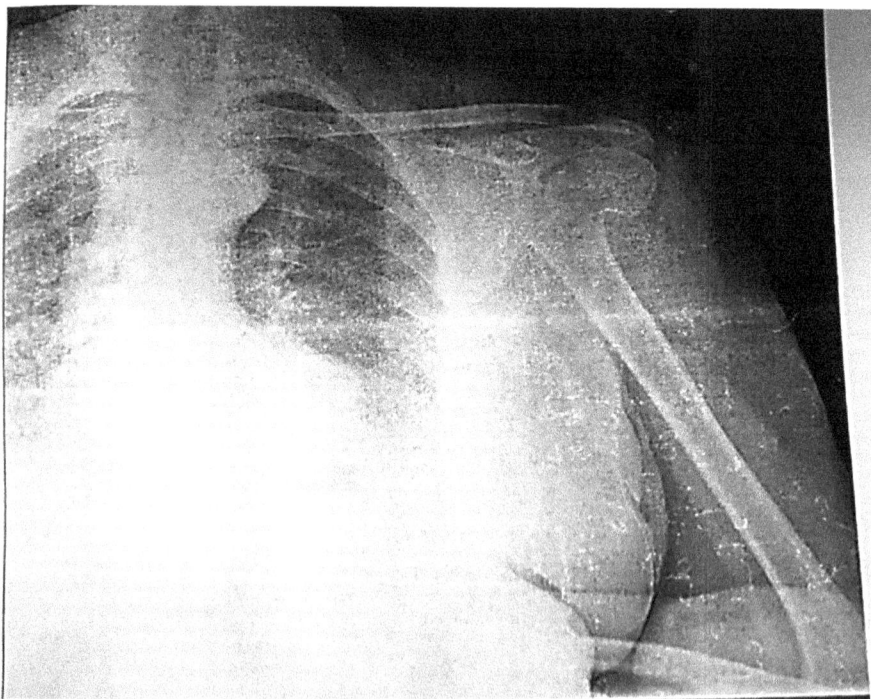

Figure 2. X-ray of left shoulder.

The patient was positioned in the dorsal decubitus position on the operating table under general anesthesia. An approximately 15 cm incision was made on the anterior aspect of the left shoulder.

Dissection was carried out between the deltoid and pectoral muscles, revealing the subscapular muscle tendon. The joint capsule was incised, exposing the fracture site.

The fracture was reduced under fluoroscopy control and stabilized with an anatomical plate secured with nine screws (Figure 3). Finally, wound closure was achieved through layered suturing with skin stitches and sterile dressing.

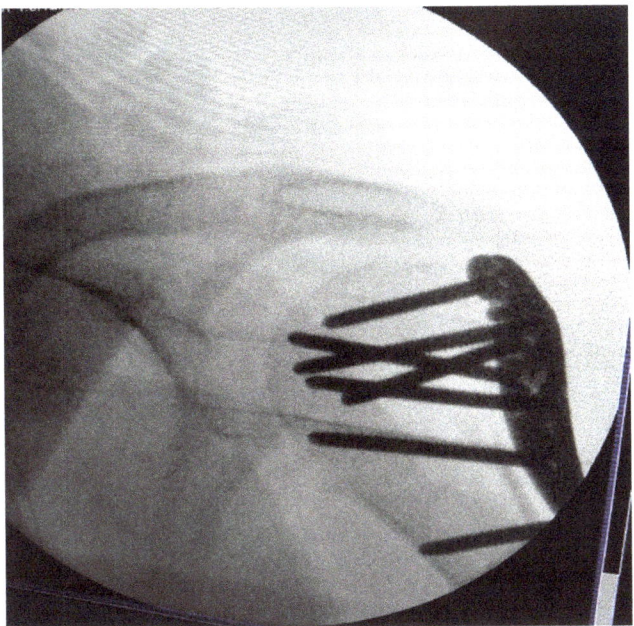

Figure 3. Post-op X-ray.

Following the completion of the intervention, a reassessment of the brachial artery pulse revealed its absence, leading the vascular surgeon to decide on a secondary surgical intervention to explore the axillary and brachial arteries.

An incision was made along the bicipital groove in the proximal 1/3 of the left arm, extending to the anterior wall of the axilla. The proximal axillary and brachial arteries were isolated, revealing non-pulsatile vessels (Figure 4).

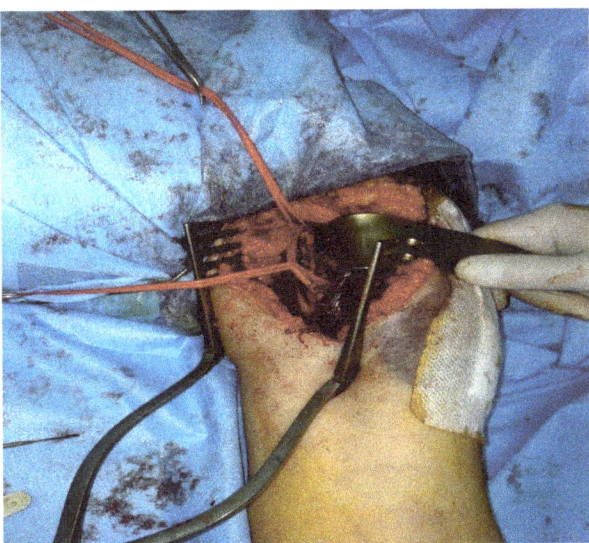

Figure 4. Exposure of the left axillary artery with highlighting of thrombosis and the underlying dissection.

A region of angulation was observed at the distal axillary artery caused by a tractioned branch, and approximately 2 cm distal to the angulated zone, a segment suggestive of arterial dissection was identified. The angulating branch was ligated and sectioned. Heparin (5000 IU) was administered, clamping ensued, and the segmentally injured arterial portion was cut, followed by anastomosis of the remaining arterial ends with 6.0 sutures (Surjet).

This procedure successfully restored functional integrity to the arterial axis, rendering the arteries pulsatile. Hemostasis was achieved, and drainage was conducted with an externalized drain tube through a counter-incision, followed by closure of the wound in anatomical layers and application of a dressing.

After the completion of the surgical procedures, the patient was closely monitored through continuous ECG, blood pressure, and pulse tracking in the affected limb. Electrolyte balance was restored, and emergency antibiotic prophylaxis with a broad-spectrum antibiotic was initiated for 48 h.

Trophic nerve medications were administered using Milgamma N capsules (three times a day) due to persistent signs suggestive of radial and musculocutaneous nerve injury. Additionally, anticoagulant treatment with intravenous Clexane was administered.

Following the improvement of the clinical condition, the patient underwent a follow-up X-ray to assess the postoperative state of the proximal humerus and the success of the osteosynthesis procedures (Figure 5).

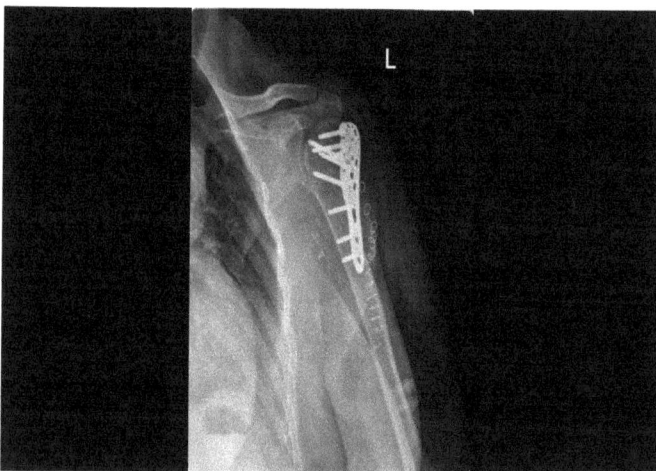

Figure 5. Post-op X-ray; Abbreviation: L—left.

Following the complete amelioration of the clinical condition, with normalization of diuresis, blood pressure, pulse, body temperature, hemodynamic, and biochemical parameters, the patient was discharged with the following recommendations:

- Bed rest for 30 days with limited arm abduction movements up to 90°;
- Sterile dressing with iodine every 2–3 days;
- Suture removal after 14 days postoperatively;
- Anticoagulant treatment with Clexane 0.6 mL two times a day for 14 days, followed by continuation with Aspenter 75 mg once daily;
- Treatment with Arcoxia 60 mg tablets twice daily and Milagamma N (benfotiamină 40 mg, clorhidrat de piridoxină 90 mg și cianocobalamină 0.250 mg.) 100 mg/g three times a day;
- Reevaluation after 30 days;

During this post-discharge period, the patient was advised to adhere to functional rest, careful wound care, and the prescribed medications.

Follow-up assessments are crucial to monitoring the progress of the healing process, assess any potential complications, and make adjustments to the treatment plan as necessary.

It is imperative for the patient to maintain open communication with the medical team and promptly report any unusual symptoms or concerns. This comprehensive postoperative care plan aims to ensure the optimal recovery and well-being of the patient.

At one year and ten months post-surgery, the patient exhibited a range of motion with internal and external rotation reaching 70 degrees. The radial pulse was palpable, indicating restored vascular perfusion. Additionally, the fracture site had achieved complete closure, and radiological assessments revealed the absence of evidence for osteonecrosis of the humeral head. These positive outcomes underscore the success of the surgical intervention and subsequent postoperative care, emphasizing the restoration of both functional mobility and vascular integrity.

The observed improvement in range of motion, palpable radial pulse, and radiological evidence of fracture site closure collectively indicate a favorable long-term outcome. Furthermore, the absence of osteonecrosis, a potential complication in such cases, reinforces the effectiveness of the chosen surgical approach and underscores the importance of diligent postoperative management.

This encouraging clinical status in the specified time frame underscores the success of the integrated treatment plan and the patient's adherence to postoperative recommendations. Continuous follow-up assessments will remain essential to monitor the sustained recovery and address any potential late-onset complications, ensuring the optimal long-term functional outcome for the patient.

Case II: 69 y old, female patient. The patient presented with pain, bony crepitus, and functional impairment in the left upper limb, with the hand displaying a "swan neck" appearance. The skin was cool to the touch, accompanied by a large bruise on the posterior aspect of the shoulder, and the pulses measured at the radial and ulnar arteries were diminished.

An emergency radiograph (Figure 6) of the left proximal humerus in two views, anteroposterior and lateral, was promptly conducted, revealing a displaced surgical neck fracture (Neer II).

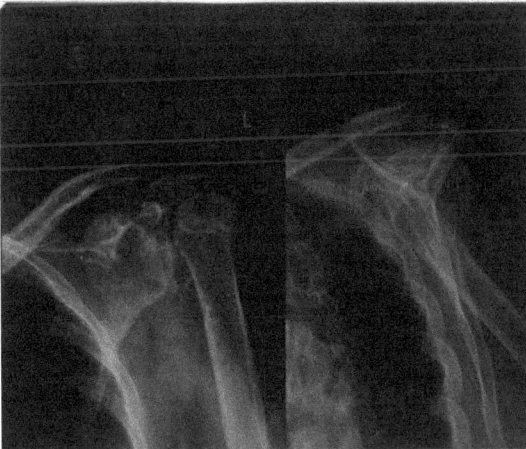

Figure 6. X-ray in ER department; Abbreviation: L—left.

The fracture was immobilized using a Dessault plaster splint in the emergency department, and the patient was admitted to the orthopedic ward for further specialized investigations and treatment.

This clinical presentation indicates a severe injury requiring urgent attention and underscores the importance of comprehensive orthopedic evaluation and intervention in managing complex fractures.

A duplex Doppler scan was performed, confirming the absence of arterial flow in the brachial and radial arteries. However, proper evaluation of the axillary artery was hindered due to sensitivity and edema in the area. The patient was urgently taken to the operating room for exploration, arterial repair, and joint stabilization.

The restoration of arterial integrity and osteosynthesis procedures were conducted on the same day by a multidisciplinary team comprising a cardiovascular surgeon, orthopedic surgeon, and an anesthesiologist.

The patient was positioned in the dorsal decubitus position on the operating table under general anesthesia. An approximately 15 cm incision was made along the bicipital groove in the proximal 1/3 of the left arm, extending to the anterior wall of the axilla.

Intraoperatively, contusion of the distal segment of the axillary artery was identified (Figure 7), along with the absence of pulsations within the vessel and a lack of distal flow. The prompt intervention of the multidisciplinary team aimed at addressing both the vascular and orthopedic aspects, underscoring the collaborative and comprehensive nature of the surgical approach.

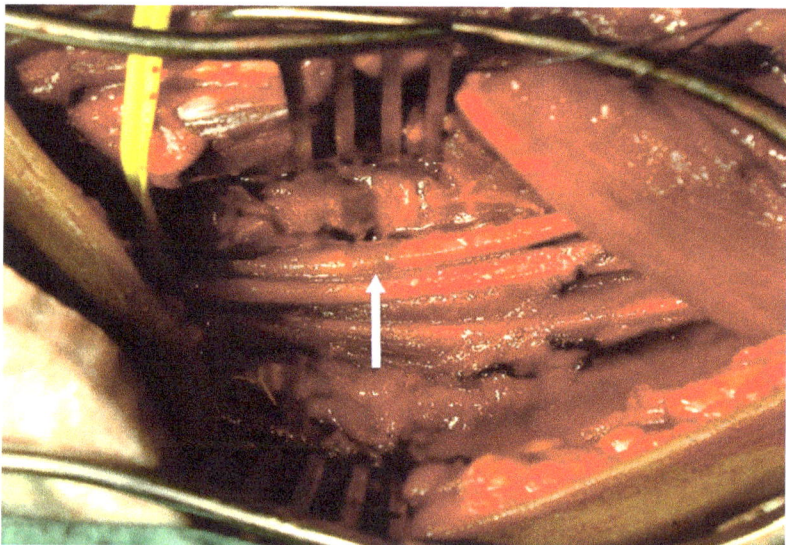

Figure 7. Exposure of the left axillary artery. The white arrow indicate the contused segment of the distal axillary artery.

The shoulder joint was stabilized using an anatomical plate secured with 11 screws, and the contused segment of the axillary artery was excised following proximal and distal control. Attempts were made to restore circulation through anastomosis using a 10 cm graft of the great saphenous vein harvested from the ipsilateral thigh.

However, due to reduced arterial flow, the biological graft was replaced with a synthetic Gore-Tex graft of 10 cm/5 mm, facilitating proper restoration of circulation.

Primary anastomoses were completed with 6/0 polypropylene sutures, successfully reestablishing pulsatile flow in the brachial and radial arteries (Figure 8). The surgical procedure concluded with hemostasis, drainage using an externalized drain tube through a counter-incision, wound closure, and application of a sterile dressing.

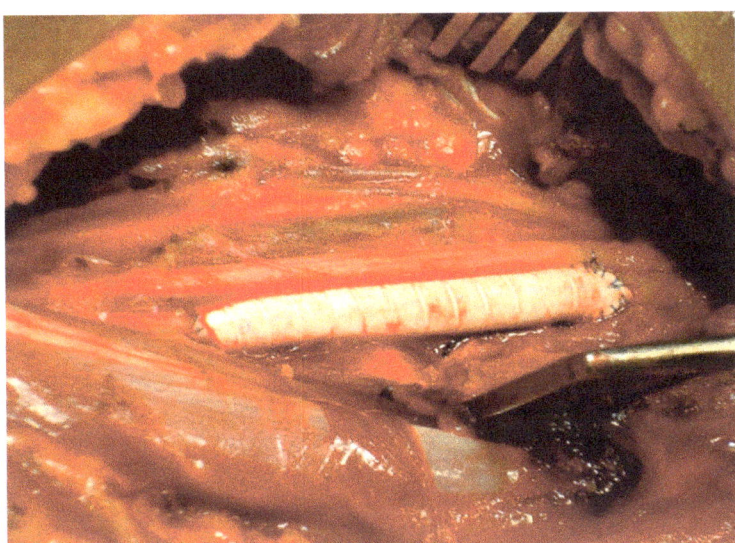

Figure 8. Intraoperative image highlighting the restoration of arterial flow through the interposition of a Gore-Tex graft.

Following the completion of the surgical procedures, the patient underwent vigilant monitoring, and emergency antibiotic prophylaxis and anticoagulant treatment with Clexane were promptly initiated. Upon complete amelioration of the clinical condition, with normalization of diuresis, blood pressure, pulse, body temperature, hemodynamic and biochemical parameters, the patient was discharged with the following recommendations:

- Bed rest for 30 days with limited arm abduction movements up to 90°. (With the thumb facing up and outwards, move the arm in a big arc out to the side. With the elbow by your side, rotate forearm outwards, keeping the elbow at about 90 degrees in flexion. We repeated all of these 3 exercises 10 times each, 4–5 times a day.);
- Sterile dressing with iodine every 2–3 days;
- Suture removal after 14 days postoperatively;
- Anticoagulant treatment with Clexane 0.6 mL 2 times a day for 14 days, followed by continuation with Aspenter 25 mg once daily;
- Treatment with Arcoxia 60 mg tablets (etoricoxib) twice daily and Milgamma N.

A reassessment was scheduled after 30 days to ensure ongoing recovery and address any emerging concerns. These postoperative guidelines are aimed at promoting optimal healing and minimizing the risk of complications during the patient's recovery period.

The postoperative recovery period has unequivocally demonstrated success. At 30 days post-intervention, the limb remained viable with normal pulses, albeit with a limitation in shoulder mobility. Over the course of 18 months following the injury, with the assistance of physical therapy, there had been a significant restoration of movements.

Notably, at the 2-year mark, the range of internal and external rotation had expanded to 90 degrees, the radial pulse was palpable, the fracture site had completely closed, and radiological assessments revealed an absence of evidence for osteonecrosis of the humeral head.

This comprehensive and positive trajectory in the recovery journey underscores the efficacy of the surgical intervention, postoperative care, and the collaborative efforts of rehabilitation specialists. The milestone achievements in shoulder mobility and vascular health are indicative of a successful and well-managed recovery process, providing the patient with a promising outlook for long-term functional well-being.

3. Discussion

Arterial injuries in the context of proximal humeral fractures represent a highly uncommon complication, often overlooked by medical personnel unless heightened attention is given to clinical signs.

The studied cases were encountered in women aged between 62 and 88 years, with a typical mechanism of injury involving proximal humeral dislocations resulting from indirect trauma, such as falls from height or at the same level.

The clinical presentation was indicative of proximal limb trauma, featuring pain, functional impairment in the left shoulder, a hand displaying a "swan neck" appearance, bony crepitus, variable paresthesias depending on the involved nerve territory, ecchymosis in the affected limb, and reduced or absent pulses in the arteries descending from the axillary artery [6–8].

In all presented cases, fracture diagnosis was established based on two-view X-rays, revealing displaced, comminuted fractures of the proximal humerus, classified as Neer II to Neer IV. Subsequent to the onset of paresthesias and the detection of a radial artery pulse deficit, arterial oxygenation was measured using a pulse oximeter, revealing a significant decrease in oxygen saturation [7–9].

Together with typical clinical signs of upper limb ischemia (cool skin and reduced arterial pulses), this led to the decision to perform an echo-Doppler scan of the upper limb, confirming the absence of arterial flow in the brachial and radial arteries, with the axillary artery not being adequately assessed due to sensitivity and edema in the area.

In light of these findings, a consultation with cardiovascular surgery was sought, and an angio-CT scan was conducted, confirming the nature of the fracture and revealing arterial flow interruption through the axillary artery due to trauma-induced arterial thrombosis.

The surgical intervention was carried out by a multidisciplinary team, including a vascular surgeon, an orthopedic surgeon, and an anesthesiologist. In cases of prolonged or critical ischemic periods, vascular repair took precedence, being performed prior to fracture stabilization. This collaborative and comprehensive approach aimed to address both the vascular and orthopedic aspects, emphasizing the intricate nature of managing such complex cases. The intricate balance of medical specialties involved underscores the nuanced care required for optimal patient outcomes in these challenging scenarios [1,9,10].

In the context of surgical intervention, the multidisciplinary team's involvement, comprising a vascular surgeon, orthopedic surgeon, and anesthesiologist, speaks to the comprehensive nature of care required for successful outcomes.

The prioritization of vascular repair in cases of prolonged or critical ischemic periods emphasizes the dynamic decision-making involved in balancing the immediate vascular concerns with the longer-term orthopedic considerations. Furthermore, the utilization of synthetic Gore-Tex grafts in vascular reconstruction demonstrates the innovative approaches employed in addressing arterial compromise [1,11,12].

As the postoperative period unfolds, the emphasis on ongoing monitoring, antibiotic prophylaxis, and anticoagulant therapy further highlights the commitment to preventing complications and promoting optimal healing. The inclusion of physical therapy in the recovery plan plays a pivotal role in restoring shoulder mobility, aligning with a patient-centered approach aimed at enhancing overall quality of life [12–14].

In conclusion, the management of arterial injuries in proximal humeral fractures is a multifaceted journey that extends beyond the operating room. It involves a careful orchestration of medical specialties, advanced diagnostic techniques, and a holistic approach to patient care. Continuous collaboration between healthcare professionals, coupled with a commitment to ongoing research and advancements, is imperative in further refining treatment protocols and improving outcomes in these rare and challenging clinical scenarios.

The examination of arterial axis lesions in proximal humeral fractures has yielded significant insights, elucidating the intricate interplay between skeletal trauma and vascular compromise. Noteworthy findings include a predominant occurrence in women aged between 62 and 88 years, commonly resulting from falls of varying heights and manifesting as Neer II to Neer IV fractures. Clinical presentations were characterized by distinctive features such as a "swan neck" appearance, bony crepitus, diverse paresthesias, ecchymosis, and a diminished pulses in the affected limb.

Diagnostic assessments, encompassing two-view X-rays, echo-Doppler scans, and angio-CT imaging, played a pivotal role in confirming fractures, identifying vascular compromise, and guiding subsequent interventions. The collaborative efforts of a multidisciplinary surgical team, comprising vascular and orthopedic surgeons, alongside an anesthesiologist, were instrumental in addressing both the skeletal and vascular dimensions of these intricate cases.

Surgical interventions entailed fracture stabilization using anatomical plates and screws, coupled with meticulous vascular repair using synthetic Gore-Tex grafts in instances of arterial compromise. Postoperative monitoring, antibiotic prophylaxis, and anticoagulant therapy were implemented to avert complications and facilitate optimal recovery. Physical therapy interventions proved effective in restoring shoulder mobility over time.

A comprehensive literature review complemented these case-specific findings, providing a broader perspective on the prevalence, mechanisms, and management strategies for arterial axis lesions in proximal humeral fractures. The existing literature underscored the rarity of such complications, emphasizing the imperative of heightened clinical awareness and thorough diagnostic evaluations.

In conclusion, the results explicate the nuanced clinical presentations, diagnostic approaches, and multidisciplinary interventions in cases of arterial axis lesions in proximal humeral fractures. The integration of case-specific outcomes with insights from the existing literature contributes to a more profound understanding of this rare and challenging clinical scenario.

4. Conclusions

This case report and literature review delves into arterial axis lesions in proximal humeral fractures, emphasizing the need to recognize and address this intricate clinical entity. The amalgamation of specific case outcomes and insights from the existing literature contributes to a nuanced understanding of the complexities associated with these challenging scenarios.

The demographic focus on women aged 62–88, predominantly experiencing falls from varying heights, underscores the necessity for targeted assessments and interventions, considering potential age-related factors in both diagnosis and treatment planning. The consistent clinical presentation, featuring the distinctive "swan neck" appearance, bony crepitus, and varied paresthesias, serves as a clinical hallmark for early recognition, emphasizing the importance of thorough clinical examinations.

Diagnostic modalities, including advanced imaging techniques such as echo-Doppler scans and angio-CT imaging, prove instrumental in confirming fractures and assessing vascular compromise. The collaboration of a multidisciplinary surgical team, led by vascular and orthopedic surgeons, along with an anesthesiologist, reflects the necessity for a holistic approach in managing these complex cases, addressing both skeletal and vascular dimensions concurrently.

Surgical interventions, encompassing fracture stabilization and innovative vascular repair using synthetic Gore-Tex grafts, demonstrate success in restoring both skeletal and arterial integrity. Postoperative care, marked by vigilant monitoring, antibiotic prophylaxis, and anticoagulant therapy, is crucial in mitigating complications and fostering optimal recovery.

The literature review contextualizes our findings within the broader landscape, highlighting the rarity of arterial axis lesions in proximal humeral fractures and emphasizing the imperative for heightened clinical awareness to avoid oversight. In summary, our investigation significantly advances the ongoing dialogue concerning the intricate interplay between proximal humeral fractures and arterial axis lesions. The synthesis of specific case findings and an extensive literature review enriches our comprehension of these infrequent complications and lays a solid groundwork for future research endeavors.

The valuable insights derived from individual cases and the broader literature underscore the pivotal role of a multidisciplinary approach, cutting-edge diagnostic methodologies, and inventive surgical interventions in enhancing outcomes for individuals navigating through the complexities of this distinctive clinical challenge. Furthermore, the study prompts a deeper reflection on the evolving landscape of orthopedic and vascular care, emphasizing the imperative for continuous collaboration among medical disciplines.

The integration of specific case outcomes into the broader context of existing knowledge not only refines our clinical acumen but also stimulates a proactive mindset towards the identification, management, and prevention of arterial axis lesions in the context of proximal humeral fractures. This holistic understanding, rooted in both empirical evidence and collective clinical wisdom, paves the way for a more informed and effective approach to patient care in the realm of orthopedic trauma.

Author Contributions: Conceptualization, A.A.-A., C.I.F. and R.N.; methodology, S.-A.A.-A.; software, C.I.F.; validation, A.A.-A., R.N. and C.T.; formal analysis, S.-A.A.-A.; investigation, C.T.; resources, A.A.-A.; data curation, C.T.; writing—original draft preparation, A.A.-A.; writing—review and editing, S.-A.A.-A.; visualization, C.T.; supervision, C.I.F.; project administration, R.N.; funding acquisition, C.T. All authors have read and agreed to the published version of the manuscript.

Funding: This research received no external funding.

Institutional Review Board Statement: The study was conducted in accordance with the Declaration of Helsinki, and approved by the Institutional Review Board of Pius Brinzeu Couty Clinical Emergency Hospital of Timisoara (ethics code 1045, 16 May 2023).

Informed Consent Statement: Informed consent was obtained from all subjects involved in the study.

Data Availability Statement: All data are included in the text.

Conflicts of Interest: The authors declare no conflict of interest.

References

1. Krasney, L.C.; Rennie, C.; Brustein, J.; Naylor, B. Rare finding of axillary artery dissection secondary to a proximal humerus fracture-dislocation: A case report. *Trauma Case Rep.* **2023**, *45*, 100828. [CrossRef] [PubMed]
2. Razaeian, S.; Rustum, S.; Sonnow, L.; Meller, R.; Krettek, C.; Hawi, N. Axillary Artery Dissection and Thrombosis after Closed Proximal Humerus Fracture—A Rare Interdisciplinary Challenge. *Z. Orthop. Unfall.* **2020**, *158*, 406–413. [CrossRef] [PubMed]
3. Mahmuti, A.; Kaya Şimşek, E.; Haberal, B. The medial cortical ratio as a risk factor for failure after surgical fixation of proximal humerus fractures in elderly patients. *Jt. Dis. Relat. Surg.* **2023**, *34*, 432–438. [CrossRef] [PubMed]
4. Schumaier, A.; Grawe, B. Proximal humerus fractures: Evaluation and management in the elderly patient. *Geriatr. Orthop. Surg. Rehabil.* **2018**, 9. [CrossRef] [PubMed]
5. Panagiotopoulou, V.C.; Varga, P.; Richards, R.G.; Gueorguiev, B.; Giannoudis, P.V. Late screw-related complications in locking plating of proximal humerus fractures: A systematic review. *Injury* **2019**, *50*, 2176–2195. [CrossRef] [PubMed]
6. Wallace, M.J.; Bledsoe, G.; Moed, B.R.; Israel, H.A.; Kaar, S.G. Relationship of cortical thickness of the proximal humerus and pullout strength of a locked plate and screw construct. *J. Orthop. Trauma* **2012**, *26*, 222–225. [CrossRef] [PubMed]
7. Peters, R.M.; Menendez, M.E.; Mellema, J.J.; Ring, D.; Smith, R.M. Axillary Artery Injury Associated with Proximal Humerus Fracture: A Report of 6 Cases. *Arch. Bone Jt. Surg.* **2017**, *5*, 52–57. [PubMed]
8. Adıyeke, L.; Geçer, A.; Bulut, O. Comparison of effective factors in loss of reduction after locking plate-screw treatment in humerus proximal fractures. *Ulus. Travma Acil Cerrahi Derg.* **2022**, *28*, 1008–1015. [CrossRef] [PubMed]
9. Passaretti, D.; Candela, V.; Sessa, P.; Gumina, S. Epidemiology of proximal humeral fractures: A detailed survey of 711 patients in a metropolitan area. *J. Shoulder Elb. Surg.* **2017**, *26*, 2117–2124. [CrossRef] [PubMed]
10. Sukeik, M.; Vashista, G.; Shaath, N. Axillary artery compromise in a minimally displaced proximal humerus fracture: A case report. *Cases J.* **2009**, *2*, 9308–9312. [CrossRef] [PubMed]
11. Menendez, M.E.; Ring, D.; Heng, M. Proximal humeral fracture with injury to the axillary artery: A population-based study. *Injury* **2015**, *46*, 1367–1371. [CrossRef] [PubMed]
12. Neuhaus, V.; Bot, A.G.; Swellengrebel, C.H.; Jain, N.B.; Warner, J.J.; Ring, D.C. Treatment choice affects inpatient adverse events and mortality in older aged inpatients with an isolated fracture of the proximal humerus. *J. Shoulder Elb. Surg.* **2014**, *23*, 800–806. [CrossRef] [PubMed]

13. Hems, T.E.J.; Mahmood, F. Injuries of the terminal branches of the infraclavicular brachial plexus: Patterns of injury, management and outcome. *J. Bone Jt. Surg. Br. Vol.* **2012**, *94*, 799–804. [CrossRef] [PubMed]
14. Hasan, S.A.; Cordell, C.L.; Rauls, R.B.; Eidt, J.F. Brachial artery injury with a proximal humerus fracture in a 10-year-old girl. *Am. J. Orthop.* **2009**, *38*, 462–466. [PubMed]

Disclaimer/Publisher's Note: The statements, opinions and data contained in all publications are solely those of the individual author(s) and contributor(s) and not of MDPI and/or the editor(s). MDPI and/or the editor(s) disclaim responsibility for any injury to people or property resulting from any ideas, methods, instructions or products referred to in the content.

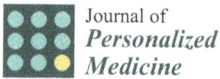

Case Report

Staged Treatment of Posttraumatic Tibial Osteomyelitis with Rib Graft and Serratus Anterior Muscle Autografts—Case Report

Bogdan Anglitoiu [1,2,3], Ahmed Abu-Awwad [1,2,3,*], Jenel-Marain Patrascu, Jr. [1,2,3], Simona-Alina Abu-Awwad [2,4], Anca Raluca Dinu [2,5,6], Alina-Daniela Totorean [2,5,6], Dan Cojocaru [2,3] and Mihai-Alexandru Sandesc [1,2,3]

[1] Department XV—Discipline of Orthopedics—Traumatology, Victor Babes University of Medicine and Pharmacy, Eftimie Murgu Square, No. 2, 300041 Timisoara, Romania; bogdananglitoiu@gmail.com (B.A.); patrascujenel@yahoo.com (J.-M.P.J.); sandesc.mihai@umft.ro (M.-A.S.)

[2] "Pius Brinzeu" Emergency Clinical County Hospital, Bld Liviu Rebreanu, No. 156, 300723 Timisoara, Romania; alina.abuawwad@umft.ro (S.-A.A.-A.); dinu.anca@umft.ro (A.R.D.); totorean.alina@umft.ro (A.-D.T.); dr_cojocaru@yahoo.com (D.C.)

[3] Research Center University Professor Doctor Teodor Șora, Victor Babes University of Medicine and Pharmacy, Eftimie Murgu Square, No. 2, 300041 Timisoara, Romania

[4] Department XII—Discipline of Obstetrics and Gynecology, Victor Babes University of Medicine and Pharmacy, Eftimie Murgu Square, No. 2, 300041 Timisoara, Romania

[5] Department XVI—Balneology, Medical Recovery and Rheumatology, Victor Babes University of Medicine and Pharmacy, Eftimie Murgu Square, No. 2, 300041 Timisoara, Romania

[6] Research Center for Assessment of Human Motion and Functionality and Disability, Victor Babes University of Medicine and Pharmacy, Eftimie Murgu Square, No. 2, 300041 Timisoara, Romania

* Correspondence: ahm.abuawwad@umft.ro

Abstract: Osteomyelitis of the tibia is a challenging condition, particularly when it occurs as a result of trauma. This abstract presents a case study detailing the successful staged treatment of posttraumatic tibial osteomyelitis utilizing a unique combination of rib graft and serratus anterior muscle. This medical abstract presents a case study of a 52-year-old male with a history of heavy smoking and obliterating arteriopathy of the lower limbs. The patient sustained a traumatic open fracture classified as Type IIIA Gustilo Anderson involving one-third of the distal right tibia diaphysis, with an associated right fibular malleolus fracture. The treatment approach comprised multiple stages, focusing on wound management, infection control, and limb salvage. The initial stage involved the application of an external fixation device in the emergency setting. Seven days later, an osteosynthesis procedure was performed using a Kuntscher nail and wire cerclage. However, complications emerged, with wound dehiscence and purulent secretion observed at 14 days postsurgery. Subsequently, secondary suturing was carried out at the 20-day mark. The second stage of the treatment involved implant removal, wide excisional debridement, pulse lavage, osteoclasia, and relaxation of the peroneal malleolus. A monoplane external fixation system was applied. As a part of postoperative care, aspiration therapy with a vacuum pump was administered, along with a 10-day course of vancomycin according to the antibiogram. Positive clinical signs of healing were noted, and sterile cultures confirmed the results. The third stage of the intervention focused on grafting the osteomuscular defect, utilizing autografts from the rib and serratus anterior muscle. The external fixator was maintained in place during this phase. In the fourth and final stage, after an 8-week integration period of the musculocutaneous flap, the external fixator was removed, and internal fixation was accomplished with a blocked Less Invasive Stabilization System (LISS) plate inserted using the Minimally Invasive Plate Osteosynthesis (MIPO) technique. This case underscores the significance of a multistage approach in managing complex limb injuries, emphasizing the importance of timely intervention, infection control, and innovative techniques for limb salvage and restoration of function.

Keywords: staged treatment; posttraumatic tibial osteomyelitis; rib graft; serratus anterior muscle; limb salvage

1. Introduction

Posttraumatic tibial osteomyelitis is a complex and often refractory condition that presents significant challenges for both patients and healthcare providers. Its genesis is frequently rooted in traumatic injuries, leading to devastating consequences for the affected limb and overall quality of life. In this context, our case report explores a compelling and innovative approach to managing posttraumatic tibial osteomyelitis, centering on the staged treatment with the novel inclusion of rib graft and serratus anterior muscle autografts. This multifaceted case report not only delves into the clinical intricacies of the case but also serves as a testament to the remarkable capabilities of modern orthopedic surgery [1–3].

Osteomyelitis, an infection of the bone, represents a formidable challenge in the realm of musculoskeletal health [4–6]. When it occurs in the tibia, it can result in substantial morbidity and potentially devastating consequences, necessitating a multifaceted approach to restore function and quality of life. While osteomyelitis can stem from various sources, posttraumatic osteomyelitis, as the name implies, arises following traumatic injuries to the bone. Such injuries often result in open fractures, which increase the risk of infection due to the exposure of the bone to external contaminants. Successful treatment of posttraumatic tibial osteomyelitis requires a delicate balance between infection control, wound management, and strategies to promote limb salvage [1,3,7–9].

This case report serves as an invaluable illustration of the critical significance of a staged approach to complex limb injuries, especially when osteomyelitis is involved. It emphasizes the pivotal role of timely intervention and the paramount importance of infection control. Furthermore, this report showcases the innovative use of rib graft and serratus anterior muscle autografts as a viable solution for addressing complex osteo-muscular defects. This case report also underscores the remarkable potential of contemporary orthopedic techniques, like MIPO, to facilitate limb salvage and restore function in the face of formidable challenges. Through a meticulous exploration of this complex case, we aim to contribute to the body of knowledge in the field of orthopedic surgery and inspire further research and innovation in the management of posttraumatic tibial osteomyelitis.

2. Case Report
2.1. Patient Selection

The subject of this case study was a 52-year-old male patient with a history of chronic heavy smoking and a confirmed diagnosis of obliterating arteriopathy affecting the lower limbs. He presented with a traumatic open fracture of the distal right tibia diaphysis, which was classified as a Type IIIA Gustilo Anderson fracture involving one-third of the tibia's length. Simultaneously, the patient had suffered a fracture of the right fibular malleolus. Informed consent was obtained from the patient for the entire course of treatment and for the subsequent publication of this case report.

In the presented clinical case, the patient exhibits a notable medical profile, including a daily cigarette consumption of one pack, a lack of surgical history, moderate alcohol intake, and a confirmed diagnosis of peripheral artery disease (PAD) with an absence of other comorbidities.

The patient at the center of this case report is a 52-year-old male who presented with a challenging clinical profile. His medical history includes chronic heavy smoking and a diagnosis of obliterating arteriopathy of the lower limbs, predisposing him to complications in the management of vascular and wound-related issues. The primary injury was a traumatic open fracture of the distal right tibia diaphysis, classified as a Type IIIA Gustilo Anderson fracture, which accounts for a substantial portion of the tibia. This fracture was further complicated by a concurrent right fibular malleolus fracture. The combination of these factors made his case particularly intricate and demanding.

The diagnosis of osteomyelitis was established through a comprehensive approach, considering the patient's clinical presentation, positive culture findings, and supportive imaging results. The convergence of these diagnostic elements collectively confirmed the presence of osteomyelitis in the patient.

The treatment approach adopted for this patient was a staged one, with distinct phases carefully designed to address the challenges posed by his condition. The initial phase involved the immediate application of an external fixation device in the emergency setting, providing stability to the fractured bone segments. Subsequently, seven days postinjury, an osteosynthesis procedure was undertaken, which included the insertion of a Kuntscher nail and wire cerclage to facilitate the alignment and fixation of the fractured tibia. However, the patient's course was marked by complications, with wound dehiscence and the emergence of purulent wound secretions observed at the 14-day mark following surgery. In response, a second-stage intervention was initiated, involving implant removal, wide excisional debridement, pulse lavage to cleanse the wound, osteoclasia for bone remodeling, and relaxation of the peroneal malleolus. To maintain bone stability and support the healing process, an external fixation device with a monoplane design was retained.

In addition to these surgical interventions, postoperative care included aspiration therapy with a vacuum pump and a 10-day course of vancomycin, a potent antibiotic agent chosen based on the antibiogram. Positive clinical signs of healing were observed, and sterile cultures confirmed the resolution of the infection.

The third phase of treatment was marked by the unique approach of grafting the osteo-muscular defect with autografts sourced from the rib and serratus anterior muscle. Throughout this stage, the external fixation device continued to provide support and stability.

The fourth and final stage, carried out after an 8-week integration period of the musculocutaneous flap, entailed the removal of the external fixation device and the implementation of internal fixation using a blocked Less Invasive Stabilization System (LISS) plate. This technique, known as Minimally Invasive Plate Osteosynthesis (MIPO), is particularly valuable for reducing the invasiveness of surgical procedures and promoting quicker recovery.

2.2. Treatment Staging

The treatment plan was divided into four distinct stages, each with specific objectives and interventions:

Stage 1: initial stabilization and osteosynthesis (Figure 1).

Objective: To provide immediate stabilization of the open tibial fracture and initiate the process of bone fixation.

Methods: The patient underwent external fixation in the emergency room.

Seven days postinjury, an osteosynthesis procedure was performed, involving the placement of a Kuntscher nail and wire cerclage (Figures 2 and 3).

Stage 2: Infection control and debridement (Figure 4).

Objective: To address complications, prevent infection, and manage the wound dehiscence.

Methods: Implants from the initial surgery were removed, wide excisional debridement of necrotic tissue was carried out, pulse lavage was performed for wound cleansing, and osteoclasia was executed to facilitate bone healing. The peroneal malleolus was also manipulated, and a monoplane external fixation system was applied. Post-operatively, aspiration therapy using a vacuum pump was employed, and antibiotic therapy with vancomycin (2 g/day) for ten days was initiated based on the results of the antibiogram.

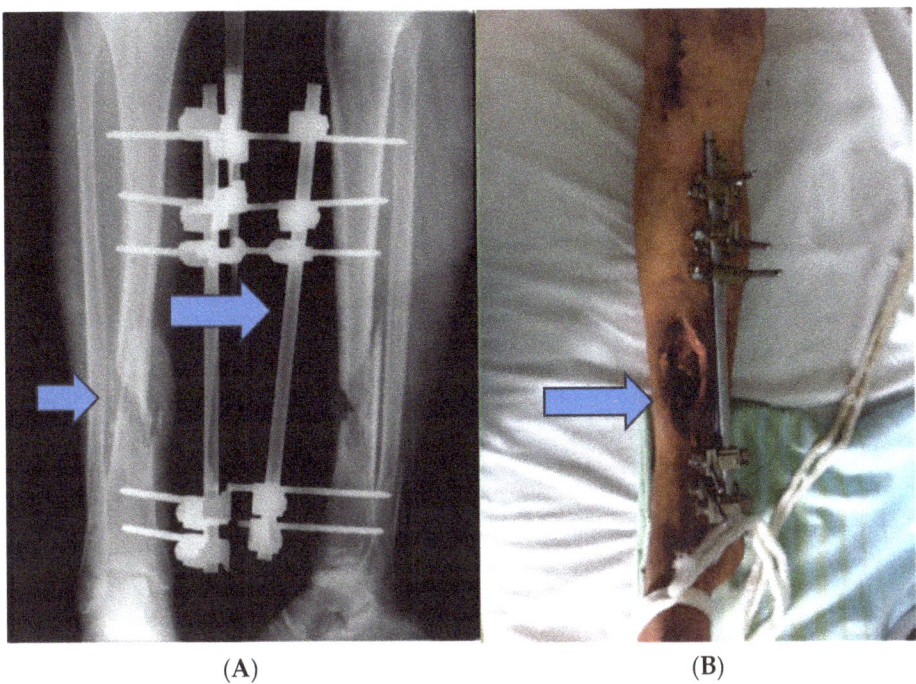

Figure 1. (**A**,**B**) External fixation in the emergency room.

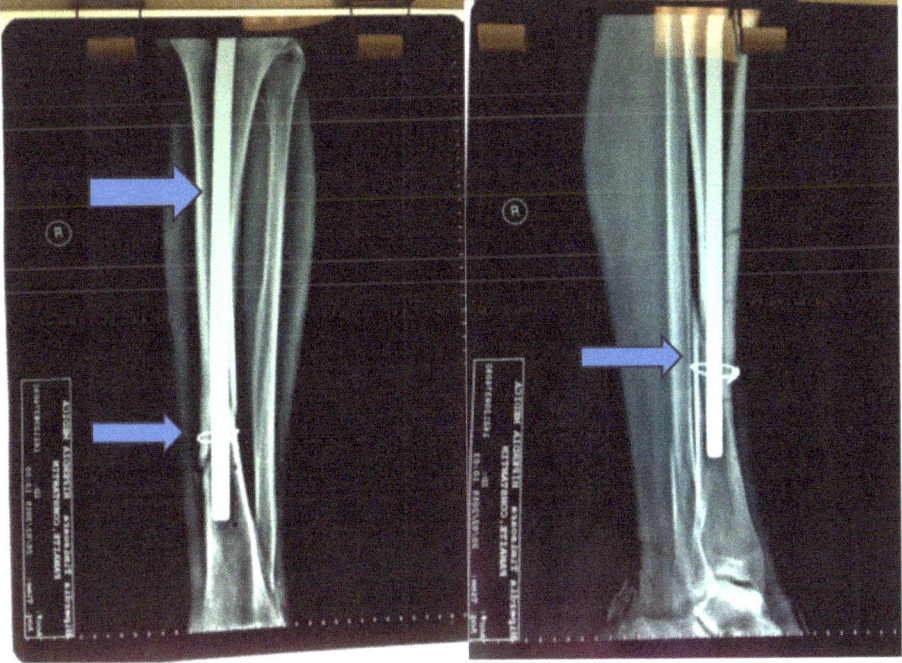

Figure 2. Kuntscher nail and wire cerclage.

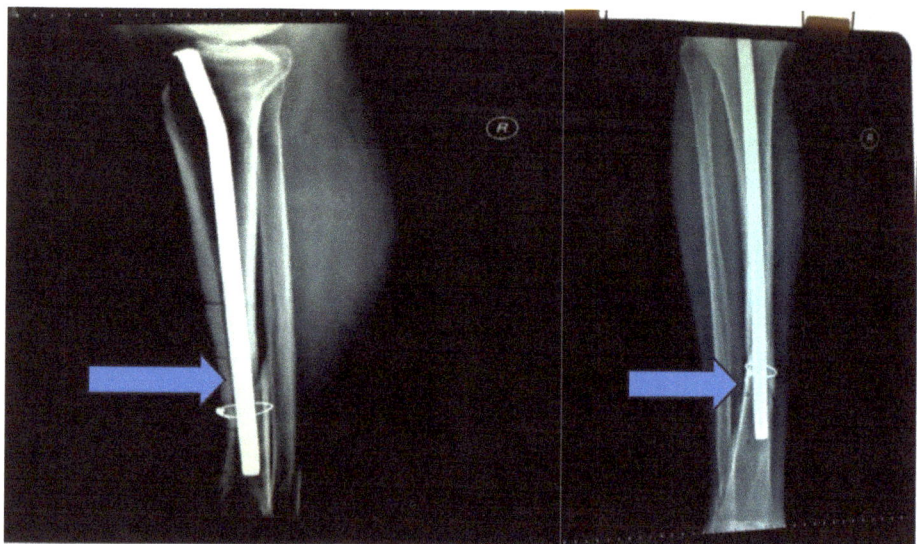

Figure 3. Postoperative X-ray—2 months.

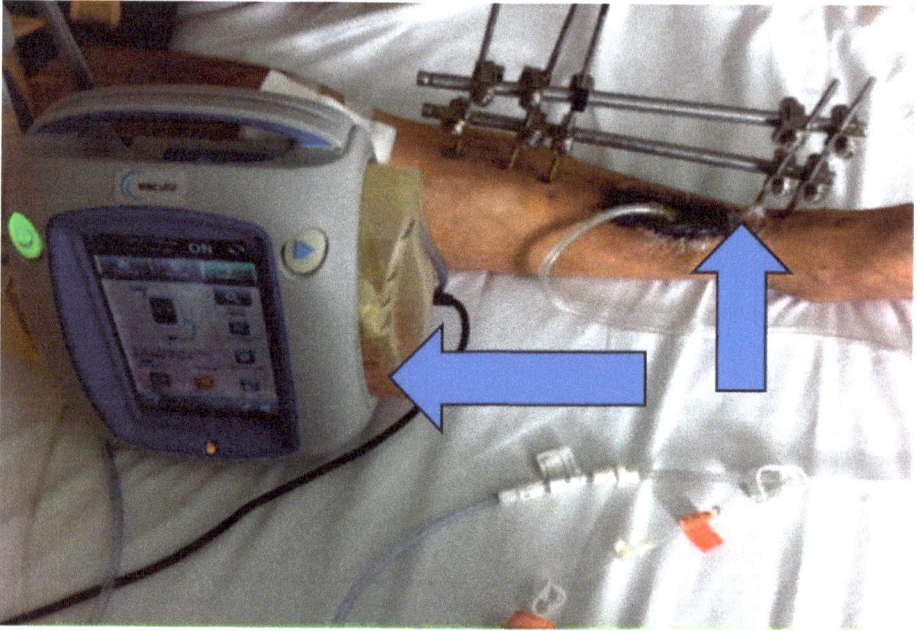

Figure 4. Vacuum pump and ex fix.

Stage 3: Grafting for osteo-muscular defect (Figure 5).
Objective: To address the osteo-muscular defect and facilitate tissue regeneration.
Methods: This stage involved grafting the osteo-muscular defect using autografts harvested from the rib and serratus anterior muscle. The external fixation device was maintained to provide support during the graft integration period.

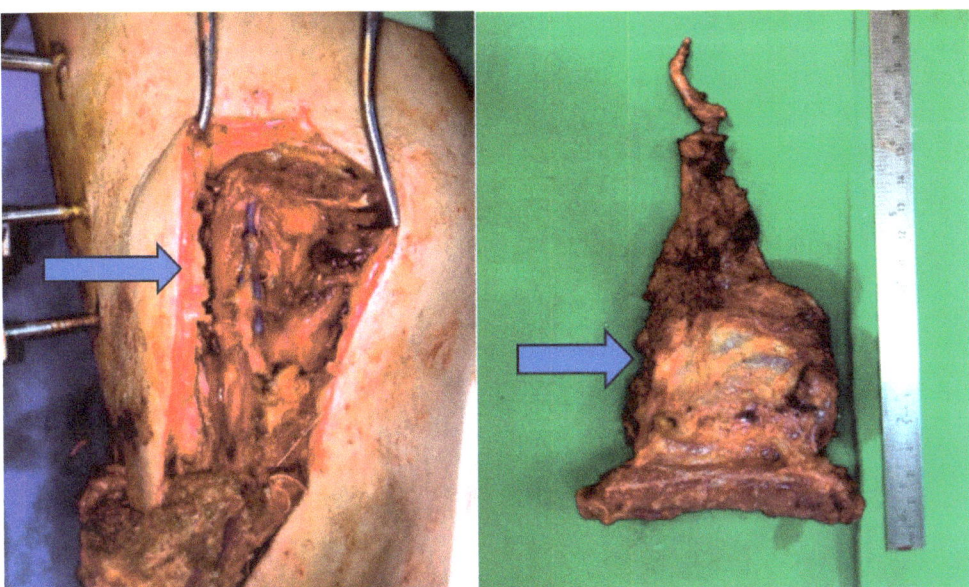

Figure 5. Osteo-muscular defect.

Stage 4: Flap integration and internal fixation (Figure 6).

Objective: To ensure the integration of the musculocutaneous flap and provide internal fixation to stabilize the tibia.

Methods: After an 8-week integration period, the musculocutaneous flap was deemed stable. The external fixator was removed, and internal fixation was achieved using a blocked Less Invasive Stabilization System (LISS) plate, which was inserted utilizing the Minimally Invasive Plate Osteosynthesis (MIPO) technique.

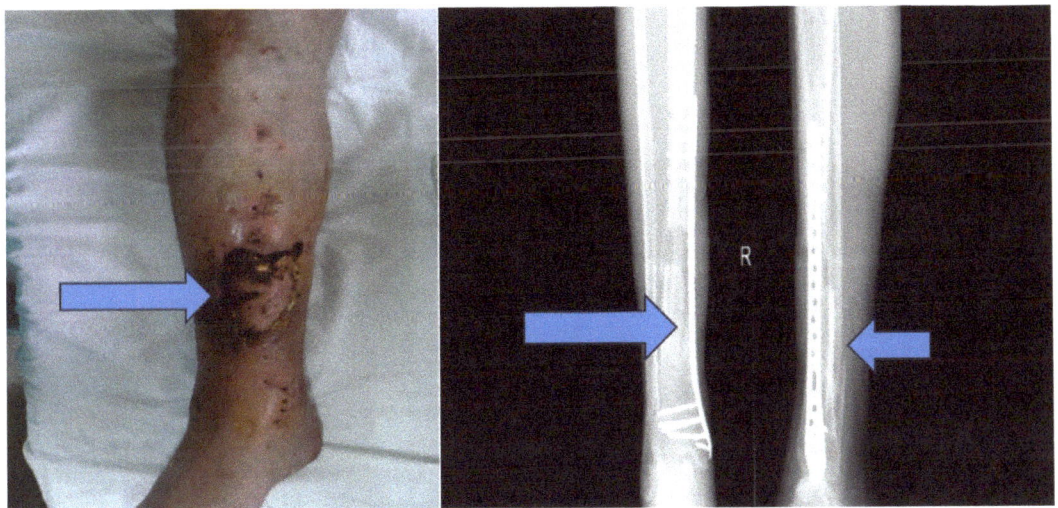

Figure 6. Musculocutaneous flap and internal fixation was achieved using a blocked Less Invasive Stabilization System (LISS) plate.

2.3. Antibiotic Therapy and Medication

Antibiotic therapy was initiated as per the results of the antibiogram, with vancomycin administered at a dosage of 2 g/day for ten days postoperatively during the second stage of treatment.

The administration of vancomycin was extended to a duration of 21 days to effectively address the osteomyelitis in accordance with hospital guidelines. This decision was guided by a systematic approach, including negative culture results. The antibiotic regimen was appropriately tailored based on the specific characteristics of the infection and in adherence to established clinical guidelines, ensuring a thorough and evidence-based treatment strategy.

The patient received anticoagulant therapy during the hospitalization period and continued the regimen postdischarge, adhering to the prescribed course for a total duration of 35 days. No alterations were identified in the patient's everyday medication regimen during the course of our assessment.

2.4. Clinical Assessment and Follow-Up

Throughout the treatment, the patient's progress was closely monitored, and clinical signs of healing were recorded. Sterile cultures were obtained to verify the resolution of the infection. The patient's overall condition, pain level, and functional status were assessed at regular intervals (Figure 7).

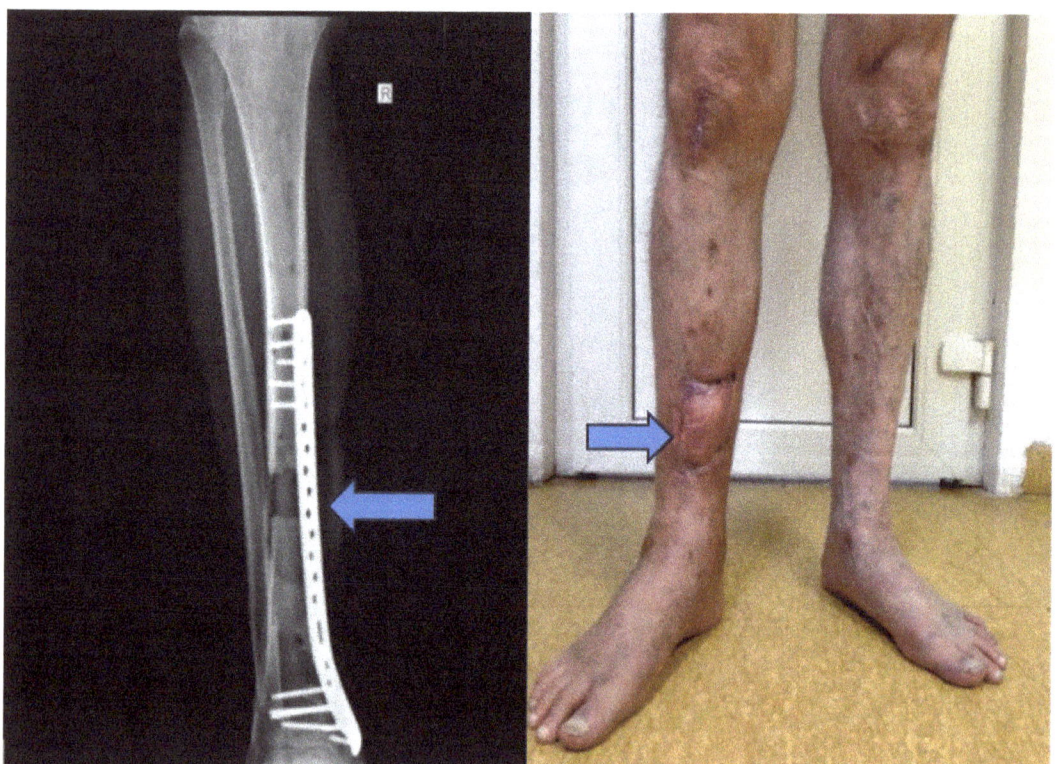

Figure 7. Six-month follow-up.

2.5. Data Analysis

Quantitative data, including laboratory results and clinical assessments, were analyzed to evaluate the progress of the patient's condition throughout the four treatment stages. The success of the staged approach was determined by the resolution of osteomyelitis, the prevention of complications, and the restoration of limb function.

2.6. Ethical Considerations

This case study was conducted in accordance with the ethical principles outlined in the Declaration of Helsinki. Informed consent was obtained from the patient for the treatment and subsequent publication of this case report, ensuring the protection of patient confidentiality and privacy.

2.7. Management of the Case

The management of posttraumatic tibial osteomyelitis is a complex and challenging endeavor, especially in cases resulting from trauma. This case study details a successful staged treatment approach in a 52-year-old male with a history of heavy smoking and obliterating arteriopathy of the lower limbs who presented with a traumatic open fracture of the right tibia and fibular malleolus. The treatment strategy consisted of multiple stages, focusing on wound management, infection control, and limb salvage.

The initial stage involved the application of an external fixation device in the emergency setting. Subsequent to this, an osteosynthesis procedure using a Kuntscher nail and wire cerclage was performed seven days later. However, complications emerged, with wound dehiscence and purulent secretion observed at 14 days postsurgery. Secondary suturing was undertaken at the 20-day mark, which resolved the wound issues.

The second stage of treatment encompassed implant removal, wide excisional debridement, pulse lavage, osteoclasia, and relaxation of the peroneal malleolus. A monoplane external fixation system was applied, followed by aspiration therapy with a vacuum pump and a 10-day course of vancomycin based on the antibiogram. Positive clinical signs of healing were noted during this phase, and sterile cultures confirmed the absence of infection.

In the third stage, the focus shifted to addressing the osteo-muscular defect through grafting. Autografts from the rib and serratus anterior muscle were utilized to reconstruct the bone and soft tissue. Throughout this stage, the external fixator was maintained to provide stability and support to the graft site.

The fourth and final stage marked the conclusion of the intervention after an 8-week integration period of the musculocutaneous flap. During this phase, the external fixator was removed, and internal fixation was achieved using a blocked Less Invasive Stabilization System (LISS) plate, inserted via the Minimally Invasive Plate Osteosynthesis (MIPO) technique.

This comprehensive approach to managing posttraumatic tibial osteomyelitis led to a successful outcome. The patient experienced significant improvements in clinical symptoms and functional recovery. The staged treatment allowed for the resolution of the infection, restoration of bone continuity, and reconstruction of the soft tissue defect, ultimately leading to limb salvage.

Throughout the entire treatment process, diligent monitoring of the patient's progress and the use of appropriate antibiotics guided by antibiogram results played a pivotal role in ensuring the success of the intervention.

This case highlights the significance of a multistage approach in managing complex limb injuries, emphasizing the importance of timely intervention, infection control, and innovative techniques for limb salvage and the restoration of function. The utilization of autografts from the rib and serratus anterior muscle represents a novel and effective approach for addressing osteo-muscular defects in such challenging cases. Overall, this case serves as a testament to the potential for successful outcomes in the management of posttraumatic tibial osteomyelitis through a systematic and innovative approach.

3. Discussion

Posttraumatic tibial osteomyelitis, especially when resulting from trauma, presents a formidable challenge for healthcare professionals. The case study presented here sheds light on the successful management of this complex condition in a 52-year-old male with a history of heavy smoking and obliterating arteriopathy of the lower limbs. The treatment strategy, involving a multistaged approach, aimed at wound management, infection control, and limb salvage, ultimately led to a positive outcome.

Posttraumatic tibial osteomyelitis poses unique difficulties due to the traumatic etiology, which often results in extensive soft tissue and bone damage [7–10]. The risk factors associated with this case, such as heavy smoking and arteriopathy, further complicated the treatment. Management strategies must be carefully planned to address these challenges and ensure a successful outcome.

The success of this case can be attributed to the staged treatment approach, which allowed for the systematic and comprehensive management of the condition. Each stage was meticulously planned and executed, with the goals of achieving infection control, promoting healing, and restoring limb function. The use of external fixation, osteosynthesis, debridement, aspiration therapy, and grafting in different stages highlights the importance of tailoring treatment to the specific needs of the patient.

Infection control played a pivotal role in this case, as infection is a common and serious complication of tibial osteomyelitis [11–13]. The initial emergence of wound complications was promptly addressed, and secondary suturing was performed to resolve the issues. Subsequently, wide excisional debridement, pulse lavage, and antibiotic therapy based on antibiogram results were employed to eradicate the infection. Monitoring for positive clinical signs of healing and sterile cultures confirmed the success of these interventions.

The innovative use of autografts from the rib and serratus anterior muscle to address the osteo-muscular defect is a noteworthy aspect of this case. This technique showcases the importance of exploring novel approaches to managing complex limb injuries. The combination of bone and soft tissue reconstruction using autografts contributed to the overall success of the treatment, ultimately leading to limb salvage.

The hallmark of this case report is the utilization of innovative techniques in the form of rib graft and serratus anterior muscle autografts. The combination of these grafts allowed for the reconstruction of both bone and soft tissue defects, addressing the complexities of posttraumatic tibial osteomyelitis. This approach exemplifies the necessity of exploring novel methods and tailoring treatment strategies to the specific needs of each patient. The multifaceted approach, consisting of multiple stages and focusing on infection control, wound management, and limb salvage, showcases the versatility and adaptability required to manage such intricate cases successfully.

This case underscores the significance of a multistage approach in the management of complex limb injuries. The timely transition from one stage to the next ensured that the patient received the necessary treatments at the right juncture of their recovery [14–16]. This approach minimizes complications and maximizes the chances of successful outcomes.

The staged treatment strategy employed in this case led to significant improvements in the patient's clinical symptoms and functional recovery. The restoration of bone continuity and reconstruction of soft tissue defects contributed to limb salvage, preserving both function and quality of life for the patient.

Posttraumatic tibial osteomyelitis is a complex and demanding condition that poses significant challenges to both patients and healthcare providers. This case report presented a unique and successful approach to managing this condition through staged treatment involving rib graft and serratus anterior muscle autografts. The intricate interplay of trauma, additional risk factors, and extent of tissue and bone involvement necessitates a comprehensive and innovative treatment strategy. In the culmination of this case, we underscore the significance of such an approach and its potential to enhance patient outcomes and advance the field of orthopedic and trauma surgery.

This case report serves as a testament to the potential for successful outcomes in the management of posttraumatic tibial osteomyelitis through innovative and multifaceted approaches. It is imperative to recognize that while the condition is complex and challenging, there are strategies that can lead to positive results. The patient in this case experienced significant improvements in clinical symptoms and functional recovery, emphasizing the effectiveness of the chosen treatment strategy.

The staged treatment of posttraumatic tibial osteomyelitis with rib graft and serratus anterior muscle is a topic that has gained attention in the recent literature. The existing body of research highlights the significance of adopting a staged approach for managing posttraumatic tibial osteomyelitis, focusing on the utilization of rib grafts and the serratus anterior muscle. Studies underscore the efficacy of this treatment strategy in achieving infection control, promoting healing, and restoring limb function.

Literature reviews indicate that the staged treatment approach allows for systematic and comprehensive management, with each stage meticulously planned to address specific aspects of the condition. The incorporation of rib grafts and the serratus anterior muscle introduces innovative techniques that contribute to the success of the treatment. These techniques not only demonstrate the adaptability of the approach but also underscore the importance of tailoring treatment to the unique needs of each patient.

Overall, the literature supports the notion that the staged treatment of posttraumatic tibial osteomyelitis with rib graft and serratus anterior muscle is a promising avenue for effective and individualized patient care. Further exploration and in-depth analysis of these innovative techniques are warranted to continually enhance our understanding and refine treatment protocols for this challenging condition.

4. Conclusions

A key takeaway from this case report is the importance of timely intervention. The staged treatment approach ensured that each aspect of the patient's condition was addressed at the most opportune moment in their recovery journey. This minimized complications and optimized the chances of a favorable outcome. Additionally, the diligent attention to infection control cannot be overstated. Promptly addressing complications; employing wide excisional debridement, aspiration therapy, and appropriate antibiotic therapy based on antibiogram results; and closely monitoring the patient for positive clinical signs of healing were all critical in eradicating the infection and achieving the ultimate goal of limb salvage.

Moving forward, further research and exploration of similar approaches are paramount. The field of orthopedic and trauma surgery continues to evolve, and innovation is essential to improving outcomes for patients with posttraumatic tibial osteomyelitis. The lessons learned from this case report, particularly the use of rib graft and serratus anterior muscle autografts, could inspire further investigations into the potential benefits of these techniques and the refinement of existing treatment protocols.

In conclusion, the staged treatment of posttraumatic tibial osteomyelitis with rib graft and serratus anterior muscle autografts represents a promising and innovative approach to addressing a challenging medical condition. This case report demonstrates that with a careful and comprehensive strategy, patients can achieve positive outcomes even in the face of complex and multifaceted clinical challenges. As the field of orthopedic and trauma surgery continues to progress, the lessons from this case serve as a reminder of the potential for innovation and improvement in patient care, particularly for those facing the daunting prospect of posttraumatic tibial osteomyelitis.

This case demonstrates the potential for successful outcomes when such an approach is implemented, highlighting the importance of innovative techniques, timely intervention, and meticulous infection control. Further research and exploration of similar approaches are essential to advance the field of orthopedic and trauma surgery and improve the outcomes for patients with posttraumatic tibial osteomyelitis.

Author Contributions: Conceptualization, A.A.-A., B.A. and M.-A.S.; methodology, S.-A.A.-A.; software, D.C.; validation, A.A.-A., A.-D.T. and A.R.D.; formal analysis, S.-A.A.-A.; investigation, D.C.; resources, M.-A.S.; data curation, B.A. and J.-M.P.J.; writing—original draft preparation, A.A.-A.; writing—review and editing, S.-A.A.-A.; visualization, A.R.D.; supervision, B.A.; project administration, M.-A.S.; funding acquisition, A.-D.T. and J.-M.P.J. All authors have read and agreed to the published version of the manuscript.

Funding: This research received no external funding.

Institutional Review Board Statement: This study was conducted in accordance with the Declaration of Helsinki and approved by the Institutional Review Board of Pius Brînzeu County Clinical Emergency Hospital of Timisoara/No 404/11.08.2023.

Informed Consent Statement: Informed consent was obtained from all subjects involved in this study.

Data Availability Statement: The data presented in this study are available on request from the corresponding author.

Conflicts of Interest: The authors declare no conflict of interest.

References

1. Tetsworth, K.; Paley, D.; Sen, C.; Jaffe, M.; Maar, D.C.; Glatt, V.; Hohmann, E.; Herzenberg, J.E. Bone transport versus acute shortening for the management of infected tibial non-unions with bone defects. *Injury* **2017**, *48*, 2276–2284. [CrossRef] [PubMed]
2. Harshwal, R.K.; Sankhala, S.S.; Jalan, D. Management of nonunion of lower-extremity long bones using mono-lateral external fixator-report of 37 cases. *Injury* **2014**, *45*, 560–567. [CrossRef] [PubMed]
3. McNally, M.; Ferguson, J.; Kugan, R.; Stubbs, D. Ilizarov treatment protocols in the management of infected nonunion of the Tibia. *J. Orthop. Trauma* **2017**, *31* (Suppl. S5), S47–S54. [CrossRef]
4. Oh, C.-W.; Apivatthakakul, T.; Oh, J.-K.; Kim, J.-W.; Lee, H.-J.; Kyung, H.-S.; Baek, S.-G.; Jung, G.-H. Bone transport with an external fixator and a locking plate for segmental tibial defects. *Bone Joint J.* **2013**, *95*, 1667–1672. [CrossRef] [PubMed]
5. Aktuglu, K.; Erol, K.; Vahabi, A. Ilizarov bone transport and treatment of critical-sized tibial bone defects: A narrative review. *J. Orthop. Traumatol.* **2019**, *20*, 22. [CrossRef] [PubMed]
6. Klosterhalfen, B.; Peters, K.M.; Tons, C.; Hauptmann, S.; Klein, C.L.; Kirkpatrick, C.J. Local and systemic inflammatory mediator release in patients with acute and chronic posttraumatic osteomyelitis. *J. Trauma* **1996**, *40*, 372–378. [CrossRef]
7. Du, B.; Su, Y.; Li, D.; Ji, S.; Lu, Y.; Xu, Y.; Yang, Y.; Zhang, K.; Li, Z.; Ma, T. Analysis of risk factors for serous exudation of biodegradable material calcium sulfate in the treatment of fracture-related infections. *Front. Bioeng. Biotechnol.* **2023**, *11*, 1189085. [CrossRef] [PubMed]
8. Morgenstern, M.; Kühl, R.; Eckardt, H.; Acklin, Y.; Stanic, B.; Garcia, M.; Baumhoer, D.; Metsemakers, W.-J. Diagnostic challenges and future perspectives in fracture-related infection. *Injury Int. J. Care Inj.* **2018**, *49*, S83–S90. [CrossRef]
9. Neut, D.; van de Belt, H.; Stokroos, I.; van Horn, J.R.; van der Mei, H.C.; Busscher, H.J. Biomaterial-associated infection of gentamicin-loaded pmma beads in orthopaedic revision surgery. *J. Antimicrob. Chemother.* **2001**, *47*, 885–891. [CrossRef]
10. Panagopoulos, P.; Drosos, G.; Maltezos, E.; Papanas, N. Local antibiotic delivery systems in diabetic foot osteomyelitis: Time for one step beyond? *Int. J. Low. Extrem. Wounds* **2015**, *14*, 87–91. [CrossRef] [PubMed]
11. Parker, A.C.; Smith, J.K.; Courtney, H.S.; Haggard, W.O. Evaluation of two sources of calcium sulfate for a local drug delivery system: A pilot study. *Clin. Orthop. Rel. Res.* **2011**, *469*, 3008–3015. [CrossRef] [PubMed]
12. Rice, O.M.; Phelps, K.D.; Seymour, R.; Askam, B.M.; Kempton, L.B.; Chen, A.; Dart, S.; Hsu, J.R. Single-stage treatment of fracture-related infections. *J. Orthop. Trauma* **2021**, *35*, S42–S43. [CrossRef]
13. Shi, X.; Wu, Y.; Ni, H.; Li, M.; Zhang, C.; Qi, B.; Wei, M.; Wang, T.; Xu, Y. Antibiotic-loaded calcium sulfate in clinical treatment of chronic osteomyelitis: A systematic review and meta-analysis. *J. Orthop. Surg. Res.* **2022**, *17*, 104. [CrossRef]
14. Simpson, A.H.; Tsang, J. Current treatment of infected non-union after intramedullary nailing. *Inj. Int. J. Care Inj.* **2017**, *48*, S82–S90. [CrossRef] [PubMed]
15. Aktuglu, K.; Günay, H.; Alakbarov, J. Monofocal bone transport technique for bone defects greater than 5 cm in tibia: Our experience in a case series of 24 patients. *Injury* **2016**, *47* (Suppl. S6), S40–S46. [CrossRef] [PubMed]
16. Tuttle, M.S.; Mostow, E.; Mukherjee, P.; Hu, F.Z.; Melton-Kreft, R.; Ehrlich, G.D.; Dowd, S.E.; Ghannoum, M.A. Characterization of bacterial communities in venous insufficiency wounds by use of conventional culture and molecular diagnostic methods. *J. Clin. Microbiol.* **2011**, *49*, 3812–3819. [CrossRef] [PubMed]

Disclaimer/Publisher's Note: The statements, opinions and data contained in all publications are solely those of the individual author(s) and contributor(s) and not of MDPI and/or the editor(s). MDPI and/or the editor(s) disclaim responsibility for any injury to people or property resulting from any ideas, methods, instructions or products referred to in the content.

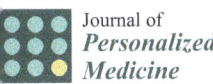

Article

Predictive Performance of Scoring Systems for Mortality Risk in Patients with Cryptococcemia: An Observational Study

Wei-Kai Liao [1,2,3,4,5,6,†], Ming-Shun Hsieh [6,7,8,†], Sung-Yuan Hu [1,2,3,4,6,*], Shih-Che Huang [2,9,10], Che-An Tsai [11], Yan-Zin Chang [1,12,*] and Yi-Chun Tsai [3]

1. Institute of Medicine, Chung Shan Medical University, Taichung 40201, Taiwan; kents90124@hotmail.com
2. School of Medicine, Chung Shan Medical University, Taichung 40201, Taiwan; cucu0214@gmail.com
3. Department of Emergency Medicine, Taichung Veterans General Hospital, Taichung 407219, Taiwan; rosa87324@gmail.com
4. Department of Post-Baccalaureate Medicine, College of Medicine, National Chung Hsing University, Taichung 402, Taiwan
5. School of Medicine, National Cheng Kung University, Tainan 701, Taiwan
6. School of Medicine, National Yang Ming Chiao Tung University, Taipei 11217, Taiwan; edmingshun@gmail.com
7. Department of Emergency Medicine, Taipei Veterans General Hospital, Taoyuan Branch, Taoyuan 330, Taiwan
8. Department of Emergency Medicine, Taipei Veterans General Hospital, Taipei 11217, Taiwan
9. Department of Emergency Medicine, Chung Shan Medical University Hospital, Taichung 40201, Taiwan
10. Lung Cancer Research Center, Chung Shan Medical University Hospital, Taichung 40201, Taiwan
11. Division of Infectious Disease, Department of Internal Medicine, Taichung Veterans General Hospital, Taichung 40705, Taiwan; lucky-sam@yahoo.com.tw
12. Department of Clinical Laboratory, Drug Testing Center, Chung Shan Medical University Hospital, Taichung 40201, Taiwan
* Correspondence: song9168@pie.com.tw (S.-Y.H.); yzc@csmu.edu.tw (Y.-Z.C.); Tel.: +886-4-23592525 (ext. 3601) (S.-Y.H.); +886-4-24730022 (ext. 11699) (Y.-Z.C.); Fax: +886-4-23594065 (S.-Y.H.)
† These authors contributed equally to this work.

Abstract: Cryptococcal infection is usually diagnosed in immunocompromised individuals and those with meningeal involvement, accounting for most cryptococcosis. Cryptococcemia indicates a poor prognosis and prolongs the course of treatment. We use the scoring systems to predict the mortality risk of cryptococcal fungemia. This was a single hospital-based retrospective study on patients diagnosed with cryptococcal fungemia confirmed by at least one blood culture collected from the emergency department covering January 2012 and December 2020 from electronic medical records in the Taichung Veterans General Hospital. We enrolled 42 patients, including 28 (66.7%) males and 14 (33.3%) females with a mean age of 63.0 ± 19.7 years. The hospital stay ranged from 1 to 170 days (a mean stay of 44.4 days), and the overall mortality rate was 64.3% (27/42). In univariate analysis, the AUC of ROC for MEWS, RAPS, qSOFA, MEWS plus GCS, REMS, NEWS, and MEDS showed 0.833, 0.842, 0.848, 0.846, 0.846, 0.878, and 0.905. In the multivariate Cox regression analysis, all scoring systems, older age, lactate, MAP, and DBP, indicated significant differences between survivor and non-survivor groups. Our results show that all scoring systems could apply in predicting the outcome of patients with cryptococcal fungemia, and the MEDS displays the best performance. We recommend a further large-scale prospective study for patients with cryptococcal fungemia.

Keywords: cryptococcus; emergency department; mortality risk; risk factors; scoring systems

1. Introduction

Cryptococcus has encapsulated yeast that lives in the natural environment, but it is rarely a pathogen in individuals with a healthy immune system. In literature reviews, *Cryptococcus neoformans* is humans' most common pathogenic cryptococcal species, usually diagnosed in immunocompromised individuals [1]. In addition, *Cryptococcus gattii* is reported as a rare pathogen in cryptococcosis cases and is predominantly a causative pathogen in immunocompetent individuals [2,3]. The central nervous system (CNS) involvement generally accounts for most cryptococcosis [4], so the clinicians suggest evaluating CNS involvement in patients with evidence of cryptococcal infection. Cryptococcal meningitis is estimated to be associated with human immunodeficiency virus (HIV), with the global occurrence of 223,100 cases in 2014 and the annual deaths of 181,100 patients [5]. Other possible infected sites of cryptococcosis, including the respiratory tract, urinary tract, skin, bone, eye, and gastrointestinal tract, have been reported in previous studies [6–15].

Cryptococcemia occurred in only 10% to 30% of all cryptococcal diseases but was often associated with prolonging the clinical course of treatment and higher mortality rates [16–20]. Unfortunately, few published articles on cryptococcemia analyzed the clinical characteristics and outcomes according to clinical presentations, comorbidities, and scoring systems. Previous studies reported the presence of an immunocompromised condition, liver cirrhosis, high Acute Physiology and Chronic Health Evaluation (APACHE) II score ($\geq$20), and severity of sepsis, and they were associated with a higher mortality rate [18,20]. Published articles did not establish the predictive factors or scoring systems to evaluate cryptococcemia.

In recent studies, they applied various simple scoring systems (Supplementary Materials), including quick the Sequential Organ Failure Assessment (qSOFA) Score, Rapid Acute Physiology Score (RPAS), Mortality in Emergency Department Sepsis (MEDS) score, Modified Early Warning Score (MEWS), National Early Warning Score (NEWS), and Rapid Emergency Medicine Score (REMS), to become the predictors of clinical outcomes for critical illness. However, they did not apply these in the survey of cryptococcemia [21–28]. Therefore, we analyzed the risk factors for patients with cryptococcemia and the impact of mortality rate by different origins of cryptococcal infection, clinical characteristics, and the performance of the abovementioned scoring systems.

2. Materials and Methods

2.1. Data Collection and Definition

The institutional review board of Taichung Veterans General Hospital (TCVGH), Taichung, Taiwan, approved our study (CE22240B). It was a single hospital-based retrospective study on patients with cryptococcal fungemia confirmed by at least one blood culture collected from the emergency department (ED) [29]. We excluded patients only presenting the positive cryptococcal antigen without the growth of cryptococcus in blood culture.Patients' data, including clinical characteristics, comorbidities, laboratory investigations, co-infection conditions, hospital course, and mortality rate, were collected between January 2012 and December 2020 from the electronic medical records (EMRs) in TCVGH. We collected patients' vital signs and laboratory data to analyze scoring systems during blood culture, which identified cryptococcal fungemia. The primary outcome was the overall in-hospital mortality rate. We excluded patients younger than 18 years old or transferring to other hospitals. We defined cryptococcosis as a positive culture of *Cryptococcus neoformans* yielded from the various specimens of the clinically involved sites, including cerebrospinal fluid (CSF), sputum/bronchial lavage, urine, ascites, and skin biopsy.We collected blood cultures and vital signs for analyses in the case of identified cryptococcal fungemia. We defined septic shock as needing inotropic agents or vasopressors to correct hypotension and lactic acidosis resulting from infection.

2.2. Scoring Systems

We collected all of the parameters for analysis in the scoring systems from the EMRs. The clinical scoring systems of this study included qSOFA, RAPS, MEDS, MEWS, NEWS, and REMS.

2.3. Statistical Analysis

We presented continuous data as mean ± standard deviation (SD). We expressed categorical data as numbers and percentages. Chi-squared tests were applied to compare categorical data. Mann–Whitney–Wilcoxon U-tests were involved to compare continuous data regarding mortality risks in survivors and non-survivors. To assess possible predictors for mortality, we conducted univariate and multivariate analyses using the Cox regression model to express results as confidence interval and hazard ratio. We used the area under the curve (AUC) receiver operating of the characteristic curve (ROC) to compare predictive power across different scoring systems. We used cut-off points of scores to stratify mortality risks in terms of sensitivity, specificity, negative predictive value (NPV), and positive predictive value (PPV). A p value < 0.05 was considered statistically significant. We analyzed the data using the Statistical Package for the Social Science (IBM SPSS version 22.0; International Business Machines Corp., New York, NY, USA) and R (Version 4.1.3, R Foundation for Statistical Computing, Vienna, Austria).

3. Results

3.1. Demographics and Clinical Characteristics

We identified 43 patients with cryptococcemia from January 2012 to December 2020, and excluded one patient due to transferring to other hospitals before being diagnosed with cryptococcal fungemia. Finally, we enrolled 42 patients in our study. There were 28 (66.7%) males and 14 (33.3%) females with a mean age of 63.0 ± 19.7 years. The total hospital stays ranged from 1 to 170 days (a mean stay of 44.4 days), and the overall mortality rate was 64.3% (27/42). Only one patient did not have immunodeficient status. Of the remaining 41 patients, there were 16 under immunosuppressants (such as steroids or immunomodulatory drugs for autoimmune disorders or organ transplants), 8 with HIV infection, 6 with liver cirrhosis, 6 with diabetes mellitus (DM), 5 with end-stage renal disease (ESRD), and 4 under chemotherapy due to neoplasms or hematologic disorders. Among all the comorbidities, the prevalence of HIV infection was higher in the survivors than in the non-survivors (40.0% vs. 7.4%, $p = 0.016$). We summarized the demographics and clinical characteristics, laboratory data, and scoring systems of 42 patients in Table 1. In the subgroup analysis of 30 patients who underwent lumbar puncture, we concluded their characteristics and laboratory investigations in Table 2.

We showed patient distribution in different seasons and the average temperature of each season. There was an increasing overall patient number according to the higher average temperature in different seasons ($p = 0.044$). Moreover, increased cases of mortalitywere also associated with increased average temperature ($p = 0.014$) and low average temperature ($p = 0.030$) in the different seasons (Figure 1).

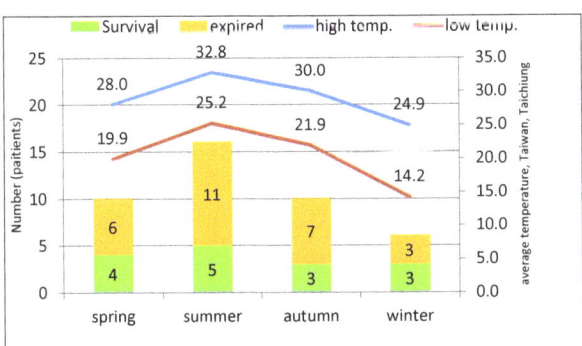

Figure 1. The trend association between the seasonal temperature and total deceased patient numbers of cryptococcemia. Trend of high temperature and total patients, $p = 0.044$. Trend of high temperature and deceased patients, $p = 0.014$; Trend of low temperature and deceased patients, $p = 0.030$.

Table 1. Demographics and laboratory data of 42 patients with fungemia of *Cryptococcus neoformans*.

General Data	Patients (n = 42)	Survivors (n = 15)	Non-Survivors (n = 27)	p-Value
Age (years)	63.0 ± 19.7	52.5 ± 19.7	68.9 ± 17.4	0.014 *
Male (%)	28 (66.7%)	12 (80%)	16 (59.3%)	0.172
Hospital stays (days)	44.4 ± 42.9	61.3 ± 46.5	35.0 ± 38.5	0.008 **
Focus of cryptococcosis				
CNS [f]	22 (52.4%)	11 (73.3%)	11 (40.7%)	0.009 **
Respiratory tract [f]	4 (9.5%)	2 (13.3%)	2 (7.4%)	0.608
Clinical conditions				
Septic shock [f]	7 (16.7%)	0 (0.0%)	7 (25.9%)	0.038 *
IICP [f]	18 (42.9%)	8 (53.3%)	10 (37.0%)	0.007 **
Concomitant infections				
Pneumonia	16 (38.1%)	5 (33.3%)	11 (40.7%)	0.746
Urinary tract [f]	8 (19.1%)	2 (13.3%)	6 (22.2%)	0.689
Bacteremia	21 (50.0%)	7 (46.7%)	14 (51.9%)	1
Comorbidities				
HIV [f]	8 (19.1%)	6 (40.0%)	2 (7.4%)	0.016 *
Liver cirrhosis [f]	6 (14.3%)	1 (6.7%)	5 (18.5%)	0.395
ESRD [f]	5 (11.9%)	0 (0.0%)	5 (18.5%)	0.142
DM [f]	6 (14.3%)	1 (6.7%)	5 (18.5%)	0.395
Immunosuppressant use	16 (38.1%)	5 (33.3%)	11 (40.7%)	0.746
Under chemotherapy [f]	4 (9.5%)	1 (6.7%)	3 (11.1%)	1
Vital signs				
SBP (mmHg)	134.6 ± 26.8	136.8 ± 20.1	133.4 ± 30.2	0.763
DBP (mmHg)	80.6 ± 19.4	79.9 ± 12.6	81.0 ± 22.5	0.937
MAP (mmHg)	98.6 ± 20.5	98.8 ± 13.5	98.4 ± 23.7	1
HR (bpm)	97.4 ± 25.5	96.2 ± 18.5	98.0 ± 29.0	0.636
RR (bpm)	20.1 ± 3.7	18.5 ± 1.6	20.9 ± 4.3	0.022 *
BT (°C)	37.7 ± 0.9	37.7 ± 1.2	37.7 ± 0.8	0.590
SpO$_2$ (%)	95.6 ± 5.4	96.1 ± 2.6	95.3 ± 6.5	0.355
O$_2$ use	26 (61.9%)	3 (20.0%)	23 (85.2%)	<0.001 **
GCS	11.6 ± 4.2	14.6 ± 1.1	10.0 ± 4.4	<0.001 **
Laboratory data				
WBC (counts/uL)	9312.9 ± 6707.0	7026.0 ± 5071.7	10,583.3 ± 7238.2	0.125
Hb (g/dL)	10.1 ± 2.4	11.0 ± 1.6	9.5 ± 2.6	0.021 *
PLT (×10^3 counts/uL)	170.2 ± 119.0	244.7 ± 124.5	128.7 ± 94.9	0.002 **
Crea (mg/dL)	1.97 ± 2.17	0.96 ± 0.42	2.56 ± 2.54	0.003 **
Lactate (mg/dL)	22.1 ± 28.6	11.6 ± 4.6	25.6 ± 32.3	0.104
pH	7.40 ± 0.07	7.42 ± 0.04	7.39 ± 0.07	0.427
Scoring systems				
qSOFA	1.0 ± 0.9	0.3 ± 0.6	1.4 ± 0.8	<0.001 **
RAPS	3.2 ± 2.2	1.5 ± 0.8	4.1 ± 2.3	<0.001 **
MEWS	3.5 ± 2.0	2.1 ± 1.4	4.3 ± 1.9	<0.001 **
MEWS with GCS	3.9 ± 2.6	2.0 ± 2.0	4.9 ± 2.2	<0.001 **
REMS	7.1 ± 3.7	4.3 ± 3.0	8.6 ± 3.1	<0.001 **
NEWS	6.1 ± 4.1	2.9 ± 3.4	8.0 ± 3.2	<0.001 **
MEDS	7.1 ± 4.8	2.9 ± 2.9	9.5 ± 4.0	<0.001 **

Chi–squared test. [f] Fisher's exact test. Mann–Whitney U-test.* p <0.05, ** p <0.01, Statistically significant. Continuous data were expressed as mean ± SD. Categorical data were expressed as number and percentage. BT, body temperature; CNS, central nervous system; Crea, Creatinine; DBP, diastolic blood pressure; DM, Diabetes Mellitus; ESRD, end–stage renal disease; GCS, Glasgow coma scale; HR, heart rate; Hb, hemoglobin; IICP, increased intracranial pressure; MAP, mean blood pressure; MEDS, Mortality in Emergency Department Sepsis Score; MEWS, Modified Early Warning Score; NEWS, National Early Warning Score; PLT, platelet; qSOFA, quick Sequential Organ Failure Assessment; RAPS, Rapid Acute Physiology Score; REMS, Rapid Emergency Medicine Score; RR, respiratory rate; SBP, systolic blood pressure; WBC, white blood cells.

Table 2. Demographics and laboratory data of 30 patients who underwent lumbar puncture and CSF examination.

General Data	Patients (n = 30)	Survivors (n = 15)	Non-Survivors (n = 15)	p-Value
Age (years)	57.5 ± 19.5	52.5 ± 19.7	62.6 ± 18.7	0.106
Male (%)	23 (76.7%)	12 (80.0%)	11 (73.3%)	1
Hospital stays (days)	53.5 ± 45.9	61.3 ± 46.5	45.7 ± 45.5	0.116
Focus of cryptococcosis				
CNS	22 (73.3%)	11 (73.3%)	11 (73.3%)	1
Respiratory tract	4 (13.3%)	2 (13.3%)	2 (13.3%)	1
Clinical conditions				
Septic shock	2 (6.7%)	0 (0.0%)	2 (13.3%)	0.483
IICP	18 (60.0%)	8 (53.3%)	10 (66.7%)	0.709
Concomitant infections				
Pneumonia	13 (38.1%)	5 (33.3%)	8 (53.3%)	0.461
Urinary tract	5 (16.7%)	2 (13.3%)	3 (20.0%)	1
Bacteremia	16 (53.3%)	7 (46.7%)	9 (60.0%)	0.714
Comorbidities				
HIV	8 (26.7%)	6 (40.0%)	2 (13.3%)	0.215
Liver cirrhosis	4 (13.3%)	1 (6.7%)	3 (20.0%)	0.598
ESRD	2 (6.7%)	0 (0.0%)	2 (13.3%)	0.483
DM	4 (13.3%)	1 (6.7%)	3 (20.0%)	0.598
Immunosuppressant use	12 (40.0%)	5 (33.3%)	7 (46.7%)	0.709
Under chemotherapy	2 (6.6%)	1 (6.7%)	1 (6.7%)	1
Vital signs				
SBP (mmHg)	139.2 ± 21.8	136.8 ± 20.1	141.5 ± 23.9	0.567
DBP (mmHg)	84.4 ± 17.9	79.9 ± 12.6	88.87 ± 21.4	0.217
MAP (mmHg)	102.6 ± 17.6	98.8 ± 13.5	106.4 ± 20.6	0.267
HR (bpm)	93.9 ± 24.3	96.2 ± 18.5	91.5 ± 29.5	0.744
RR (bpm)	19.0 ± 2.6	18.5 ± 1.6	19.4 ± 3.3	0.187
BT (°C)	37.7 ± 1.1	37.7 ± 1.2	37.8 ± 1.0	0.870
SpO_2 (%)	96.2 ± 2.8	96.1 ± 2.6	96.3 ± 3.0	0.838
O_2 use	14 (46.7%)	3 (20.0%)	11 (73.3%)	<0.001 **
GCS	12.6 ± 4.0	14.6 ± 1.1	10.5 ± 4.7	0.019 *
Laboratory data				
WBC (counts/uL)	7574.0 ± 4616.7	7026.0 ± 5071.7	8122.0 ± 4217.2	0.412
Hb (g/dL)	10.4 ± 2.5	11.0 ± 1.6	9.7 ± 3.0	0.098
PLT ($\times 10^3$ counts/uL)	181.3 ± 124.3	244.7 ± 124.5	117.9 ± 88.8	0.002
Crea (mg/dL)	1.63 ± 2.10	0.96 ± 0.42	2.34 ± 2.87	0.026 *
Lactate (mg/dL)	14.1 ± 8.8	11.6 ± 4.6	15.6 ± 10.5	0.313
pH	7.42 ± 0.04	7.42 ± 0.04	7.41 ± 0.05	0.681
Scoring systems				
qSOFA	0.6 ± 0.8	0.3 ± 0.6	1.0 ± 0.8	0.011 *
RAPS	2.7 ± 2.1	1.5 ± 0.8	3.9 ± 2.3	0.002 **
MEWS	2.8 ± 1.6	2.1 ± 1.4	3.4 ± 1.5	0.013 *
MEWS GCS	3.0 ± 2.1	2.0 ± 2.0	4.1 ± 1.6	0.004 **
REMS	6.0 ± 3.3	4.3 ± 3.0	7.6 ± 2.8	0.005 **
NEWS	4.4 ± 3.1	2.9 ± 3.4	5.9 ± 1.8	0.001 **
MEDS	5.5 ± 4.3	2.9 ± 2.9	8.2 ± 3.8	<0.001 **

Chi–squared test. Mann–Whitney U-test. * $p < 0.05$, ** $p < 0.01$, Statistically significant. BT, body temperature; CNS, central nervous system; Crea, Creatinine; DBP, diastolic blood pressure; DM, Diabetes Mellitus; ESRD, end–stage renal disease; GCS, Glasgow coma scale; HR, heart rate; Hb, hemoglobin; IICP, increased intracranial pressure; MAP, mean blood pressure; MEDS, Mortality in Emergency Department Sepsis Score; MEWS, Modified Early Warning Score; NEWS, National Early Warning Score; PLT, platelet; qSOFA, quick Sequential Organ Failure Assessment; RAPS, Rapid Acute Physiology Score; REMS, Rapid Emergency Medicine Score; RR, respiratory rate; SBP, systolic blood pressure; WBC, white blood cells.

3.2. Laboratory Data and Scoring Systems

We showed laboratory data and scoring systems in Table 1. The non-survivors had lower hemoglobin (Hb) (11.0 ± 1.6 vs. 9.5 ± 2.6, $p = 0.021$), lower platelet (PLT) counts (244.7 ± 124.5 vs. 128.7 ± 94.9, $p = 0.002$), and a higher level of creatinine (1.0 ± 0.4 vs. 2.6 ± 2.5, $p = 0.003$) than the survivors. In addition, all scoring systems showed significantly higher scores in the non-survivors than in the survivors.

3.3. Microbiology

Our study identified no other cryptococcal species but *Cryptococcus neoformans* in patients with cryptococcal fungemia. We suggested that all patients undergo an examination of CSF once the diagnosis of cryptococcemia was confirmed. However, only 22 patients confirmed diagnosis of cryptococcosis with CNS involvement. Additionally, *Cryptococcus neoformans* was isolated from urine in four patients, the respiratory tract in two, skin biopsy in one, and peritoneal fluid in one. We confirmed 12 patients with a diagnosis of primary cryptococcemia. Another 12 patients, assumed as primary cryptococcemia, passed away before undergoing an examination of CSF or declining lumbar puncture.

3.4. Clinical Outcomes and Co-Infections Related to Other Pathogens

Twenty-seven patients passed away during hospitalization, with an overall in-hospital mortality rate of 64.3%. We found co-infections of urinary tract infections in 8 patients, pneumonia in 16, and primary bacteremia in 21.

3.5. Univariate and Multivariate Analysis of Risk Factors

In the univariate analysis, older age, no CNS involvement, female gender, high respiratory rate, oxygen (O_2) use, low scores of Glasgow Coma Scale (GCS), combined lower respiratory tract infection (LRTI), elevated white blood cell (WBC) counts, low PLT counts, high levels of lactate and creatinine, high scores of qSOFA, RAPS, MEDS, MEWS, MEWS GCS, REMS, and NEWS were associated with a higher overall in-hospital mortality rate (Table 3). In the multivariate analysis, MEDS presented a higher in-hospital mortality rate (HR: 1.21, 95% CI: 1.03–1.41, $p = 0.018$) (Table 4).

Table 3. Univariate Cox regression analyses for predisposing factors on clinical outcomes in 42 patients of cryptococcal fungemia.

Characteristics	Hazard Ratios	95% Confidence Interval	*p*-Value
Age (years)	1.03	(1.00–1.06)	0.023 *
Female	2.45	(1.11–5.42)	0.027 *
		Focus of cryptococcosis	
CNS	0.36	(0.16–0.85)	0.013 *
Concomitant infection			
LRTI	2.59	(1.15–5.81)	0.021 *
		Vital signs	
RR (bpm)	1.18	(1.06–1.32)	0.002 **
GCS	0.92	(0.84–0.97)	0.008 **
Laboratory data			
WBC (counts/uL)	1.00	(1.00–1.00)	0.028 *
PLT ($\times 10^3$ counts/uL)	1.00	(0.99–1.00)	0.026 *
Crea (mg/dL)	1.17	(1.03–1.32)	0.016 *
Lactate (mg/dL)	1.03	(1.00–1.05)	0.004 **
		Clinical management	
O_2 use	4.74	(1.64–13.73)	0.004 **
		Scoring systems	
REMS	1.18	(1.06–1.32)	0.003 **
RAPS	1.30	(1.11–1.53)	0.001 **
MEWS	1.37	(1.14–1.66)	0.001 **
MEWS with GCS	1.29	(1.12–1.48)	<0.001 **
MEDS	1.18	(1.08–1.28)	<0.001 **
NEWS	1.19	(1.09–1.30)	<0.001 **
qSOFA	2.11	(1.47–3.02)	<0.001 **

Cox regression analysis. * $p < 0.05$, ** $p < 0.01$, Statistically significant. BT, body temperature; CNS, central nervous system; Crea, Creatinine; DBP, diastolic blood pressure; DM, Diabetes Mellitus; ESRD, end–stage renal disease; GCS, Glasgow coma scale; HR, heart rate; Hb, hemoglobin; IICP, increased intracranial pressure; MAP, mean blood pressure; MEDS, Mortality in Emergency Department Sepsis Score; MEWS, Modified Early Warning Score; NEWS, National Early Warning Score; PLT, platelet; qSOFA, quick Sequential Organ Failure Assessment; RAPS, Rapid Acute Physiology Score; REMS, Rapid Emergency Medicine Score; RR, respiratory rate; SBP, systolic blood pressure; WBC, white blood cells.

Table 4. Univariate and multivariate Cox regression analyses for scoring systems on the in-hospital mortality rate in 42 patients of cryptococcal fungemia.

Variables	Univariate			Multivariate		
	HR	95% CI	p-Value	HR	95% CI	p-Value
MEDS	1.18	(1.08–1.28)	<0.001 **	1.20	(1.03–1.40)	0.018 *
NEWS	1.19	(1.09–1.30)	<0.001 **	1.03	(0.77–1.39)	0.813
MEWS with GCS	1.29	(1.12–1.48)	<0.001 **	1.09	(0.59–2.04)	0.766
MEWS	1.37	(1.14–1.66)	0.001 **	0.84	(0.40–1.75)	0.647
RAPS	1.30	(1.11–1.53)	0.001 **	1.24	(0.88–1.74)	0.211
REMS	1.18	(1.06–1.32)	0.003 **	0.84	(0.65–1.09)	0.196
qSOFA	2.11	(1.47–3.02)	<0.001 **	1.73	(0.61–4.88)	0.298

Cox regression analysis. * $p < 0.05$, ** $p < 0.01$, statistically significant. GCS, Glasgow coma scale; MEDS, Mortality in Emergency Department Sepsis Score; MEWS, Modified Early Warning Score; NEWS, National Early Warning Score; qSOFA, quick Sequential Organ Failure Assessment; RAPS, Rapid Acute Physiology Score; REMS, Rapid Emergency Medicine Score.

3.6. Receiver Operating Characteristic Curve (ROC)

The AUC of ROC for MEWS, RAPS, qSOFA, MEWS plus GCS, REMS, NEWS, and MEDS showed 0.833, 0.842, 0.848, 0.846, 0.846, 0.878, and 0.905, respectively. They performed well in predicting the in-hospital mortality risk of patients with cryptococcal fungemia. The MEDS showed the best performance in predicting the mortality risk, and the AUC of ROC was 0.905 at the cut-off points of 4 in Figure 2. The sensitivity and specificity of the MEDS in predicting the mortality risk were 93% and 80% (Table 5).

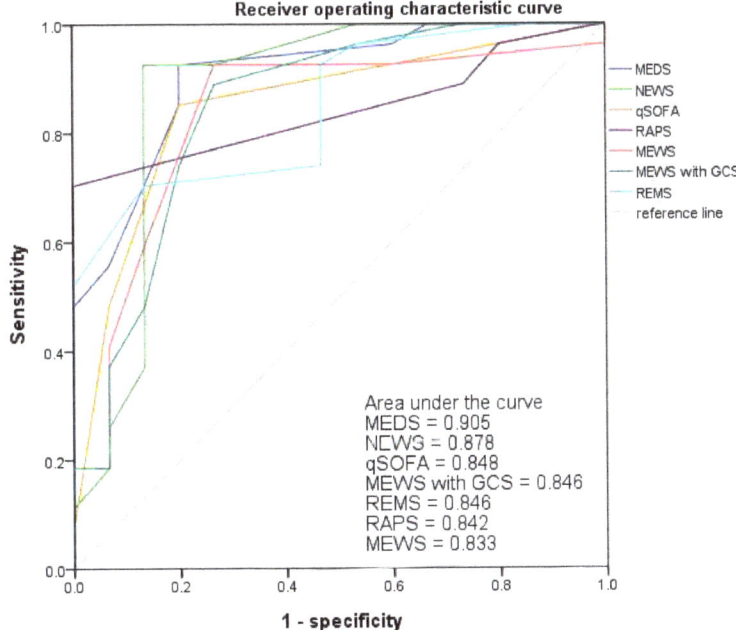

Figure 2. The AUC of ROC for MEDS, NEWS, qSOFA, MEWS plus GCS, REMS, RAPS, and MEWS indicated 0.905, 0.878, 0.848, 0.846, 0.846, 0.842, and 0.833 to predict the mortality risks of patients with cryptoccemia. AUC, area under the curve; GCS, Glasgow coma scale; MEDS, Mortality in Emergency Department Sepsis Score; MEWS, Modified Early Warning Score; NEWS, National Early Warning Score; qSOFA, quick Sequential Organ Failure Assessment; RAPS, Rapid Acute Physiology Score; REMS, Rapid Emergency Medicine Score; ROC, receiver operating characteristic curve.

Table 5. The AUC of ROC, COP, sensitivity, specificity, PPV, NPV, accuracy, and SE of scoring systems to predict mortality risk.

Scores	AUC	COP	Sensitivity	Specificity	PPV	NPV	Accuracy	SE	p-Value
MEDS	0.905	4	93%	80%	89%	86%	88%	0.047	<0.001 **
NEWS	0.878	5	93%	87%	93%	87%	91%	0.069	<0.001 **
qSOFA	0.848	1	85%	80%	89%	75%	83%	0.064	<0.001 **
MEWS with GCS	0.846	3	89%	73%	86%	79%	83%	0.069	<0.001 **
REMS	0.846	8	70%	87%	91%	62%	76%	0.059	<0.001 **
RAPS	0.842	3	70%	100%	100%	65%	81%	0.061	<0.001 **
MEWS	0.833	3	93%	73%	86%	85%	86%	0.071	<0.001 **

** $p < 0.01$, Statistically significant. AUC, area under the curve; COP, cut-off point; GCS, Glasgow coma scale; MEDS, Mortality in Emergency Department Sepsis Score; MEWS, Modified Early Warning Score; NEWS, National Early Warning Score; NPV, negative predictive value; PPV, positive predictive value; qSOFA, quick Sequential Organ Failure Assessment; RAPS, Rapid Acute Physiology Score; REMS, Rapid Emergency Medicine Score; ROC, receiver operating characteristic curve; SE, standard error.

3.7. Cumulative Survival Rates Using Kaplan–Meier and Discrimination Plots

We calculated the cumulative survival rates of patients with cryptococcemia to predict the 30-day mortality rate using Kaplan–Meier analyses (Figure 3). The cut-off points of MEDS, NEWS, qSOFA, MEWS plus GCS, REMS, RAPS, and MEWS were 4, 5, 1, 3, 8, 3, and 3, respectively. Furthermore, the overall mortality case numbers of MEDS, NEWS, qSOFA, MEWS plus GCS, REMS, RAPS, and MEWS were 25, 22, 13, 20, 14, 15, and 16, with the overall mortality rate of 89.3%, 91.7%, 92.9%, 87.0%, 100%, 100%, and 88.9% if the cut-off points were more than 4, 5, 1, 3, 8, 3, and 3, respectively, which is shown in the discrimination plots in Figure 4.

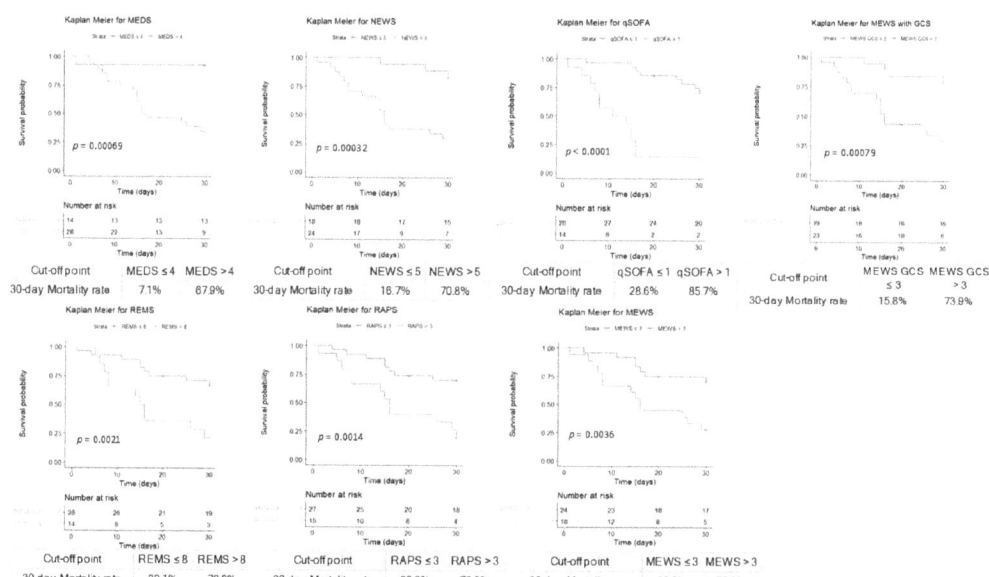

Figure 3. The cumulative survival rates of patients with cryptococcemia were calculated to predict the 30-day mortality rate using Kaplan–Meier analyses. The cut-off point of MEDS, NEWS, qSOFA, MEWS plus GCS, REMS, RAPS, and MEWS was 4, 5, 1, 3, 8, 3, and 3, respectively. GCS, Glasgow coma scale; MEDS, Mortality in Emergency Department Sepsis Score; MEWS, Modified Early Warning Score; NEWS, National Early Warning Score; qSOFA, quick Sequential Organ Failure Assessment; RAPS, Rapid Acute Physiology Score; REMS, Rapid Emergency Medicine Score.

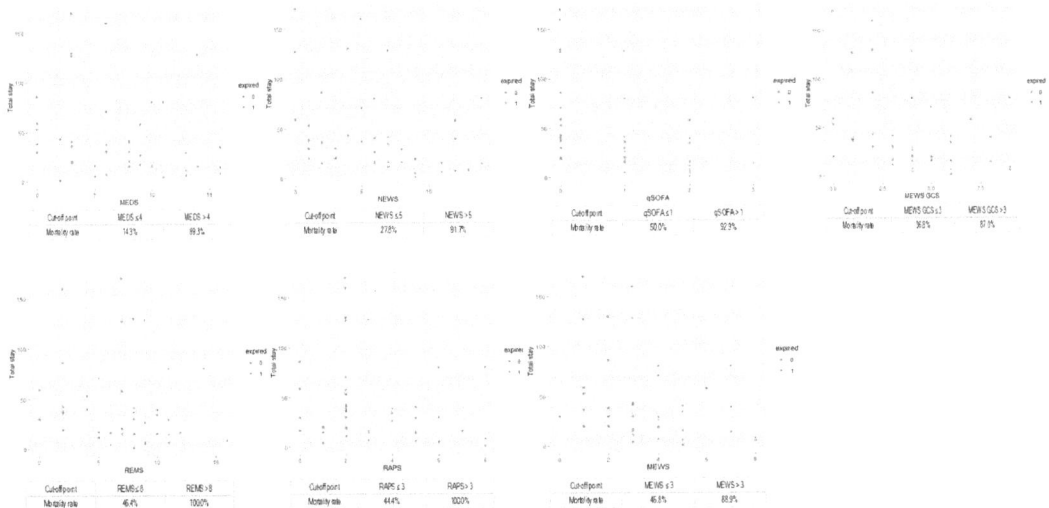

Figure 4. The overall mortality case numbers of MEDS, NEWS, qSOFA, MEWS plus GCS, REMS, RAPS, and MEWS were 25, 22, 13, 20, 14, 15, and 16, with the overall mortality rate of 89.3%, 91.7%, 92.9%, 87.0%, 100%, 100%, and 88.9% if the cut-off point was more than 4, 5, 1, 3, 8, 3, and 3, respectively. GCS, Glasgow coma scale; MEDS, Mortality in Emergency Department Sepsis Score; MEWS, Modified Early Warning Score; NEWS, National Early Warning Score; qSOFA, quick Sequential Organ Failure Assessment; RAPS, Rapid Acute Physiology Score; REMS, Rapid Emergency Medicine Score.

4. Discussion

In the literature, this is the first study of applying scoring systems in predicting the mortality risk of patients with cryptococcemia and identifying higher scores associated with a significantly higher mortality rate in patients with cryptococcemia.

In this study, the overall in-hospital mortality rate of cryptococcemia was 64.3% (27/42), and the 30-day mortality rate was 47.6% (20/42), which was higher compared to the previously reported 30-day mortality rate of 35% [18–20]. This may be related to higher age, with a mean age of 63 years, compared to a mean age of 40–50 years in previous studies [18–20]. We also found a higher incidence of primary cryptococcemia (12/42, 28.6%), which may be related to a higher incidence of patients' mortality. Meningeal involvement could account for most cryptococcosis. The higher incidence of cryptococcosis made physicians aware of cryptococcal infections in the HIV population. Hence, all patients with HIV infection received an examination for CSF during hospitalization in our study. Of all the 30 patients who received an analysis for CSF, 22 patients were diagnosed with cryptococcal meningitis through a positive culture of CSF or positive findings of India ink. We found 73.3% CNS involvement in 30 patients with cryptococcemia, similar to the previous report of 71.0–89.3% with CNS involvement in patients with cryptococcemia [18,20].

Cryptococcus neoformans distribute worldwide, and the optimal temperature of *Cryptococcus neoformans* is 30 °C in laboratory conditions [29]. The published literature report showed a relatively higher growth rate in the planktonic type at 30 °C compared to 35 °C, but better biofilm growth at 35 °C [30]. A systemic investigation in Colombia showed *Cryptococcus neoformans* to be more easily isolated in cold temperate climates and related to higher humidity or lower sunshine [31]. In our research, we found an increasing trend in the prevalence of cryptococcemia in the summer, and the average summer temperature in Taiwan was also closest to 30 °C. Additionally, we also found the tendency of a positive relationship between mortality case numbers and both high and low average temperatures. However, there was no significant difference in mortality rate in different seasons, which may be related to the few case numbers. Therefore, the possibility of a positive relationship between temperature and cryptococcal infection is worthy of further investigation.

The risk factors of mortality in cryptococcal fungemia of this study were higher age, being female, no CNS involvement, higher respiratory rate, O_2 use, lower GCS level, combined LRTI, higher WBC counts, lower PLT counts, more elevated lactate and creatinine levels, and higher scores of qSOFA, RAPS, MEDS, MEWS, MEWS GCS, REMS, and NEWS. In addition, we found patients with CNS involvement with a lower mortality rate in the univariate analysis of all populations but a non-significant difference in the subgroup analysis of 30 patients who underwent an examination of CSF (Table 2). We supposed the possibility that patients who died before undergoing a test of CSF were classified into the non-CNS involvement group, resulting in a higher mortality rate of the non-CNS involvement group.

Generally, amphotericin B, liposomal amphotericin, and azoles (including fluconazole and itraconazole) were considered effective antifungal agents for cryptococcosis [20,32]. However, nine patients passed away without being prescribed effective antifungal agents, and only one patient receiving amphotericin B passed away within 24 h in our study. Although the abovementioned patients were diagnosed with cryptococcemia by blood culture after mortality, all received amphotericin B according to the positive cryptococcal antigen in the examination for CSF.

These clinical scoring systems have been a clinical tool applied to evaluate the mortality risk in the ED or general ward. The qSOFA was first created in 2016 as a measuring tool to determine critical conditions in septic patients [21]. Still, it was considered to have a lower prognostic accuracy for in-hospital mortality or risk of intensive care unit (ICU) admission than the SOFA score [22]. The RAPS, as an abbreviated version of the APECHE-II score, was developed in 1987 as a severity scale in critical care transport and was considered for its predictive ability regarding mortality risk by only using simple parameters available on transported patients. The RAPS is further applied to evaluate the mortality risk of the patients in the ED or other different categories of patients [23]. The MEWS was investigated in 2001 and was created to identify patients in busy areas with a risk of deterioration. A reported score of 5 or more was associated with a higher risk of death or depravation [24]. The NEWS, created by teams at the Royal College of Physicians in London, was recommended as an early discriminating tool for patients at risk of cardiac arrest, with unplanned admission to the ICU, or in the case of death within 24 h with a high AUROC [25]. In 2004, the REMS extended the RAPS by adding the patient's age and peripheral oxygen saturation to predict the in-hospital mortality of the non-surgical ED patients.

Further investigation demonstrated its superior predictive value in comparison to the RAPS [26]. Shapiro et al. developed the MEDS score initially according to the odds ratio of mortality risk in ED patients with a chance of sepsis in 2003. In Taiwan, many authors applied the MEDS score to predict the severity and mortality rate of patients with bacteremia [27,28,33].

In our study, higher scores in all the abovementioned scoring systems were associated with a substantially higher mortality rate, and the MEDS presented the best predictive performance. In general, the MEDS is composed of clinical manifestations and laboratory data, including age >65 years (3 points), nursing home residence (2 points), terminal illness (6 points), altered mental status (2 points), tachypnea or hypoxia (3 points), septic shock (3 points), LRTI (2 points), PLT counts <150,000 (3 points), and band portion >5% (3 points) with a maximum of 27 points. The AUC of ROC of MEDS was 0.905 at the cut-off point of 4, with a sensitivity of 92.6% (25/27) and specificity of 80% (12/15), respectively. However, we found a lower cut-off point than other studies [27,28,34]. The possible causes were the presence of no patients with nursing home residence or terminal illness conditions and no band portion >5% in our study.

5. Limitations

First, our study had some limitations due to the retrospective nature and small sample size. For example, the possible time lag between collecting the first blood culture to identify cryptococcemia and the records of vital signs or laboratory data—or missing data, presented in some cases—such as relating to lumbar puncture. Second, antifungal agents or other management procedures, after diagnosis of cryptococcemia, were not standardized, so we cannot compare the clinical outcomes according to those treatments. Third, the enrolled patients had high rates of comorbidities and co-infections. Fourth, cryptococcemia is a rare disease. Therefore, there is a lack of awareness in patients initially presented in the ED. Also, the long inoculation time of cryptococcus species' growth makes it difficult to conduct a prospective study and to standardize the treatment protocol for patients with cryptococcemia.

6. Conclusions

Cryptococcemia is a rare entity, but it is life-threatening with a high mortality rate, so physicians should maintain suspicion in high-risk patients. An examination for CSF in patients with cryptococcemia is strongly recommended, due to the fact that the majority of patients with cryptococcemia present CNS involvement. Age, gender, respiratory rate, O_2 use, GCS level, LRTI, WBC counts, PLT counts, lactate, creatinine, and high points of scoring systems are associated with poor prognosis in patients with cryptococcemia. The MEDS (≥ 4) performs best in predicting mortality risk. We recommend further large-scale studies on early detection through the biomarkers of cryptococcemia and the appropriate use of scoring systems to predict the mortality risk in order to improve clinical outcomes.

Supplementary Materials: The following supporting information can be downloaded at: https://www.mdpi.com/article/10.3390/jpm13091358/s1, Table S1: Scoring systems.

Author Contributions: Conceptualization, S.-Y.H.; methodology, M.-S.H., S.-Y.H. and Y.-C.T.; data curation, W.-K.L., S.-Y.H., S.-C.H., C.-A.T. and Y.-C.T.; writing—original draft preparation, W.-K.L. and S.-Y.H.; writing—review and editing, M.-S.H., S.-C.H., Y.-Z.C. and S.-Y.H.; project administration, S.-Y.H.; funding acquisition, S.-Y.H. All authors have read and agreed to the published version of the manuscript.

Funding: This work was supported by grants from the Taichung Veterans General Hospital (TCVGH), Taichung, Taiwan (TCVGH-1107202C, TCVGH-1127203C, and TCVGH-T1127801), and the Taipei Veterans General Hospital, Taoyuan branch, Taoyuan, Taiwan (TYVH-10808, TYVH-10809, and TYVH-10902). The funders had no role in the study design, data collection, analysis, decision to publish, or preparation of the manuscript. No additional external funding was received for this study.

Institutional Review Board Statement: The institutional review board of the Taichung Veterans General Hospital approved this study. (Study period ranged from 1 July 2021 to 30 June 2022) (IRB file number: CE22240B).

Informed Consent Statement: Patient consent was waived because this study was retrospective, observational, and anonymous.

Data Availability Statement: Readers can access the data and material supporting the study's conclusions by contacting Sung-Yuan Hu at song9168@pie.com.tw.

Acknowledgments: We thank the Clinical Informatics Research and Development Center and the Biostatistics Task Force of the Taichung Veterans General Hospital.

Conflicts of Interest: The authors declare no conflict of interest.

References

1. Maziarz, E.K.; Perfect, J.R. Cryptococcosis. *Infect. Dis. Clin. N. Am.* **2016**, *30*, 179–206. [CrossRef]
2. Bicanic, T.; Harrison, T.S. Cryptococcal meningitis. *Br. Med. Bull.* **2005**, *72*, 99–118. [CrossRef]

3. Kidd, S.E.; Hagen, F.; Tscharke, R.L.; Huynh, M.; Bartlett, K.H.; Fyfe, M.; Macdougall, L.; Boekhout, T.; Kwon-Chung, K.J.; Meyer, W. A rare genotype of *Cryptococcus gattii* caused the cryptococcosis outbreak on Vancouver Island (British Columbia, Canada). *Proc. Natl. Acad. Sci. USA* **2004**, *101*, 17258–17263. [CrossRef]
4. Williamson, P.R.; Jarvis, J.N.; Panackal, A.A.; Fisher, M.C.; Molloy, S.F.; Loyse, A.; Harrison, T.S. Cryptococcal meningitis: Epidemiology, immunology, diagnosis and therapy. *Nat. Rev. Neurol.* **2017**, *13*, 13–24. [CrossRef]
5. Rajasingham, R.; Smith, R.M.; Park, B.J.; Jarvis, J.N.; Govender, N.P.; Chiller, T.M.; Denning, D.W.; Loyse, A.; Boulware, D.R. Global burden of disease of HIV-associated cryptococcal meningitis: An updated analysis. *Lancet Infect. Dis.* **2017**, *17*, 873–881. [CrossRef]
6. Chang, C.C.; Sorrell, T.C.; Chen, S.C. Pulmonary Cryptococcosis. *Semin. Respir. Crit. Care Med.* **2015**, *36*, 681–691. [CrossRef]
7. Setianingrum, F.; Rautemaa-Richardson, R.; Denning, D.W. Pulmonary cryptococcosis: A review of pathobiology and clinical aspects. *Med. Mycol.* **2019**, *57*, 133–150. [CrossRef]
8. Sobel, J.D.; Vazquez, J.A. Fungal infections of the urinary tract. *World J. Urol.* **1999**, *17*, 410–414. [CrossRef]
9. Noguchi, H.; Matsumoto, T.; Kimura, U.; Hiruma, M.; Kusuhara, M.; Ihn, H. Cutaneous Cryptococcosis. *Med. Mycol. J.* **2019**, *60*, 101–107. [CrossRef]
10. Dumenigo, A.; Sen, M. Cryptococcal Osteomyelitis in an Immunocompetent Patient. *Cureus* **2022**, *14*, e21074. [CrossRef]
11. Zainal, A.I.; Wong, S.L.; Pan, K.L.; Wong, O.L.; Tzar, M.N. Cryptococcal osteomyelitis of the femur: A case report and review of literature. *Trop. Biomed.* **2011**, *28*, 444–449. [PubMed]
12. Amphornphruet, A.; Silpa-Archa, S.; Preble, J.M.; Foster, C.S. Endogenous Cryptococcal Endophthalmitis in Immunocompetent Host: Case Report and Review of Multimodal Imaging Findings and Treatment. *Ocul. Immunol. Inflamm.* **2018**, *26*, 518–522. [CrossRef] [PubMed]
13. Sheu, S.J.; Chen, Y.C.; Kuo, N.W.; Wang, J.H.; Chen, C.J. Endogenous cryptococcal endophthalmitis. *Ophthalmology* **1998**, *105*, 377–381.
14. Jean, S.S.; Wang, J.L.; Wang, J.T.; Fang, C.T.; Chen, Y.C.; Chang, S.C. *Cryptococcus neoformans* peritonitis in two patients with liver cirrhosis. *J. Formos. Med. Assoc.* **2005**, *104*, 39–42.
15. Gushiken, A.C.; Saharia, K.K.; Baddley, J.W. Cryptococcosis. *Infect. Dis. Clin. N. Am.* **2021**, *35*, 493–514. [CrossRef]
16. Chen, Y.C.; Chang, S.C.; Shih, C.C.; Hung, C.C.; Luhbd, K.T.; Pan, Y.S.; Hsieh, W.C. Clinical features and in vitro susceptibilities of two varieties of *Cryptococcus neoformans* in Taiwan. *Diagn. Microbiol. Infect. Dis.* **2000**, *36*, 175–183. [CrossRef]
17. Archibald, L.K.; McDonald, L.C.; Rheanpumikankit, S.; Tansuphaswadikul, S.; Chaovanich, A.; Eampokalap, B.; Banerjee, S.N.; Reller, L.B.; Jarvis, W.R. Fever and human immunodeficiency virus infection as sentinels for emerging mycobacterial and fungal bloodstream infections in hospitalized patients >/=15 years old, Bangkok. *J. Infect. Dis.* **1999**, *180*, 87–92. [CrossRef]
18. Jean, S.S.; Fang, C.T.; Shau, W.Y.; Chen, Y.C.; Chang, S.C.; Hsueh, P.R.; Hung, C.C.; Luh, K.T. Cryptococcaemia: Clinical features and prognostic factors. *QJM* **2002**, *95*, 511–518. [CrossRef] [PubMed]
19. Pasqualotto, A.C.; BittencourtSevero, C.; de Mattos Oliveira, F.; Severo, L.C. Cryptococcemia. An analysis of 28 cases with emphasis on the clinical outcome and its etiologic agent. *Rev. Iberoam. Micol.* **2004**, *21*, 143–146. [PubMed]
20. Fu, Y.; Xu, M.; Zhou, H.; Yao, Y.; Zhou, J.; Pan, Z. Microbiological and clinical characteristics of cryptococcemia: A retrospective analysis of 85 cases in a Chinese hospital. *Med. Mycol.* **2020**, *58*, 478–484. [CrossRef]
21. Singer, M.; Deutschman, C.S.; Seymour, C.W.; Shankar-Hari, M.; Annane, D.; Bauer, M.; Bellomo, R.; Bernard, G.R.; Chiche, J.D.; Coopersmith, C.M.; et al. The Third International Consensus Definitions for Sepsis and Septic Shock (Sepsis-3). *JAMA* **2016**, *315*, 801–810. [CrossRef] [PubMed]
22. Raith, E.P.; Udy, A.A.; Bailey, M.; McGloughlin, S.; MacIsaac, C.; Bellomo, R.; Pilcher, D.V.; Australian and New Zealand Intensive Care Society (ANZICS) Centre for Outcomes and Resource Evaluation (CORE). Prognostic Accuracy of the SOFA Score, SIRS Criteria, and qSOFA Score for In-Hospital Mortality Among Adults With Suspected Infection Admitted to the Intensive Care Unit. *JAMA* **2017**, *317*, 290–300. [CrossRef]
23. Rhee, K.J.; Fisher, C.J., Jr.; Willitis, N.H. The rapid acute physiology score. *Am. J. Emerg. Med.* **1987**, *5*, 278–282. [CrossRef] [PubMed]
24. Subbe, C.P.; Kruger, M.; Rutherford, P.; Gemmel, L. Validation of a modified Early Warning Score in medical admissions. *QJM* **2001**, *94*, 521–526. [CrossRef]
25. Smith, G.B.; Prytherch, D.R.; Meredith, P.; Schmidt, P.E.; Featherstone, P.I. The ability of the National Early Warning Score (NEWS) to discriminate patients at risk of early cardiac arrest, unanticipated intensive care unit admission, and death. *Resuscitation* **2013**, *84*, 465–470. [CrossRef] [PubMed]
26. Olsson, T.; Terent, A.; Lind, L. Rapid Emergency Medicine score: A new prognostic tool for in-hospital mortality in nonsurgical emergency department patients. *J. Intern. Med.* **2004**, *255*, 579–587. [CrossRef]
27. Hsieh, C.C.; Yang, C.Y.; Lee, C.H.; Chi, C.H.; Lee, C.C. Validation of MEDS score in predicting short-term mortality of adults with community-onset bacteremia. *Am. J. Emerg. Med.* **2020**, *38*, 282–287. [CrossRef]
28. Huang, S.H.; Hsieh, M.S.; Hu, S.Y.; Huang, S.C.; Tsai, C.A.; Hsu, C.Y.; Lin, T.C.; Lee, Y.C.; Liao, S.H. Performance of Scoring Systems in Predicting Clinical Outcomes in Patients with Bacteremia of *Listeria monocytogenes*: A 9-Year Hospital-Based Study. *Biology* **2021**, *10*, 1073. [CrossRef]
29. Doering, T.L. A unique α-1,3 mannosyltransferase of the pathogenic fungus *Cryptococcus neoformans*. *J. Bacteriol.* **1999**, *181*, 5482–5488. [CrossRef] [PubMed]

30. Pettit, R.K.; Repp, K.K.; Hazen, K.C. Temperature affects the susceptibility of *Cryptococcus neoformans* biofilms to antifungal agents. *Med. Mycol.* **2010**, *48*, 421–426. [CrossRef] [PubMed]
31. Serna-Espinosa, B.N.; Guzmán-Sanabria, D.; Forero-Castro, M.; Escandón, P.; Sánchez-Quitian, Z.A. Environmental status of *Cryptococcus neoformans* and *Cryptococcus gattii* in Colombia. *J. Fungi* **2021**, *7*, 410. [CrossRef] [PubMed]
32. Perfect, J.R.; Dismukes, W.E.; Dromer, F.; Goldman, D.L.; Graybill, J.R.; Hamill, R.J.; Harrison, T.S.; Larsen, R.A.; Lortholary, O.; Nguyen, M.H.; et al. Clinical practice guidelines for the management of cryptococcal disease: 2010 update by the Infectious Diseases Society of America. *Clin. Infect. Dis.* **2010**, *50*, 291–322. [CrossRef] [PubMed]
33. Zhang, G.; Zhang, K.; Zheng, X.; Cui, W.; Hong, Y.; Zhang, Z. Performance of the MEDS score in predicting mortality among emergency department patients with a suspected infection: A meta-analysis. *Emerg. Med. J.* **2020**, *37*, 232–239. [CrossRef] [PubMed]
34. Shapiro, N.I.; Wolfe, R.E.; Moore, R.B.; Smith, E.; Burdick, E.; Bates, D.W. Mortality in Emergency Department Sepsis (MEDS) score: A prospectively derived and validated clinical prediction rule. *Crit. Care Med.* **2003**, *31*, 670–675. [CrossRef]

Disclaimer/Publisher's Note: The statements, opinions and data contained in all publications are solely those of the individual author(s) and contributor(s) and not of MDPI and/or the editor(s). MDPI and/or the editor(s) disclaim responsibility for any injury to people or property resulting from any ideas, methods, instructions or products referred to in the content.

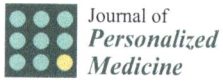

Article

Resilience in Emergency Medicine during COVID-19: Evaluating Staff Expectations and Preparedness

Mariusz Goniewicz [1,*], Anna Włoszczak-Szubzda [2], Ahmed M. Al-Wathinani [3] and Krzysztof Goniewicz [4]

1. Department of Emergency Medicine, Medical University of Lublin, 20-081 Lublin, Poland
2. Faculty of Human Sciences, University of Economics and Innovation, 20-209 Lublin, Poland; anna.wloszczak-szubzda@wsei.lublin.pl
3. Department of Emergency Medical Services, Prince Sultan Bin Abdulaziz College for Emergency Medical Services, King Saud University, Riyadh 11451, Saudi Arabia; ahmalotaibi@ksu.edu.sa
4. Department of Security, Polish Air Force University, 08-521 Deblin, Poland; k.goniewicz@law.mil.pl
* Correspondence: mariusz.goniewicz@umlub.pl

Abstract: Introduction: The COVID-19 pandemic brought about significant challenges for health systems globally, with medical professionals at the forefront of this crisis. Understanding their organizational expectations and well-being implications is crucial for crafting responsive healthcare environments. Methods: Between 2021 and 2022, an online survey was conducted among 852 medical professionals across four provinces in Poland: Mazovia, Łódź, Świętokrzyskie, and Lublin. The survey tool, based on a comprehensive literature review, comprised dichotomous questions and specific queries to gather explicit insights. A 5-point Likert scale was implemented to capture nuanced perceptions. Additionally, the Post-Traumatic Stress Disorder Checklist-Civilian (PCL-C) was utilized to ascertain the correlation between workplace organization and post-traumatic stress symptoms. Results: A noteworthy 84.6% of participants believed their employers could enhance safety measures, highlighting a discrepancy between healthcare workers' expectations and organizational implementations. Major concerns encompassed the demand for improved personal protective equipment (44.6%), structured debriefing sessions (40%), distinct building entrances and exits (38.8%), and psychological support (38.3%). Statistical analyses showcased significant variations in 'Avoidance' and 'Overall PTSD Score' between individuals who had undergone epidemic safety procedure training and those who had not. Conclusions: The results illuminate the imperative for healthcare organizations to remain agile, attentive, and deeply compassionate, especially during worldwide health emergencies. Despite showcasing remarkable resilience during the pandemic, medical professionals ardently seek an environment that underscores their safety and mental well-being. These findings reinforce the call for healthcare institutions and policymakers to champion a forward-thinking, employee-focused approach. Additionally, the data suggest a potential avenue for future research focusing on specific demographic groups, further enriching our understanding and ensuring a more comprehensive readiness for impending health crises.

Keywords: COVID-19; healthcare professionals; organizational expectations; personal protective equipment (PPE); post-traumatic stress disorder (PTSD); workplace safety; epidemic preparedness; debriefing

Citation: Goniewicz, M.; Włoszczak-Szubzda, A.; Al-Wathinani, A.M.; Goniewicz, K. Resilience in Emergency Medicine during COVID-19: Evaluating Staff Expectations and Preparedness. *J. Pers. Med.* **2023**, *13*, 1545. https://doi.org/10.3390/jpm13111545

Academic Editor: Ovidiu Alexandru Mederle

Received: 17 September 2023
Revised: 19 October 2023
Accepted: 25 October 2023
Published: 28 October 2023

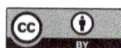

Copyright: © 2023 by the authors. Licensee MDPI, Basel, Switzerland. This article is an open access article distributed under the terms and conditions of the Creative Commons Attribution (CC BY) license (https://creativecommons.org/licenses/by/4.0/).

1. Introduction

The COVID-19 pandemic, which began in late 2019, swiftly transformed into a global health crisis, significantly impacting the dynamics of healthcare systems worldwide [1]. As emergency departments bore the brunt of rising case numbers, the on-ground staff—comprising nurses, medical rescuers, doctors, and healthcare caregivers—faced an unprecedented surge in patient volume and acuity [2]. In these challenging circumstances, the expectations and safety concerns of these medical professionals regarding organizational support emerged as pivotal in ensuring the efficient management of the crisis.

Central to this narrative was the relationship between healthcare professionals and their employers. While literature [3–6] emphasizes the importance of protective equipment, adequate training, and psychological support for healthcare workers during pandemics, how effectively were these requirements met during the COVID-19 crisis? Moreover, what were the tangible and immediate expectations of these professionals, and how did they align with organizational provisions? A failure to address these questions and concerns in real time may lead to increased vulnerabilities, not only for healthcare workers but also for the patients relying on them.

Adding a layer of immediacy to this discourse is the realization that the challenges thrown up by the pandemic are not merely localized. Instead, the implications of these challenges resonate on a global scale [7]. From a hospital in New York to a clinic in New Delhi, the narrative of medical professionals battling the pandemic, armed with their skills, resilience, and expectations from their employers, remains a shared story.

The universal impact of the COVID-19 pandemic was felt in every corner of the world. However, the organizational responses to these challenges displayed significant regional variations, influenced by a myriad of factors ranging from governmental policies to available resources and the socio-economic landscape.

For instance, countries like South Korea and New Zealand quickly became models of effective employer support [8,9]. In South Korea, medical professionals were promptly provided with an abundance of personal protective equipment (PPE), and a robust testing system was put in place [10]. This not only protected the healthcare workers but also ensured that patients received timely and safe treatment. Meanwhile, in New Zealand, clear communication between healthcare employers and their staff, coupled with the government's early action, significantly alleviated the pressures faced by frontline workers [11].

Conversely, in other regions, medical professionals battled not only the virus but also systemic issues, ranging from a lack of adequate PPE to insufficient training on the ever-evolving treatment protocols. For many, their organizational expectations were rooted more in hope than in the assurance of support [12–14].

These regional disparities underscore the importance of understanding the diverse organizational expectations of medical professionals across the globe. By highlighting best practices and learning from the challenges faced in various regions, the global healthcare community can foster a more collaborative and effective response to future health crises.

Given the intricate web of global challenges and the varied responses of healthcare systems worldwide, there is an undeniable need to scrutinize the specific expectations medical professionals held during the peak of the pandemic. This examination goes beyond simply documenting reactions; it seeks to inform and better prepare healthcare systems for potential future crises.

This research aims to elucidate the organizational expectations of medical professionals during the COVID-19 pandemic, with a focus on its implications for emergency medicine. By analyzing variations among different healthcare settings and evaluating if these expectations were met, we hope to foster a global discourse on strengthening healthcare systems for future emergencies.

2. Materials and Methods

2.1. Location of the Study

The research was conducted from 2021 to 2022. Owing to the constraints of the pandemic, the study was executed online, with the survey link disseminated to medical facilities in four provinces of Poland: Mazovia, Łódź, Świętokrzyskie, and Lublin. The choice of these specific provinces was multi-faceted. They were strategically chosen to provide a balanced geographical representation, capturing key regions of the country. Additionally, historical epidemiological trends and healthcare engagement levels in these provinces demonstrated a level of consistency that dovetailed neatly with our research objectives. The logistical feasibility of focusing on these areas, especially during the challenges posed by the pandemic, ensured streamlined communication with local medical facilities and professionals. Furthermore, pre-existing collaborations and contacts within these provinces' medical communities facilitated the efficient distribution and management of the survey, ensuring that we acquired a comprehensive yet representative sample of healthcare professionals.

2.2. Study Population

The study encompassed 852 medical professionals from diverse healthcare settings. While the participants represented a variety of roles, including paramedics, doctors, and medical caregivers, a significant majority (82.6%) identified as nurses. The gender distribution was notably skewed, with females constituting 88.1% of the cohort. The diverse array of healthcare entities from which these professionals hailed includes Primary Healthcare, Specialist Ambulatory Care, Emergency Departments (ED), Care and Treatment Institutions, Social Welfare Homes, and various hospital departments. These departments differentiated themselves based on the nature of the patients they catered to—either primarily those diagnosed with conditions other than COVID-19 or those suspected/confirmed as having COVID-19. Additionally, the study included Ambulance teams, which were categorized based on their dispatch specifics—catering either to non-suspected or suspected/confirmed COVID-19 patients.

2.3. Questionnaire

The survey was meticulously designed to capture a holistic understanding of the healthcare professionals' experiences during the pandemic. It commenced with collecting demographic data, which was pivotal in understanding the diverse backgrounds and expertise of the respondents. This section included items such as age, gender, years of experience, and specific roles within the healthcare sector.

Subsequent sections dived deeper into the main crux of the research. These segments aimed to excavate the expectations and perceptions healthcare workers harbored regarding their employers' role in organizing work amidst the pandemic. To ensure comprehensive coverage of opinions and experiences, a mix of question types was used. Dichotomous questions provided clear binary perspectives, while open-ended queries allowed respondents to share detailed insights. Moreover, to capture the nuanced gradations of opinions, a 5-point Likert scale was incorporated, ranging from 'Strongly Disagree' to 'Strongly Agree', providing a spectrum of agreement for various statements.

A robust foundation for the survey was laid by a literature review. This entailed a systematic investigation of published works that touched upon work organization during the pandemic and medical personnel's associated expectations. It ensured that our tool was grounded in existing research while addressing gaps and evolving challenges.

However, a survey is not just about questions; its efficacy lies in its clarity and relevance. To this end, we employed a qualitative method to verify the tool's effectiveness. A pilot test was conducted on a sample of 10 individuals from diverse medical backgrounds. Their primary role was to evaluate the clarity, relevance, and comprehensiveness of our questions. Feedback from this initial group was instrumental, highlighting areas for refinement. It is worth noting that to maintain data purity, the results from these dual-role participants were deliberately kept separate, ensuring that they did not influence the main study's findings.

Furthermore, in our bid to cement the tool's credibility, we subjected the survey to the scrutiny of expert judges. These individuals, with their vast academic and practical experience, evaluated our questionnaire for clarity, comprehensiveness, and relevancy to the current pandemic backdrop.

Additionally, understanding the potential psychological impact of the pandemic on healthcare workers was vital. Thus, we incorporated the PCL-C into our research. This standardized tool is recognized for its accuracy in gauging post-traumatic stress disorder (PTSD) symptoms. With its inclusion, we aimed to establish any correlations between the organization and expectations in medical units with the manifestation of PTSD symptoms among healthcare professionals.

2.4. Statistical Analysis

To answer the research questions and test the hypotheses, statistical analyses were conducted using the IBM SPSS Statistics software, version 26. Basic descriptive statistics, Pearson's r correlation analyses, independent *t*-tests, and Mann–Whitney U tests were performed. A classic threshold of $\alpha = 0.05$ was adopted for statistical significance.

2.5. Ethical Considerations

While the study does not qualify as a medical experiment under Polish law and thus did not necessitate a Bioethics Committee's oversight, it still followed rigorous ethical standards. Participants were briefed about the research objectives, assured of confidentiality, and reminded of their participation's voluntary nature. Data storage protocols adhered to strict privacy guidelines, and informed consent was acquired from all participants.

3. Results

Our study had strong representation from females, who made up 88.1% of the participants, while males accounted for only 11.9%. This gender and professional role skewness, particularly the overrepresentation of nurses (82.6%), underscores a specific demographic dynamic in our data collection, which we have further elucidated in the limitations section. The age range of the participants spanned from 20 to 59 years, averaging at 39 years. In terms of professional experience, participants reported an average of 12 years, with durations as brief as a month and as lengthy as 41 years.

Diving deeper into their job roles, after the prominent presence of nurses (82.6%), paramedics followed at 8.9%. The dataset recorded fewer representations from professions like medical caregivers and physicians, with other job roles constituting the remaining 6% of responses.

When exploring their professional involvement during the SARS-CoV-2 pandemic, a significant 91.8% affirmed their active participation in healthcare duties. The primary work setting for 40.3% was non-COVID-19 hospital wards. In contrast, 21.9% were deployed in COVID-designated wards. Other crucial segments included 14% stationed in primary healthcare and 14.4% working from unspecified locations. Interestingly, nearly one in five participants disclosed affiliations with more than one workplace, as detailed in Table 1.

Table 1. Demographic data.

Gender		N	%
Women		751	88.1
Men		101	11.9
Age (average ± SD)	39.02 ± 10.02 years (20–59 years)		
Work experience (average ± SD):	12.90 ± 11.44 years (0.08–41 years)		
Profession:		N	%
Nurse		704	86.6
Paramedic		75	8.9
Physician		8	0.9
Medical caregiver		14	1.6
Other		51	6.0
Workplace:		N	%
Primary Healthcare		119	14
Specialist Ambulatory Care		34	4.0
Emergency Department		70	8.2

Table 1. Cont.

Admissions Room	47	5.5
Care and Treatment Institution	39	4.6
Social Welfare Home	36	4.2
Hospital, non-COVID-19 ward	343	40.3
Hospital, COVID-19 ward	187	21.9
Ambulance, non-COVID cases	36	4.2
Ambulance, COVID cases	48	5.6
Other	123	14.4
Worked in healthcare during the pandemic?	N	%
Yes	782	91.8
No	70	8.2
Total	852	100

SD means standard deviation; N means the total number of individuals or observations in the sample.

3.1. Training and Pandemic Preparedness

Upon exploring their exposure to training, we discerned that a considerable majority (73.2%) had received training at their respective workplaces, specifically targeting adherence to safety measures during epidemics/pandemics. Contrarily, 26.8% lacked such training. Further insight into the facilities' pandemic preparedness revealed that participants, on average, rated their workplace's readiness level at 3.19 (with a standard deviation of 0.97). A moderate level of preparedness was the consensus for 43.8% of the respondents. These findings are detailed in Table 2.

Table 2. Assessment of Pandemic Preparedness, Training, and Employee Safety Assurance.

Question/Category	N	%
Underwent safety training during pandemic		
Yes	624	73.2%
No	228	26.8%
Organization's pandemic preparedness level		
1—Unprepared	38	4.5%
2	141	16.5%
3—Neutral	373	43.8%
4	220	25.8%
5—Fully Prepared	80	9.4%
Employer could improve in ensuring employee safety		
Yes	721	84.6%
No	131	15.4%
Total respondents	852	100%

3.2. Evaluation of Employers' Safety Measures

Participants evaluated the safety measures implemented by their employers during the pandemic. A striking 84.6% believed that their employers had potential areas of improvement regarding the implementation of safety measures. In contrast, 15.4% felt that their employers had already maximized safety precautions. When discussing improvements, a significant 44.6% emphasized the need for an enhancement in both the quality and quantity of personal protective equipment provided. Close behind, about 40% highlighted the importance of organized debriefings. Such sessions would allow staff to collaboratively discuss challenging situations, identify areas of concern, and refine their approach. In a similar vein, 38.8% believed that establishing distinct building entry and exit points for personnel directly attending to COVID-19 patients would bolster safety by segregating them from the rest of the staff. Additionally, 38.3% underscored the critical need for psychological support, suggesting that access to counseling and related services was indispensable during these challenging times (Table 3).

Table 3. Assessment of Employer Effectiveness in Ensuring Employee Safety and Suggested Improvements.

Questions/Measures	N	%
Employer's Effectiveness in Ensuring Employee Safety		
Could your employer improve in ensuring employee safety?		
Yes	721	84.6%
No	131	15.4%
Suggested Measures for Improving Employee Safety *		
Reorganize work structure	42	4.9%
Provide separate entrances and exits for staff directly working with COVID-19 patients and other personnel	331	38.8%
Ensure a higher quantity and quality of personal protective equipment	380	44.6%
Provide employees with psychological support, contact with a psychologist	326	38.3%
Organize debriefings to discuss challenging situations, assess mistakes, and refine procedures	341	40.0%
Other measures not mentioned in the survey	34	4.0%
Total respondents	852	100%

* This mean multiple answers were allowed.

3.3. PTSD Symptoms and Their Association with Training and Preparedness

Our investigation illuminated a dichotomy in PTSD symptomatology predicated on participants' training pedigree. Specifically, individuals devoid of prior training on epidemic safety protocols exhibited heightened symptoms in the 'Avoidance' and 'Overall PTSD Score' metrics. It is intriguing to note that parametric tests affirmed these differences as statistically significant. However, when these findings were juxtaposed against the results from the non-parametric Mann–Whitney U test, the differences in the aforementioned indices were not mirrored. Notably, for other scales, such as 'Intrusion' and 'Hyperarousal', the dichotomy remained elusive, with no discernible differences arising from either testing methodology. Further, a correlation analysis revealed a negative, albeit weak, relationship between PTSD symptoms and the assessment of an organization's pandemic preparedness. This indicates that as the perceived preparedness of the workplace increased, the intensity of PTSD symptoms reported by participants decreased (Table 4).

Table 4. PTSD Symptoms in Relation to Training Participation and Organizational Preparedness for Pandemics.

Measures/Criteria	Trained (n = 624)	Not Trained (n = 227)	r Pearson [Org. Preparedness Rating]	Significance
Intrusion	M: 9.94, SD: 3.73	M: 10.57, SD: 4.35	−0.16	<0.001
Avoidance	M: 14.79, SD: 5.52	M: 15.73, SD: 6.02	−0.17	<0.001
Hyperarousal (Increased Arousal)	M: 12.58, SD: 4.57	M: 13.15, SD: 4.73	−0.18	<0.001
PTSD—Overall Score	M: 37.30, SD: 12.44	M: 39.44, SD: 13.92	−0.19	<0.001

Note: The t-test results for 'Avoidance' and 'Overall Score' were statistically significant with weak effects. This highlights higher PTSD symptom intensity among those who did not receive training compared to those who did. However, the Mann–Whitney U test did not show significant differences for these indices. Importantly, both tests found no differences for the 'Intrusion' and 'Hyperarousal' measures. The correlation analysis indicated that as the preparedness rating of the workplace for a pandemic increased, the PTSD symptoms' intensity experienced by participants decreased. This suggests that training and preparedness can influence PTSD symptoms among professionals.

4. Discussion

The findings of our study shed critical light on the organizational expectations of medical professionals during the height of the COVID-19 pandemic, especially in the context of emergency medicine. A majority (84.6%) believed that their employer could further enhance safety measures, pointing towards a perceptual gap between healthcare workers' expectations and organizational practices. Such a significant percentage underscores the necessity for institutions to continually evaluate and adapt their safety measures in line with the evolving needs of their staff.

While our study had a dominant representation of female participants, it is essential to understand the unique challenges and perspectives brought by gender dynamics in healthcare during the pandemic. It is also worth noting that perceptions related to healthcare delivery, especially in emergency settings, may vary significantly based on factors such as gender and education. For instance, studies like the one by Tiziana Ciarambino et al. have highlighted that older and less-educated females can have distinct experiences and evaluations of care during the pandemic [15]. Given our study's significant representation of female professionals, predominantly nurses, further studies should consider these intersections of age, gender, and education to provide a more nuanced understanding of expectations and perceptions in healthcare settings during emergencies.

Previous studies have shown gender-based disparities in stress perception, workload, and even access to protective measures in healthcare settings [16,17]. Additionally, with a varied age range, understanding how different age groups perceived organizational support, especially considering factors like risk perception and familial responsibilities, would offer a richer context.

While the primary focus of our study was on the direct experiences and perceptions of medical professionals, it is crucial to recognize the role of socio-economic disparities.

Beyond socio-economic factors, demographic characteristics, particularly age and education, have been shown to play an integral role in shaping the experiences of medical professionals. It is essential to understand how these dynamics influence perceptions of preparedness, especially when considering the diverse workforce engaged during the pandemic. Such an understanding could provide valuable insights for healthcare institutions and policymakers to tailor strategies that cater to the varied needs and perspectives of their staff.

Medical professionals working in underfunded or resource-scarce institutions may have different expectations and challenges compared to those in better-funded environments. Disparities in funding, infrastructure, and access to resources can lead to varied levels of satisfaction, trust, and even perceptions of safety [18]. Recognizing these socio-economic divides is essential for a holistic understanding of the healthcare landscape during the pandemic.

One of the salient expectations voiced by participants was the desire for improved quality and quantity of personal protective equipment. With 44.6% of respondents emphasizing this, it reaffirms the global narrative surrounding PPE shortages and the resultant vulnerabilities faced by healthcare professionals [19,20]. The shortage of PPE not only jeopardizes the safety of medical staff but can also impact the quality of care provided, potentially exacerbating the health crisis.

Furthermore, the emphasis placed by 40% of the participants on organizing debriefings signals an inherent need for communicative feedback loops within medical institutions. Debriefings provide a platform for collective reflection, error identification, and procedural refinement. Such practices are integral, especially during health emergencies, ensuring the adaptability and resilience of healthcare systems [21,22].

Drawing parallels with previous health crises, such as the SARS or MERS outbreaks, reveals recurring themes in healthcare workers' expectations. The demand for adequate protective measures, clear communication, and psychological support has been consistent [23,24]. However, the unprecedented scale of the COVID-19 pandemic might have intensified these needs, making it imperative for organizations to learn from the past while innovatively addressing the present challenges.

As the world grappled with the pandemic, technology and digital health emerged as crucial allies. While our study touched upon the tangible needs of healthcare professionals, it might be worth exploring if there was an underlying expectation or desire for better technological support. Enhanced telehealth platforms, digital tracking of resources, or even AI-driven patient management tools could offer additional layers of support and efficiency, reducing the strain on our frontline heroes [25,26].

The pivotal role of leadership during such crises cannot be understated. Strong leadership and transparent communication influence not only the operations but also the morale and confidence of medical professionals [27]. When leadership is decisive, communicative, and supportive, it creates an environment where professionals feel valued, heard, and reassured [28]. The impact of leadership styles and strategies during the COVID-19 pandemic might be an invaluable area for further investigation, especially in understanding its influence on healthcare workers' perceptions.

The call by 38.8% of participants for separate building entrances and exits also brings forth an essential aspect of infection control, which often goes beyond the immediate scope of personal protection. Such measures, while logistically challenging, can significantly reduce cross-contamination risks, protecting both healthcare workers and patients.

The implications of meeting or failing to meet the expectations of medical professionals stretch beyond their personal well-being. Patient care, the crux of the medical profession, is intrinsically tied to the conditions under which professionals operate [28]. When healthcare workers' needs are not addressed, it could lead to reduced efficiency, heightened stress, and potential lapses in care quality [29,30]. Addressing the expectations of healthcare professionals is, by extension, a commitment to ensuring optimal patient care and outcomes.

A concerning aspect of our findings is the apparent psychological toll the pandemic has exerted on medical professionals. With 38.3% underscoring the need for psychological support and counseling access, it is evident that the crisis has had profound mental health implications. Previous studies during past health crises have similarly emphasized the psychological vulnerabilities of frontline healthcare workers, necessitating robust mental health support structures [31–34].

Our study underscores the importance of regular feedback mechanisms. Institutions should consider periodic surveys, town hall meetings, or even anonymous feedback platforms. These mechanisms will ensure that the evolving needs of healthcare workers are promptly addressed, fostering an environment of trust and proactive adaptability.

Our statistical analyses also provide a nuanced perspective on the significance of training. While parametric tests revealed stark differences in 'Avoidance' and 'Overall PTSD Score' between those trained in safety procedures during epidemics and those not, non-parametric tests did not corroborate this entirely. This dichotomy indicates the multifaceted nature of psychological responses to crises and underscores the need for more comprehensive research in this area.

Our findings are not just significant for medical institutions but hold substantial policy implications. Decision-makers at governmental or institutional levels could benefit from integrating these insights into their policy formulations. Addressing the gaps between healthcare workers' expectations and the realities on the ground could lead to policies that prioritize not only immediate safety and resources but also long-term well-being and resilience. Ensuring that the voice of the frontline resonates in policy can streamline the response to future health crises and strengthen the healthcare sector at large [35,36].

While our study highlighted the significance of training, it is imperative to delve deeper into the content and quality of these programs. Are our current training modules adequately equipped to handle the unique challenges posed by pandemics like COVID-19? Given the varied psychological responses noted, there might be a need to incorporate a blend of technical, psychological, and crisis-management skills in training regimens. Such a holistic approach could ensure that medical professionals are not just technically adept but also mentally fortified for unprecedented challenges.

In light of the expectations voiced by medical professionals, there are broader implications for healthcare infrastructure. An adaptive response to immediate challenges, such as those posed by the COVID-19 pandemic, offers a blueprint for handling future health crises. By integrating robust feedback mechanisms, addressing the holistic well-being of healthcare workers, and ensuring adequate resources, medical institutions can be better equipped not just to manage crises but to foster a culture of continual improvement and resilience [37]. This proactive approach could also be pivotal in attracting and retaining talent in the healthcare sector, ensuring that our medical institutions remain robust and reliable in the face of any future challenges.

Building upon our findings, healthcare institutions can take proactive measures to bridge the perceptual gap between organizational practices and workers' expectations.

Firstly, periodic training sessions could be organized that are tailored to the unique challenges of pandemics like COVID-19. These should not only focus on technical skills but also emphasize psychological readiness and coping strategies. Secondly, the establishment of a centralized digital platform can streamline communications, resource tracking, and feedback collection, ensuring that immediate needs and concerns are promptly addressed. Recognizing socio-economic disparities, resource allocation should be prioritized for underfunded institutions to ensure equity in safety measures and care quality. Lastly, fostering transparent communication from leadership can be achieved through regular updates, town hall meetings, and open forums, ensuring that all staff members feel valued, informed, and heard. These suggestions, when implemented, could lead to an environment that is not only safer but also more supportive for healthcare workers during global health emergencies.

Moreover, understanding the intricate role of demographics, particularly age, gender, and education, can help institutions develop tailored programs and interventions. For example, specific training modules for older professionals or those with varied educational backgrounds could be beneficial. Recognizing and addressing these nuances ensure that all medical professionals, irrespective of their demographic backgrounds, feel adequately supported and prepared.

Based on the insights from this study, there is a compelling case for further research that narrows its focus to specific demographic groups. Investigating the perceptions of older and less-educated females concerning healthcare delivery and PTSD symptoms during the COVID-19 pandemic could offer valuable contributions to the field.

In sum, our findings provide a holistic insight into the organizational expectations of medical professionals during the COVID-19 pandemic. The study reiterates the importance of adaptive, responsive, and supportive organizational structures, especially during global health emergencies. Ensuring that these expectations are met is not just about securing the present but also about fortifying the future, preparing healthcare systems for similar challenges that lie ahead.

5. Limitations

Our study, while comprehensive in its approach, bears certain limitations that are crucial to acknowledge. First and foremost, the geographical focus on four specific provinces in Poland might not encapsulate the broader experiences and expectations of medical professionals throughout the country or in varied global settings. The unique characteristics of these provinces could introduce biases not present in other areas, and thus, extrapolation to a larger context requires caution. The demographic makeup of our participants is heavily skewed towards female representation, with a dominant 88.1% being women. Moreover, a significant 86.6% of our respondents identified as nurses. This raises concerns about the generalizability of our findings, as the experiences and expectations of male healthcare professionals and other medical roles might be underrepresented or overlooked entirely in our dataset. This overrepresentation could inadvertently lead to a bias in our findings that primarily echo the experiences and concerns of nurses, particularly female nurses.

An important limitation to note is the noticeable underrepresentation of physicians in our study. While nurses formed a significant majority of respondents, physicians—key medical decision-makers during the pandemic—were limited in number. Several factors could explain this discrepancy: physicians' intense workloads during the pandemic might have hindered participation, the channels used for survey dissemination might not have reached physicians as effectively, or there might be a difference in survey participation inclination between professions. This lack of physician perspectives could affect the depth of insights drawn, especially relating to decision-making and organizational expectations during the crisis.

Moreover, we did not stratify our findings based on education levels or specific age brackets, particularly among older participants. Existing literature, including the study by Tiziana Ciarambino et al., indicates that perceptions related to healthcare delivery, particularly in emergency settings during the COVID-19 pandemic, can vary significantly based on demographic factors such as age and education. Specifically, older and less-educated females might have distinct perceptions that could deviate from the general trend identified in our research. By not considering these stratifications, we might be overlooking critical nuances in the experiences and perceptions of certain demographic subgroups.

The decision to conduct the research exclusively online—a necessity given the pandemic restrictions—might have introduced a selection bias. This mode could exclude potential respondents who might have been more accessible or responsive to traditional survey methodologies. Furthermore, given the emotionally charged nature of the subject, there was potential for response bias. Participants with particularly strong opinions or feelings, whether positive or negative, might have been more inclined to respond, possibly sidelining more neutral or indifferent perspectives.

Another aspect worth noting is the scope of our inquiry. While our questionnaire was thorough and rooted in existing literature, it is conceivable that certain nuanced or intangible facets of participants' experiences were not fully explored. This can always be a challenge in quantitative research, where open-ended, qualitative insights are limited. Lastly, the timeline of the pandemic introduced the possibility of recall bias. As participants reflected on experiences spanning a significant period, their memories of events or feelings from earlier stages might not have been entirely precise.

6. Conclusions

Surveying 852 medical professionals across four provinces in Poland, our study offers compelling insights into their organizational expectations during the pandemic. A clear majority voiced concerns about workplace safety, emphasizing the necessity for enhanced protective measures, distinct facility access routes, structured debriefings, and bolstered psychological support. The notable correlation between adequate safety training and decreased post-traumatic symptoms further underscores the importance of professional training during such crises.

These findings resonate beyond Poland's borders, encapsulating a global plea for healthcare establishments to be adaptable, attentive, and deeply empathetic. Medical professionals have showcased tremendous dedication and adaptability, and in turn, they seek an environment that prioritizes their safety, acknowledges their contributions, and upholds their mental well-being.

One area for further exploration, as suggested by the data, is to delve deeper into the experiences of specific demographic groups, particularly older and less-educated females. Their perceptions concerning healthcare delivery and PTSD symptoms during pandemics like COVID-19 could offer additional layers of understanding and contribute significantly to the broader knowledge base.

In anticipating future health challenges, it is crucial for global healthcare entities and leaders to internalize and act on these insights. An anticipatory, worker-centric approach, coupled with targeted research initiatives, can invigorate the medical community and fortify our health infrastructures against subsequent challenges.

In essence, our study underscores the profound significance of active listening, timely adaptation, and unwavering support. As the world navigates towards recuperation, embracing these tenets will be central to forging a more inclusive, resilient, and compassionate tomorrow.

Author Contributions: M.G. and A.W.-S. provided the main framework, identified, and organized primary materials, and collaborated on writing the manuscript. K.G. identified appropriate references and collaborated on the writing of the manuscript. A.M.A.-W. contributed to drafting sections of the manuscript. All authors have read and agreed to the published version of the manuscript.

Funding: This research received no external funding.

Institutional Review Board Statement: Not applicable.

Informed Consent Statement: Not applicable.

Data Availability Statement: The datasets used and/or analyzed during the current study are available from the corresponding author on reasonable request.

Acknowledgments: The authors would like to extend their appreciation to King Saud University for funding this work through the Researchers Supporting Project number (RSPD2023R649), King Saud University, Riyadh, Saudi Arabia.

Conflicts of Interest: The authors declare no conflict of interest.

References

1. Mayer, J.D.; Lewis, N.D. An inevitable pandemic: Geographic insights into the COVID-19 global health emergency. *Eurasian Geogr. Econ.* **2020**, *61*, 404–422. [CrossRef]
2. Uppal, A.; Silvestri, D.M.; Siegler, M.; Natsui, S.; Boudourakis, L.; Salway, R.J.; Parikh, M.; Agoritsas, K.; Cho, H.J.; Gulati, R.; et al. Critical Care and Emergency Department Response at the Epicenter of the COVID-19 Pandemic: New York City's public health system response to COVID-19 included increasing the number of intensive care units, transferring patients between hospitals, and supplementing critical care staff. *Health Aff.* **2020**, *39*, 1443–1449.
3. Catania, G.; Zanini, M.; Hayter, M.; Timmins, F.; Dasso, N.; Ottonello, G.; Aleo, G.; Sasso, L.; Bagnasco, A. Lessons from Italian front-line nurses' experiences during the COVID-19 pandemic: A qualitative descriptive study. *J. Nurs. Manag.* **2021**, *29*, 404–411. [CrossRef] [PubMed]
4. Park, S.H. Personal protective equipment for healthcare workers during the COVID-19 pandemic. *Infect. Chemother.* **2020**, *52*, 165. [CrossRef] [PubMed]
5. Zaçe, D.; Hoxhaj, I.; Orfino, A.; Viteritti, A.M.; Janiri, L.; Di Pietro, M.L. Interventions to address mental health issues in healthcare workers during infectious disease outbreaks: A systematic review. *J. Psychiatr. Res.* **2021**, *136*, 319–333. [CrossRef]
6. Goniewicz, K.; Goniewicz, M.; Włoszczak-Szubzda, A.; Burkle, F.M.; Hertelendy, A.J.; Al-Wathinani, A.; Molloy, M.S.; Khorram-Manesh, A. The importance of pre-training gap analyses and the identification of competencies and skill requirements of medical personnel for mass casualty incidents and disaster training. *BMC Public Health* **2021**, *21*, 114. [CrossRef]
7. Cuadros, D.F.; Xiao, Y.; Mukandavire, Z.; Correa-Agudelo, E.; Hernández, A.; Kim, H.; MacKinnon, N.J. Spatiotemporal transmission dynamics of the COVID-19 pandemic and its impact on critical healthcare capacity. *Health Place* **2020**, *64*, 102404. [CrossRef] [PubMed]
8. Connor, S. Is it time to ration access to acute secondary care health services to save the Aotearoa health system? *N. Z. Med. J.* **2022**, *135*, 7–12.
9. Naga, S. The struggle of mental health care delivery in South Korea and Singapore. *Harv. Int. Rev.* **2022**, *43*, 39–43.
10. Tang, K.H. Medical waste during COVID-19 pandemic: Its types, abundance, impacts and implications. *Ind. Domest. Waste Manag.* **2022**, *2*, 71–83. [CrossRef]
11. Holroyd, E.; Long, N.J.; Appleton, N.S.; Davies, S.G.; Deckert, A.; Fehoko, E.; Laws, M.; Martin-Anatias, N.; Simpson, N.; Sterling, R.; et al. Community healthcare workers' experiences during and after COVID-19 lockdown: A qualitative study from Aotearoa New Zealand. *Health Soc. Care Community* **2022**, *30*, e2761-71. [CrossRef] [PubMed]
12. Youssef, F.E.; Fathallah, S. Enhancing Hospital Operations Through the Analysis of SARS-CoV-2 Drug Interactions Using TylerADE. *J. Adv. Anal. Healthc. Manag.* **2023**, *7*, 163–187.
13. Nyashanu, M.; Pfende, F.; Ekpenyong, M.S. Triggers of mental health problems among frontline healthcare workers during the COVID-19 pandemic in private care homes and domiciliary care agencies: Lived experiences of care workers in the Midlands region, UK. *Health Soc. Care Community* **2022**, *30*, e370-6. [CrossRef] [PubMed]
14. Kasdovasilis, P.; Cook, N.; Montasem, A.; Davis, G. Healthcare support workers' lived experiences and adaptation strategies within the care sector during the COVID-19 pandemic. A meta-ethnography review. *Home Health Care Serv. Q.* **2022**, *41*, 267–290. [CrossRef]
15. Ciarambino, T.; Palmiero, L.; Bottone, R.; Schettini, F.; Adinolfi, L.E.; Giordano, M. Older female relatives of Covid-19 patients have an un-satisfactory perception of emergency room performance by clinical staff. *Aging Pathobiol. Ther.* **2021**, *3*, 37–38. [CrossRef]
16. Cole, A.; Ali, H.; Ahmed, A.; Hamasha, M.; Jordan, S. Identifying patterns of turnover intention among Alabama frontline nurses in hospital settings during the COVID-19 pandemic. *J. Multidiscip. Healthc.* **2021**, *14*, 1783–1794. [CrossRef]
17. Mersha, A.; Shibiru, S.; Girma, M.; Ayele, G.; Bante, A.; Kassa, M.; Abebe, S.; Shewangizaw, M. Perceived barriers to the practice of preventive measures for COVID-19 pandemic among health professionals in public health facilities of the Gamo zone, southern Ethiopia: A phenomenological study. *BMC Public Health* **2021**, *21*, 199. [CrossRef]
18. Zhu, Y.; Li, Y.; Wu, M.; Fu, H. How do Chinese people perceive their healthcare system? Trends and determinants of public satisfaction and perceived fairness, 2006–2019. *BMC Health Serv. Res.* **2022**, *22*, 22. [CrossRef]

19. Omar, I.A.; Debe, M.; Jayaraman, R.; Salah, K.; Omar, M.; Arshad, J. Blockchain-based supply chain traceability for COVID-19 personal protective equipment. *Comput. Ind. Eng.* **2022**, *167*, 107995. [CrossRef]
20. Huffman, E.M.; Athanasiadis, D.I.; Anton, N.E.; Haskett, L.A.; Doster, D.L.; Stefanidis, D.; Lee, N.K. How resilient is your team? Exploring healthcare providers' well-being during the COVID-19 pandemic. *Am. J. Surg.* **2021**, *221*, 277–284. [CrossRef]
21. Capolongo, S.; Rebecchi, A.; Buffoli, M.; Appolloni, L.; Signorelli, C.; Fara, G.M.; D'Alessandro, D. COVID-19 and cities: From urban health strategies to the pandemic challenge. A decalogue of public health opportunities. *Acta Bio Medica Atenei Parm.* **2020**, *91*, 13.
22. Khalil, M.; Mataria, A.; Ravaghi, H. Building resilient hospitals in the Eastern Mediterranean Region: Lessons from the COVID-19 pandemic. *BMJ Glob. Health* **2022**, *7* (Suppl. S3), e008754. [CrossRef] [PubMed]
23. Carmassi, C.; Foghi, C.; Dell'Oste, V.; Cordone, A.; Bertelloni, C.A.; Bui, E.; Dell'Osso, L. PTSD symptoms in healthcare workers facing the three coronavirus outbreaks: What can we expect after the COVID-19 pandemic. *Psychiatry Res.* **2020**, *292*, 113312. [CrossRef]
24. Curtin, M.; Richards, H.L.; Fortune, D.G. Resilience among health care workers while working during a pandemic: A systematic review and meta synthesis of qualitative studies. *Clin. Psychol. Rev.* **2022**, *95*, 102173. [CrossRef] [PubMed]
25. Lawry, T. *Hacking Healthcare: How AI and the Intelligence Revolution Will Reboot an Ailing System*; CRC Press: Boca Raton, FL, USA, 2022.
26. Nathoo, H.; Gurayah, T.; Naidoo, D. Life during Covid-19: An Explorative Qualitative Study of Occupational Therapists in South Africa. *Occup. Ther. Ment. Health* **2023**, *39*, 211–239. [CrossRef]
27. Goniewicz, K.; Burkle, F.M.; Hall, T.F.; Goniewicz, M.; Khorram-Manesh, A. Global public health leadership: The vital element in managing global health crises. *J. Glob. Health* **2022**, *12*, 03003. [CrossRef]
28. Goniewicz, K.; Hertelendy, A.J. Adaptive Leadership in a Post-Pandemic World: The Urgent Need for Transformative Change. *Prehospital Disaster Med.* **2023**, *38*, 530–531. [CrossRef]
29. Sullivan, W.M. Work and integrity: The crisis and promise of professionalism in America. *J. Am. Coll. Dent.* **2018**, *85*, 8–21.
30. Anaraki, N.R.; Mukhopadhyay, M.; Jewer, J.; Patey, C.; Norman, P.; Hurley, O.; Etchegary, H.; Asghari, S. A Qualitative Study of the Barriers and Facilitators Impacting the Implementation of a Quality Improvement Program for Emergency Departments. *BMC Health Serv. Res.* **2023**, Under Review.
31. Bender, A.E.; Berg, K.A.; Miller, E.K.; Evans, K.E.; Holmes, M.R. "Making sure we are all okay": Healthcare workers' strategies for emotional connectedness during the COVID-19 pandemic. *Clin. Soc. Work. J.* **2021**, *49*, 445–455. [CrossRef]
32. Pai, S.; Patil, V.; Kamath, R.; Mahendra, M.; Singhal, D.K.; Bhat, V. Work-life balance amongst dental professionals during the COVID-19 pandemic—A structural equation modelling approach. *PLoS ONE* **2021**, *16*, e0256663. [CrossRef]
33. Mediavilla, R.; Monistrol-Mula, A.; McGreevy, K.R.; Felez-Nobrega, M.; Delaire, A.; Nicaise, P.; Palomo-Conti, S.; Bayón, C.; Bravo-Ortiz, M.F.; Rodríguez-Vega, B.; et al. Mental health problems and needs of frontline healthcare workers during the COVID-19 pandemic in Spain: A qualitative analysis. *Front. Public Health* **2022**, *10*, 956403. [CrossRef]
34. Al-Wathinani, A.M.; Almusallam, M.A.; Albaqami, N.A.; Aljuaid, M.; Alghamdi, A.A.; Alhallaf, M.A.; Goniewicz, K. Enhancing Psychological Resilience: Examining the Impact of Managerial Support on Mental Health Outcomes for Saudi Ambulance Personnel. *InHealthcare* **2023**, *11*, 1277. [CrossRef] [PubMed]
35. Leng, C.; Challoner, T.; Hausien, O.; Filobbos, G.; Baden, J. From chaos to a new norm: The Birmingham experience of restructuring the largest plastics department in the UK in response to the COVID-19 pandemic. *J. Plast. Reconstr. Aesthetic Surg.* **2020**, *73*, 2136–2141. [CrossRef]
36. Núñez, A.; Madison, M.; Schiavo, R.; Elk, R.; Prigerson, H.G. Responding to healthcare disparities and challenges with access to care during COVID-19. *Health Equity* **2020**, *4*, 117–128. [CrossRef] [PubMed]
37. Søvold, L.E.; Naslund, J.A.; Kousoulis, A.A.; Saxena, S.; Qoronfleh, M.W.; Grobler, C.; Münter, L. Prioritizing the mental health and well-being of healthcare workers: An urgent global public health priority. *Front. Public Health* **2021**, *9*, 679397. [CrossRef] [PubMed]

Disclaimer/Publisher's Note: The statements, opinions and data contained in all publications are solely those of the individual author(s) and contributor(s) and not of MDPI and/or the editor(s). MDPI and/or the editor(s) disclaim responsibility for any injury to people or property resulting from any ideas, methods, instructions or products referred to in the content.

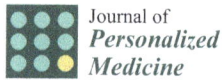

Article

Non-Ventilated Patients with Spontaneous Pneumothorax or Pneumomediastinum Associated with COVID-19: Three-Year Debriefing across Five Pandemic Waves

Adina Maria Marza [1,2], Alexandru Cristian Cindrea [3], Alina Petrica [1,4], Alexandra Valentina Stanciugelu [2,5,*], Claudiu Barsac [1,6], Alexandra Mocanu [7], Roxana Critu [5], Mihai Octavian Botea [8], Cosmin Iosif Trebuian [1] and Diana Lungeanu [9,10]

1. Department of Surgery, "Victor Babes" University of Medicine and Pharmacy, 300041 Timisoara, Romania; marza.adina@umft.ro (A.M.M.); alina.petrica@umft.ro (A.P.); trebuian.cosmin@umft.ro (C.I.T.)
2. Emergency Department, Emergency Clinical Municipal Hospital, 300079 Timisoara, Romania
3. Faculty of Medicine, "Victor Babes" University of Medicine and Pharmacy, 300041 Timisoara, Romania; alexandru.cindrea.umfvbt@gmail.com
4. Emergency Department, "Pius Brinzeu" Emergency Clinical County Hospital, 300736 Timisoara, Romania
5. Doctoral School, "Victor Babes" University of Medicine and Pharmacy, 300041 Timisoara, Romania
6. Clinic of Anaesthesia and Intensive Care, "Pius Brinzeu" Emergency Clinical County Hospital, 300736 Timisoara, Romania
7. Department of Infectious Diseases, "Victor Babes" University of Medicine and Pharmacy, 300041 Timisoara, Romania; alexandra.mocanu@umft.ro
8. Department of Surgery, Faculty of Medicine and Pharmacy, University of Oradea, 410087 Oradea, Romania
9. Center for Modeling Biological Systems and Data Analysis, "Victor Babes" University of Medicine and Pharmacy, 300041 Timisoara, Romania; dlungeanu@umft.ro
10. Department of Functional Sciences, "Victor Babes" University of Medicine and Pharmacy, 300041 Timisoara, Romania
* Correspondence: alexandra.stanciugelu@umft.ro; Tel.: +40-76-204-1933

Abstract: Spontaneous pneumothorax and pneumomediastinum (SP–SPM) are relatively rare medical conditions that can occur with or independently of COVID-19. We conducted a retrospective analysis of SP–SPM cases presented to the emergency departments (EDs) of two University-affiliated tertiary hospitals from 1 March 2020 to 31 October 2022. A total of 190 patients were identified: 52 were COVID-19 cases, and 138 were non-COVID-19 cases. The primary outcome we were looking for was in-hospital mortality. The secondary outcomes concerned the disease severity assessed by (a) days of hospitalization; (b) required mechanical ventilation (MV); and (c) required intensive care (IC). All were investigated in the context of the five pandemic waves and the patients' age and comorbidities. The pandemic waves had no significant effect on the outcomes of these patients. Logistic regression found age (OR = 1.043; 95%CI 1.002–1.085), COVID-19 (OR = 6.032; 95%CI 1.757–20.712), number of comorbidities (OR = 1.772; 95%CI 1.046–3.001), and ground-glass opacities over 50% (OR = 5.694; 95%CI 1.169–27.746) as significant risk predictors of in-hospital death while controlling for gender, smoking, the pandemic wave, and the extension of SP–SPM. The model proved good prediction performance (Nagelkerke R-square = 0.524) and would hold the same significant predictors for MV and IC.

Keywords: COVID-19; non-ventilated patients; spontaneous pneumothorax; spontaneous pneumomediastinum; complications; in-hospital mortality; emergency presentation; waves severity

1. Introduction

Spontaneous pneumothorax (SP) and spontaneous pneumomediastinum (SPM) have been frequently reported as complications associated with severe acute respiratory syndrome-coronavirus 2 (SARS-CoV-2) infection [1–3] and are defined as the presence of air in the pleural space or mediastinum without any history of trauma or other known cause. While the certain mechanisms for the development of these conditions in the context of coronavirus disease 2019 (COVID-19) pneumonia are not fully understood, it is believed that the virus may induce an excessive inflammatory response, making it more susceptible to the alveolar fragility and the occurrence of SP or SPM [4], denoted by SP–SPM hereafter.

Mechanical ventilation emerged as the primary contributing factor with a higher frequency of SP reported among patients with COVID-19 receiving mechanical ventilation compared to other cases of acute respiratory distress syndrome (ARDS) or viral causes [4]. Additionally, positive pressure ventilation was linked to increased mortality in intubated patients with COVID-19 [5].

The incidence of SP–SPM in patients with COVID-19 is still under research. A high occurrence of 18.4% (13–25.3%) has been reported by Shrestha et al. among patients admitted to the intensive care unit (ICU) who underwent mechanical ventilation [6]. Nevertheless, the incidence among non-ventilated patients is lower with reported rates below 1% [2,7]. A multicenter study conducted by Miro et al. that included non-ventilated patients with SP reported a low frequency of SP associated with SARS-CoV-2 infection (0.56‰). However, this frequency was still higher than in non-COVID-19 cases (0.28‰), and they had worse outcomes compared to SP in non-COVID-19 cases and sole COVID-19 cases [1].

SP–SPM in non-ventilated patients with COVID-19 is frequently diagnosed in the ED and associated with symptoms characteristic of SARS-CoV-2 infection, such as mild symptoms (e.g., fever, fatigue, and cough), severe symptoms (e.g., chest pain and dyspnea), respiratory distress, or even acute respiratory distress syndrome. Such cases would experience extended hospital stays, elevated probability of ICU admission, and increased risk of mortality, particularly among the elderly population [7,8].

During the COVID-19 pandemic, the SARS-CoV-2 virus underwent a series of mutations, resulting in multiple variants. Their virulence and level of transmissibility, and vaccine development and deployment in the population influenced COVID-19 evolution, affecting the severity of the disease, its clinical presentations, and mortality.

Palumbo et al. conducted the first study that compared the frequency and characteristics of SP–SPM in non-ventilated patients hospitalized with SARS-CoV-2 infection during the first two pandemic waves. They identified 14 patients with SP–SPM, reporting a 29% admission rate to the ICU and a 50% mortality rate. The study also revealed a significantly higher frequency of this complication during the second wave of the pandemic. However, it is important to note that the study included only two waves, which resulted in a limited number of patients, particularly from the first wave where they observed only one patient [9]. Furthermore, Tacconi et al. also reported a higher frequency of pneumomediastinum during the second wave compared to the first one, but their study also included mechanically ventilated patients in both waves [10].

We conducted a retrospective analysis of the SP–SPM cases presented between 1 March 2020 and 31 October 2022 to the emergency departments (EDs) of Emergency Clinical Municipal Hospital and "Pius Brinzeu" Emergency Clinical County Hospital, two tertiary hospitals affiliated with "Victor Babes" University of Medicine and Pharmacy from Timisoara.

The main objective of our research was to investigate the risk of in-hospital mortality in ED patients with SP–SPM during the COVID-19 pandemic. Specifically, we sought to observe a hypothesized relation of an increased risk of mortality with the SARS-CoV-2 infection and any possible patterns across the five pandemic waves. The secondary objectives concerned the SP–SPM disease severity assessed by (a) days of hospitalization; (b) required mechanical ventilation; and (c) required intensive care. All three secondary outcomes were also considered in the context of the five pandemic waves.

2. Materials and Methods

2.1. Study Design and Patients

A retrospective analysis of the electronic medical records (EMRs) was conducted, and 206,097 patients who presented at EDs were retrieved. The inclusion criteria were age above 18 years, presence of SP–SPM confirmed with chest X-ray or computed tomography (CT), and rapid antigenic testing and/or reverse transcription–polymerase chain reaction (RT–PCR) test for SARS-CoV-2 infection. The exclusion criteria were age below 18 years, post-traumatic SP–SPM, and iatrogenic or post-mechanical ventilation SP–SPM.

A keyword-based automated search in the hospital computer system identified 743 cases of SP–SPM. The diagnosis was determined based on the medical records at the time of hospital discharge and defined in accordance with the International Classification of Diseases, 10th Revision, Clinical Modification (ICD-10-CM). The diagnosis code U07.1 was used to identify cases of COVID-19, while J93.11 (SP) or J98.2 (SPM) were employed to designate cases of SP–SPM. Several cases were excluded as they did not meet the study protocol criteria: six patients were under the age of 18 years, 12 patients had iatrogenic (post-procedural) SP, 508 patients had post-traumatic SP–SPM, and 27 cases were associated with mechanical ventilation (e.g., following cardiopulmonary resuscitation). The remaining 190 cases of SP–SPM were manually reviewed to ensure compliance with the inclusion criteria and completeness of the relevant medical data. Figure 1 presents the study flow diagram.

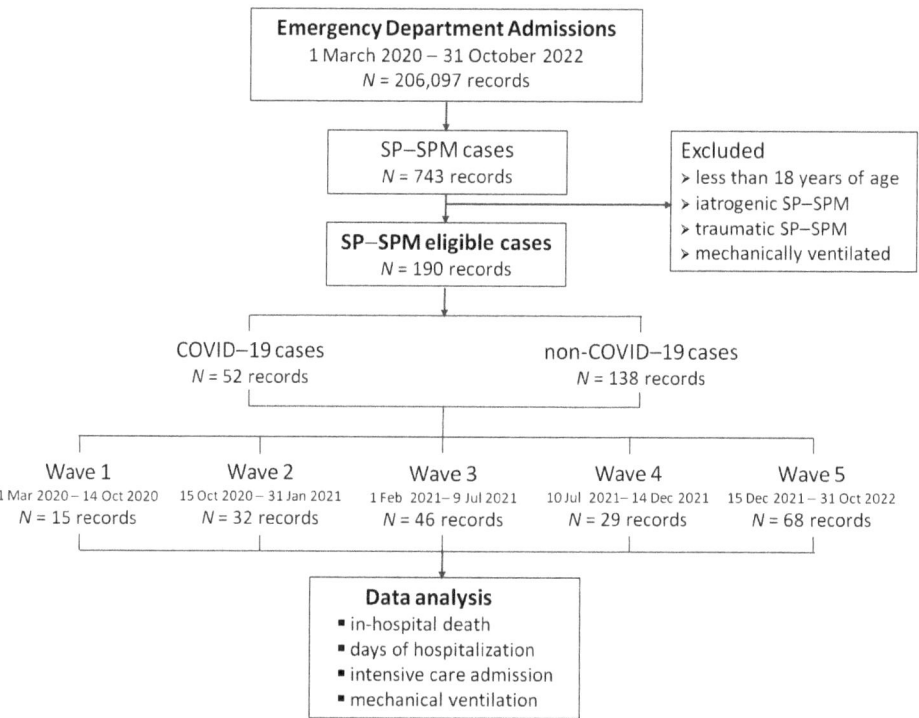

Figure 1. Study flow diagram. SP–SPM stands for spontaneous pneumothorax or spontaneous pneumomediastinum.

Public data regarding the daily number of COVID-19 cases were retrieved from the Centre for Transmissible Disease Control of Timisoara City Council website [11]. The time spells corresponding to the pandemic waves were determined based on the reports from the National Institute of Public Health [12] and corroborated with the results from a recently published study conducted in "Victor Babes" Clinical Hospital for Infectious Diseases and Pulmonology in Timisoara [13]. We were, thus, able to document the wide range of cumulative cases over the five pandemic waves. Nevertheless, it should be noted that, during the first two waves, there were no standard protocols for the management of patients suspected or confirmed to have COVID-19. Table 1 and Figure 2 show the details of the five pandemic waves.

Table 1. The time periods corresponding to the pandemic waves in Timisoara, the prominent variants of concern involved, and the number of SP–SPM cases.

	Wave 1	Wave 2	Wave 3	Wave 4	Wave 5	
Wave period	1 Mar 2020–14 Oct 2020	15 Oct 2020–31 Jan 2021	1 Feb 2021–09 Jul 2021	10 Jul 2021–14 Dec 2021	15 Dec 2021–31 Oct 2022	
Wave spike(s)	–	22 Oct 2020–4 Jan 2021	16 Feb 2021–7 Apr 2021	15 Sep 2021–14 Nov 2021	5 Jan 2022–13 Feb 2022	19 Jul 2022–13 Sep 2022
Spike duration (in days)	–	74	50	60	39	56
Frequent VOC	Wuhan-Hu-1 NC_045512.2	Clade S:D614G	Alpha B.1.1.7	Delta B.1.617.2	Omicron B.1.1.529	
Daily average case count during the spike	–	143.16	164.64	236.71	608.61	137.32
SP–SPM cases	15	32	46	29	68	
SP–SPM and COVID-19 cases	–	18 (55.9%)	15 (31.1%)	6 (20.7%)	13 (19.1%)	

Abbreviations: VOC, variant of concern; SP–SPM, spontaneous pneumothorax and/or spontaneous pneumomediastinum.

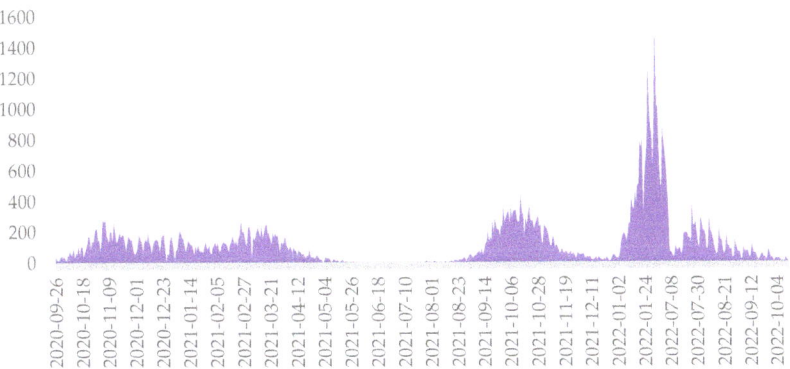

Figure 2. Daily case count in Timisoara from September 2020 to October 2022.

From March 2020, rapid antigenic testing and/or reverse transcription-polymerase chain reaction (RT-PCR) for SARS-CoV-2, along with chest imaging (X-ray or chest computed tomography, depending on the patient's diagnosis) were mandatory, according to the hospitals' internal protocols, regardless of the symptoms of the admitted patients (either on the ward or ICU) through the ED.

In Romania, the initial wave did not have a significant increase in the number of cases due to the authorities' restrictions, leading to a remarkably low count of infections. As a result, no spike could be identified during the first wave. There was not any distinct demarcation between the second and third waves, as the spikes in these two waves were very close in terms of timing (Figure 2). This could be explained by the lack of compliance with the restrictions imposed by the authorities during that period and the growing public mistrust of the healthcare system [14]. The patients infected between the two waves were categorized as belonging to the preceding wave, while those infected after the fifth wave were classified as part of that wave.

2.2. Data Collection

The EMR retrieved data comprised demographics, date of admission to the ED, patient medical history (symptoms, SpO2 value upon arrival in ED, comorbidities including smoking status, history of SARS-CoV-2 infection), paraclinical investigations (laboratory tests, radiological findings on X-ray or chest-CT), decided treatments (observation or chest tube), hospitalization days, ICU admission, need for mechanical ventilation (in hospital, after SP–SPM diagnosis), and discharge outcome. All records were de-identified.

For the present analysis, the laboratory tests on the first day of presentation in the ED (the first 24 h) were taken into consideration; some patients had additional blood tests (e.g., C-reactive protein, procalcitonin) collected at the time of ward admission; some patients stayed for several days in the ED (due to a shortage of beds in COVID-19 support hospitals), and therefore, several sets of laboratory tests were processed.

2.3. Data Analysis

The normality of the data was tested using the Shapiro–Wilk test. The descriptive statistics for the categorical variables were frequency counts and corresponding percentages. The numerical variables were described by the mean with standard deviation, irrespective of their distribution. The rank variables with less than four values were treated as categorical. The statistical significance of the associations between the categorical variables was tested with the chi-square test (either asymptotic or Monte Carlo simulation with 10,000 samples). The significance of the numerical variables' distributions across the pandemic waves was tested with the nonparametric Kruskal–Wallis statistical test, separately for COVID-19 positive and negative cases.

Logistic regression was employed to identify the significant independent predictors of the binary outcomes, namely in-hospital death, required mechanical ventilation, and required intensive care. The medically meaningful predictors that were statistically significant in the univariate analysis were progressively introduced, and the candidate regression models were compared based on the Akaike information criterion (AIC) and Nagelkerke R-square coefficient.

The reported probability values were two-tailed, and the statistical significance was conducted at a 5% level (95% level of confidence). The data analysis was conducted with the statistical software IBM SPSS v. 20 and R v. 4.3.1 packages.

2.4. Ethics

This study was conducted in accordance with the Declaration of Helsinki, and the protocol was approved by the Ethics Committees of the Emergency Clinical Municipal Hospital Timisoara (number I-1831/31 March 2023) and "Pius Brinzeu" Emergency Clinical County Hospital Timisoara (number 387/22 March 2023). The collected data were de-identified before conducting the statistical analysis. Considering the retrospective nature of the study as well as the importance of obtaining new important data regarding the consequences of the novel coronavirus infection, the patient's informed consent was waived.

3. Results

3.1. Characteristics of Patients with SP–SPM

Out of all presentations (206,097 patients) for any cause in the two emergency departments, the patients with pneumothorax and/or pneumomediastinum accounted for 0.03%, while SP–SPM represented 0.009% of the cases. A total of 190 eligible SP–SPM cases were identified: 52 were positive, and 138 were negative for SARS-CoV-2 infection. Seven patients denied hospitalization (four in Wave 5, two in Wave 4, and one in Wave 3). Out of these, three patients had both SP and SPM (one confirmed with COVID-19), one patient had isolated SPM, and three patients had isolated SP (one confirmed with COVID-19). Only one patient experienced an extensive pneumothorax (exceeding 50% of the lung), while the remaining cases had a pneumothorax extent below 10%.

The male gender was predominant (72.63%). The prevailing comorbidities among all patients in the study included hypertension as the most frequent, followed by COPD and diabetes mellitus. In Wave 5, a higher number of cancer cases were registered. Table 2 synthesizes the patients' general characteristics.

Table 2. Descriptive statistics for demographics and number of most frequent comorbidities for each pandemic wave.

Variable			All Patients (N = 190)	Wave 1 (N = 15)	Wave 2 (N = 32)	Wave 3 (N = 46)	Wave 4 (N = 29)	Wave 5 (N = 68)	p-Value [a],[b]
Age [a]		+ COVID-19	63.37 ± 13.9	-	60.4 ± 12.56	71 ± 13.5	51.83 ± 9.58	63.92 ± 13.96	0.019 *
		− COVID-19	48.83 ± 18.51	46.67 ± 16.41	53.64 ± 12.51	44.45 ± 19.27	46.13 ± 17.19	51.78 ± 20.12	0.314
Gender (male) [b]		+ COVID-19	40 (21%)	-	14 (35%)	9 (22.5%)	5 (12.5%)	12 (30%)	<0.001 **
		− COVID-19	98 (51.57%)	13 (13.3%)	7 (7.1%)	23 (23.5%)	14 (14.3%)	41 (41.8%)	
Active smoker [b]		+ COVID-19	10 (5.26%)	-	3 (30%)	3 (30%)	1 (10%)	3 (30%)	<0.001 **
		− COVID-19	59 (31.05%)	12 (20.3%)	8 (13.6%)	14 (23.7%)	5 (8.5%)	20 (33.9%)	
Comorbidities [b]									
	none	+ COVID-19	19 (21.3%)	-	5 (26.3%)	4 (21.1%)	5 (26.3%)	5 (26.3%)	
		− COVID-19	70 (78.7%)	7 (10%)	4 (5.7%)	19 (27.1%)	13 (18.6%)	27 (38.6%)	
	one	+ COVID-19	10 (22.2%)	-	5 (50%)	1 (10%)	-	4 (40%)	
		− COVID-19	35 (77.8%)	3 (8.6%)	3 (8.6%)	6 (17.1%)	8 (22.9%)	15 (42.9%)	0.043 *
	two	+ COVID-19	12 (36.4%)	-	7 (58.3%)	3 (25%)	-	2 (16.7%)	
		− COVID-19	21 (63.6%)	2 (9.5%)	4 (19%)	3 (14.3%)	2 (9.5%)	10 (47.6%)	
	three or more	+ COVID-19	11 (47.8%)	-	1 (9.1%)	7 (63.6%)	1 (9.1%)	2 (18.2%)	
		− COVID-19	12 (52.2%)	3 (25%)	3 (25%)	3 (25%)	-	3 (25%)	

[a] Mean ± SD, Kruskal–Wallis nonparametric test (separate tests for COVID-19 positive and negative patients).
[b] Observed frequency (percent); chi-square test. Calculation of percentages: "All patients" column shows percentages based on the total number of patients presenting each symptom or comorbidity; all other columns show percentages based on the row total. *, ** Statistical significance, $p < 0.05$, $p < 0.01$.

Tables 3 and 4 show the main radiological findings encountered in the patients with SP–SPM, the treatment administered in the ED, as well as the extent of GGO involvement in the patients with COVID-19 with SP–SPM. The most common imagistic findings were GGOs, lung infiltrates, and pneumomediastinum, both in the COVID-19 and non-COVID-19 cases. Chest tube insertion as an emergency treatment for pneumothorax was more frequent during the early waves of the pandemic. The majority of the patients with COVID-19 with GGOs exceeding 50% were observed during the third wave, aligning with the decreased oxygen saturation levels in that same period. The detailed descriptive statistics for the medical information retrieved from the patients' records are presented in the Supplementary Material: Tables S1–S3.

Table 3. Radiological findings (computed tomography and/or chest radiography) and preferred treatment during each successive wave of the pandemic.

Variable [a]		All Patients (N = 190)	Wave 1 (N = 15)	Wave 2 (N = 32)	Wave 3 (N = 46)	Wave 4 (N = 29)	Wave 5 (N = 68)	p-Value [a]
Lung infiltrates	+ COVID-19	20 (71.4%)	-	8 (40%)	8 (40%)	1 (5%)	3 (15%)	<0.001 ** [a]
	− COVID-19	8 (28.6%)	1 (12.5%)	2 (25%)	3 (37.5%)	1 (12.5%)	1 (12.5%)	
Ground-glass opacities	+ COVID-19	32 (84.2%)	-	16 (50%)	10 (31.3%)	2 (6.3%)	4 (12.5%)	<0.001 ** [a]
	− COVID-19	6 (15.8%)	-	1 (16.7%)	1 (16.7%)	1 (16.7%)	3 (50%)	
Pneumomediastinum	+ COVID-19	23 (60.5%)	-	9 (39.1%)	8 (34.8%)	1 (4.3%)	5 (21.7%)	<0.001 ** [a]
	− COVID-19	15 (39.5%)	-	1 (6.7%)	4 (26.7%)	3 (20%)	7 (46.7%)	
Subcutaneous emphysema	+ COVID-19	16 (53.3%)	-	7 (43.8%)	6 (37.5%)	1 (6.3%)	2 (12.5%)	<0.001 ** [a]
	− COVID-19	14 (46.7%)	1 (7.1%)	2 (14.3%)	-	4 (28.6%)	7 (50%)	
Observation	+ COVID-19	22 (64.7%)	-	7 (30.4%)	6 (26.1%)	2 (8.7%)	8 (34.8%)	<0.001 ** [b]
	− COVID-19	14 (37.8%)	-	-	3 (21.4%)	2 (14.3%)	9 (64.3%)	
Chest tube	+ COVID-19	29 (19%)	-	11 (37.9%)	9 (31%)	4 (13.8%)	5 (17.2%)	
	− COVID-19	124 (81%)	15 (12.1%)	14 (11.3%)	28 (22.6%)	21 (16.9%)	46 (37.1%)	

[a] Observed frequency (percent); chi-square test. Calculation of percentages: "All patients" column shows percentages based on the total number of patients presenting each symptom or comorbidity; all other columns show percentages based on the row total. [b] Mean ± SD. ** Statistical significance, $p < 0.01$.

Table 4. Extension of ground-glass opacities and SpO2 values for the patients with COVID-19.

Variable		All Patients N = 52 [#]	Wave 2 N = 18	Wave 3 N = 15	Wave 4 N = 6 [#]	Wave 5 N = 13	p-Value [a],[b]
GGO [a]							
	no GGO	17 (33.3%)	2 (11.8%)	5 (29.4%)	2 (11.8%)	8 (47.1%)	0.035 *
	GGO < 20%	4 (7.8%)	3 (75%)	-	1 (25%)	-	
	GGO 20–50%	10 (19.6%)	4 (40%)	4 (40%)	-	2 (20%)	
	GGO > 50%	20 (39.2%)	9 (45%)	6 (30%)	2 (10%)	3 (15%)	
SpO2 on room air [b]		80.55 ± 13.81	75.72 ± 16.37	82.27 ± 10.96	84.67 ± 14.81	83.58 ± 11.75	0.363

[a] Observed frequency (percent); chi-square test. Calculation of percentages: "All patients" column shows percentages based on the total number of patients presenting each symptom or comorbidity; all other columns show percentages based on the row total. [b] Mean ± SD, Kruskal–Wallis nonparametric test. * Statistical significance, $p < 0.05$. [#] One patient refused to be admitted to the hospital and denied CT for further evaluation. Abbreviations: CT, computed tomography; GGO, ground-glass opacity; SD, standard deviation; SpO2, peripheral oxygen saturation at hospital admittance.

Across these five waves, we observed 11 non-COVID-19 cases with SP–SPM that presented with a history of SARS-CoV-2 infection. Out of these patients, two were suffering from SPM alone and one from both SP and SPM. One patient died due to a massive SP after two days of hospitalization while being admitted to the ICU and after he had a chest tube inserted. None of these patients had significant comorbidities, 64% were males, their average age was 60 years (24–88), and their clinical feature was dominated by cough and chest pain. Six of them had the C-reactive protein checked; out of these, five had elevated values (average 121 mg/L with a 277 mg/L uppermost value). In addition, there were five patients with persistent ground-glass opacities: three of them exceeded 50% of the pulmonary surface, and two were between 10% and 50%.

Table 5 synthesizes the outcomes related to the study objectives. Figure 3 shows the box-plot diagram of the length of hospitalization across the five waves. There are many outliers and extreme values (open bullets and stars, respectively) in all waves, but there is a particularly high extreme value in Wave 2 for a COVID-19 case. The lack of a distinctive pattern is easily observable.

Table 5. Outcomes for the COVID-19 and non-COVID-19 cases across the five pandemic waves.

Variable		All Patients (N = 190)	Wave 1 (N = 15)	Wave 2 (N = 32)	Wave 3 (N = 46)	Wave 4 (N = 29)	Wave 5 (N = 68)	p-Value (a),(b)
Deceased [a]	+ COVID-19	24 (77.4%)	-	7 (29.2%)	9 (37.5%)	3 (12.5%)	5 (20.8%)	<0.001 **
	− COVID-19	7 (22.6%)	-	2 (28.6%)	4 (57.1%)	-	1 (14.3%)	
Hospitalization days [b]	+ COVID-19	17.63 ± 20.82	-	24.72 ± 30.38	18.27 ± 12.58	7.83 ± 11.39	11.08 ± 10.04	0.035 *
	− COVID-19	9.88 ± 7.58	12.07 ± 7	9.5 ± 5.19	10.81 ± 9.09	12 ± 10.02	7.94 ± 5.62	0.285
Required ICU [a]	+ COVID-19	23 (71.9%)	-	9 (39.1%)	6 (26.1%)	2 (8.7%)	6 (26.1%)	<0.001 **
	− COVID-19	9 (28.1%)	-	2 (22.2%)	2 (22.2%)	2 (22.2%)	3 (33.3%)	
Required MV [a]	+ COVID-19	19 (65.5%)	-	6 (31.6%)	5 (26.3%)	2 (10.5%)	6 (31.6%)	<0.001 **
	− COVID-19	10 (34.5%)	-	2 (20%)	2 (20%)	3 (30%)	3 (30%)	

[a] Observed frequency (percent); chi-square test. Calculation of percentages: "All patients" column shows percentages based on the total number of patients presenting each symptom or comorbidity; all other columns show percentages based on the row total. [b] Mean ± SD, Kruskal–Wallis nonparametric test. *, ** Statistical significance, $p < 0.05$, $p < 0.01$. Abbreviations: ICU, intensive care unit; MV, mechanical ventilation; SD, standard deviation.

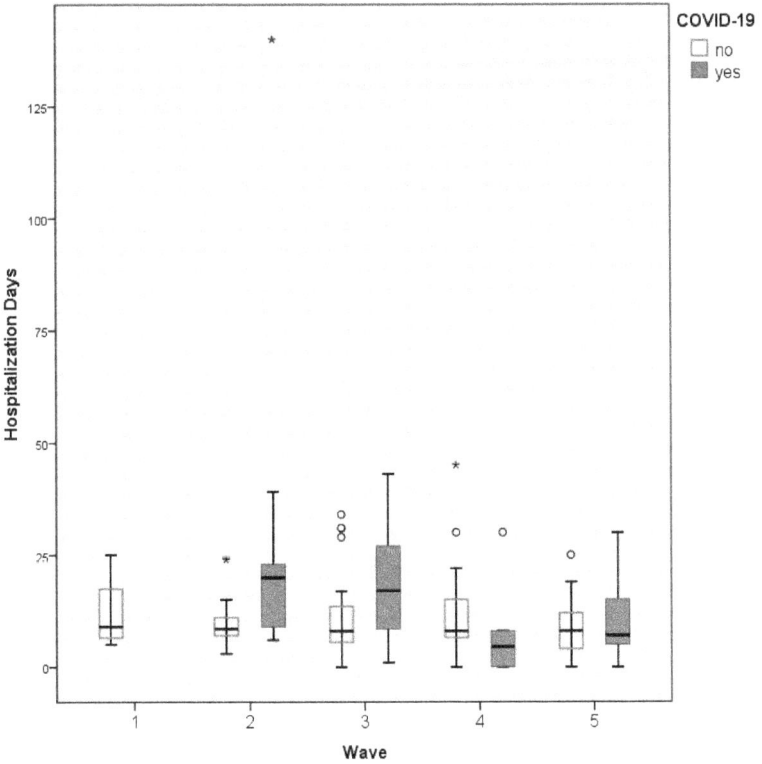

Figure 3. Box-plot diagram with length of hospitalization for COVID-19 and non-COVID-19 cases. The boxes are proportional to the interquartile range (IQR) with medians marked in-between, and the whiskers are proportional to 1.5 * IQR. (or trimmed to the minimum or maximum values).

3.2. Logistic Regression Models of the Binary Outcomes

The pandemic waves had no significant effect on the risk of death. Table 6 summarizes the results of the logistic regression analysis related to in-hospital mortality as the outcome:

the mortality was highly dependent on the presence of COVID-19, the increased number of comorbidities, and the presence of ground-glass opacities over 50%. The odds ratio (OR) values of the significant predictors and their corresponding confidence intervals on a logarithmic scale are depicted in Figure 4. Although some of these intervals are large (such as those for COVID-19 condition and the presence of ground-glass opacities), implying imprecision, the Nagelkerke R-square value (i.e., R-square = 0.524) demonstrates the model's good prediction performance: these four predictors would explain more than 50% of the SP–SPM mortality when controlling for gender, smoking habits, pandemic wave, and extension of SP–SPM. On the other hand, the OR value for age is very close to 1 with a highly tight confidence interval, thus implying little impact on the outcome (statistically significant nonetheless).

Table 6. The logistic regression model for in-hospital mortality. Exp (B) is equivalent to the odds ratio (OR), a measure of a relationship's strength between the predictor and the binary outcome.

Model: Deceased ~ Age + COVID-19 + N comorbidities + Ground glass opacities over 50%
Controlling for: GenderM + ActiveSmoker + pandemicWave (categorical) + extension of SP–SPM (categorical)

Predictor	B ± Std. err	p-Value	Exp (B) (95% CI)
Age	0.042 ± 0.02	0.039 *	1.043 (1.002–1.085)
COVID-19	1.797 ± 0.629	0.004 **	6.032 (1.757–20.712)
N comorbidities	0.572 ± 0.269	0.033 *	1.772 (1.046–3.001)
Ground glass opacities over 50%	1.739 ± 0.808	0.031 *	5.694 (1.169–27.746)
	Nagelkerke R-square = 0.524		

Abbreviations: B ± Std. err, coefficient of regression ± standard error; CI, confidence interval. *, ** Statistical significance, $p < 0.05$, $p < 0.01$.

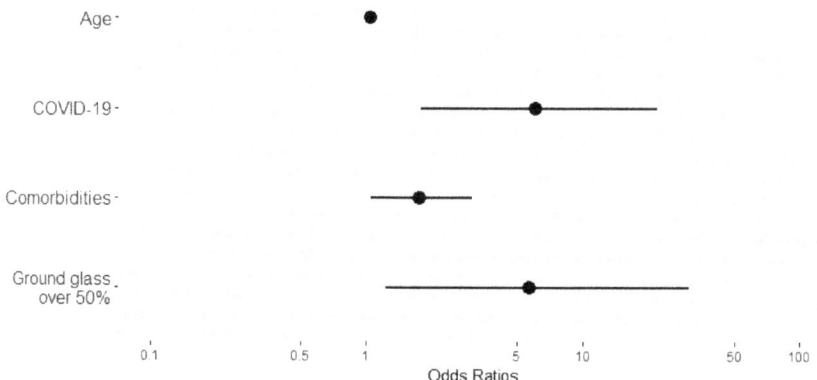

Figure 4. The independent predictors for in-hospital mortality as resulted from the logistic regression analysis. The dots correspond to the estimated OR values (shown in Table 6), and the lines depict the 95%CI intervals. The horizontal axis employs a logarithmic scale.

Tables 7 and 8 present the results of the logistic regression analyses with required intensive care and required mechanical ventilation as the outcomes, respectively. In both models, age was non-significant, and the increase in the number of comorbidities raised the risk of an unfavorable outcome. The presence of COVID-19 and extensive ground-glass opacities were both significant predictors with a high impact on the outcomes in each of these two risk models. Their different relative influence on the outcomes should be noted in Figure 5: COVID-19 had a significant impact on the ICU risk and halved the odds for mechanical ventilation, while extended ground-glass opacities were found to increase the odds of mechanical ventilation almost seven times and close to five times for the ICU. The Nagelkerke R-square values are smaller for these two models (0.419 and 0.373, respectively), implying that there are additional predictors and covariates influencing the outcomes.

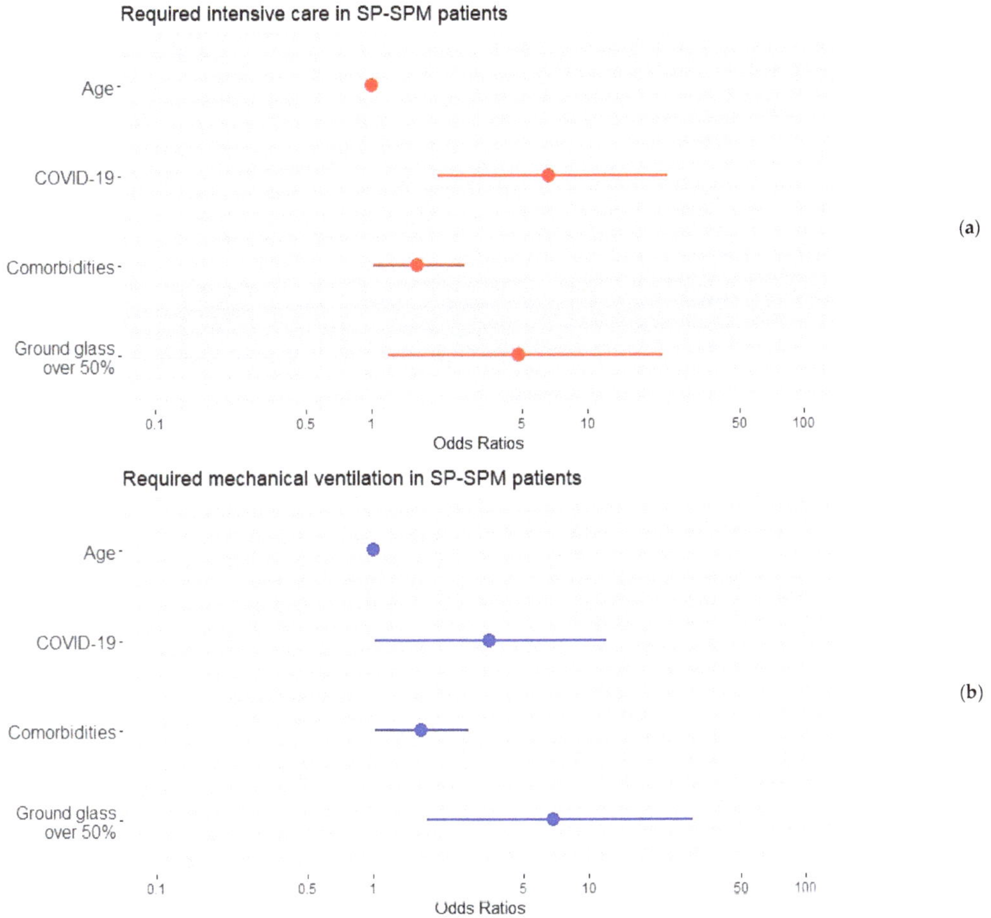

Figure 5. The independent predictors for required intensive care (**a**) and mechanical ventilation (**b**) in patients with SP–SPM as resulted from the logistic regression analysis. The dots correspond to the estimated OR values (shown in Tables 7 and 8, respectively), and the lines depict the 95%CI intervals. The horizontal axes employ a logarithmic scale.

Table 7. The logistic regression model for required intensive care. Exp (B) is equivalent to the odds ratio (OR), a measure of a relationship's strength between the predictor and the binary outcome.

Model: ICU ~ Age + COVID-19 + N comorbidities + Ground glass opacities over 50%
Controlling for: GenderM + ActiveSmoker + pandemicWave (categorical) + extension of SP–SPM (categorical)

Predictor	B ± Std. err	p-Value	Exp (B) (95% CI)
Age	0.011 ± 0.016	0.511	1.011 (0.979–1.043)
COVID-19	1.901 ± 0.613	0.002 **	6.693 (2.013–22.261)
N comorbidities	0.504 ± 0.246	0.041 *	1.656 (1.022–2.683)
Ground glass opacities over 50%	1.570 ± 0.736	0.033 *	4.807 (1.137–20.326)
Nagelkerke R-square = 0.419			

Abbreviations: B ± Std. err, coefficient of regression ± standard error; CI, confidence interval; ICU, intensive care unit. *, ** Statistical significance, $p < 0.05$, $p < 0.01$.

Table 8. The logistic regression model for required mechanical ventilation. Exp (B) is equivalent to the odds ratio (OR), a measure of a relationship's strength between the predictor and the binary outcome.

Model: MV ~ Age + COVID-19 + N comorbidities + Ground glass opacities over 50%
Controlling for: GenderM + ActiveSmoker + pandemicWave (categorical) + extension of SP–SPM (categorical)

Predictor	B ± Std. err	p-Value	Exp (B) (95% CI)
Age	0.012 ± 0.016	0.454	1.012 (0.981–1.044)
COVID-19	1.249 ± 0.622	0.045 *	3.488 (1.031–11.801)
N comorbidities	0.519 ± 0.254	0.041 *	1.681 (1.022–2.766)
Ground glass opacities over 50%	1.928 ± 0.712	0.007 *	6.876 (1.704–27.735)
Nagelkerke R-square = 0.373			

Abbreviations: B ± Std. err, coefficient of regression ± standard error; CI, confidence interval; MV, mechanical ventilation. * Statistical significance, $p < 0.05$.

4. Discussion

Each pandemic wave presented unique challenges both to the medical professionals involved in treating the patients with COVID-19 and to the healthcare system itself, thus entailing continuous research aimed at optimizing patient care. Our retrospective analysis investigated SP–SPM as a medical condition in the five waves of the COVID-19 pandemic between 1 March 2020 and 31 October 2022. The objective of this debriefing was to identify possible patterns of disease and the risk factors associated with in-hospital mortality (primary outcome) and high disease severity (secondary outcomes). Although the patients with COVID-19 were at a significantly higher risk, there were no distinct patterns across the pandemic waves.

In December 2021, the Omicron variant became the predominant lineage of SARS-CoV-2 in several European countries and was associated with significantly lower clinical severity, reduced oxygen requirements, lower rates of hospitalization, and decreased mortality rates [15]. Amodio et al. presented evidence indicating a general decrease in viral virulence from the wild-type to Omicron variants and a higher risk of MV and severe outcomes for the corresponding Delta and wild-type waves [16]. Our findings were similar regarding the hospitalization length for patients with SP–SPM with SARS-CoV-2 infection, which was longer during the second and third waves compared to that of the non-COVID cases. During the second wave, the increase in the average hospitalization was partially attributed to a single patient who required hospitalization for 140 days as a result of septic complications that arose from both COVID-19 pneumonia and the chest tube insertion. However, the hospital stay would slowly decrease in subsequent waves.

In our investigation, most of the SP–SPM cases associated with SARS-CoV-2 infection (55.9% of the total number) were identified during the second wave. These patients presented with the lowest SpO2 levels upon their arrival in the emergency department and had the longest stay in the hospital, prolonged MV (due to extensive lung damage), and a higher admission rate to the ICU. Unfortunately, they also experienced a significant mortality rate of 29.2%. These patients were at risk of developing ventilator-associated pneumonia and other nosocomial infections due to their extended hospitalization, which could have contributed to the observed increase in mortality. A systematic review and meta-analysis conducted by Shrestha et al. reported an increased occurrence of barotrauma in patients with severe forms of the disease, implying a direct connection between barotrauma and disease severity [6]. Regarding the virulence of the virus corresponding to each wave, a study conducted in 2021 by Zawbaa et al. examined the severity of the SARS-CoV-2 virus in 12 countries and revealed that the third and fourth waves were associated with higher mortality [17].

4.1. Mortality and Severity of Disease across the Five Pandemic Waves

In our data, the logistic regression analysis found that the presence of COVID-19 increased the in-hospital mortality risk more than six times (namely with an OR = 6.032) for patients with SP–SPM of the same age, gender, smoking status, pandemic wave, and severity of GGOs and comorbidities. Moreover, GGOs exceeding 50% increased the risk of death by approximately six times (OR = 5.694), and an increased number of comorbidities almost doubled the risk (OR = 1.772). In contrast, the pandemic wave had no significant effect on the risk of death in patients with SP–SPM. As other studies reported, the Omicron variant had substantially increased transmissibility and resulted in higher rates of prolonged hospitalization and mortality in unvaccinated patients [15]. Considering that Romania had a consistently low vaccination rate, this could explain the increased mortality in the subsequent waves despite the less aggressive virus strains. However, it is important to also acknowledge the role of natural immunity and the fact that better outcomes in some healthcare systems could be attributed to the improved clinical and therapeutical practices that resulted from increased knowledge and experience over time [16].

In a recent study, Akyil et al. reported no mortality difference in patients with SP–SPM with COVID-19 when compared to non-COVID-19 cases. However, it is also important to note that, in their study, the patients with COVID-19 were asymptomatic and did not have underlying lung lesions or GGOs. The only notable difference was a prolonged recovery time in the COVID-19 group [18].

Starting from the second wave, the proportion of SP–SPM cases associated with COVID-19 diminished, but it surged in the fifth wave, which was characterized by the Omicron variant. This pattern may suggest a significant susceptibility to SP or SPM among individuals who either had or might have experienced a prior SARS-CoV-2 infection, considering that this complication has already been described in several studies [19–22]. Despite all that, the PCR test for detecting SARS-CoV-2 infection may yield false-negative results if it is performed too early or too late in the course of the disease. This is especially relevant since it was frequently performed as a mandatory test upon admission, even in cases where patients did not exhibit COVID-19 symptoms.

4.2. Medical History and Comorbities of Patients with SP–SPM

In our study, the mean age of the entire group of patients with SP–SPM was 52.8 ± 18.5 years, and it was higher among those with COVID-19 (63.37 ± 13.9 years), particularly during the third wave of the pandemic (71 ± 13.5 years). This might explain the high mortality rate observed during this wave in the patients with SP–SPM with associated SARS-CoV-2 infection, considering that elder age was frequently associated with increased mortality [1,3]. In our analysis concerning in-hospital mortality, age had the least influence on the outcome. Additionally, in the secondary outcomes' investigation, age was no longer significant after accounting for the risks associated with mechanical ventilation and ICU admission.

Most of the patients who contracted SARS-CoV-2 and subsequently developed SP–SPM were males and non-smokers, aligning with the findings in the current literature [7], where smoking was not identified as a risk factor for SP in patients with COVID-19 but was associated with greater disease severity. Regardless of the virus variant's severity or of the pulmonary damage, the patients' comorbidities directly influenced mortality, as evidenced in our study. For instance, in the patients infected with SARS-CoV-2 during the fourth wave of the COVID-19 pandemic (with the Delta strain), ischemic heart disease was associated with greater disease severity and increased mortality rates, surpassing those observed in the earlier waves [23].

The most frequent comorbidities among all patients included hypertension, followed by COPD and diabetes mellitus, as observed in Supplementary material Table S1. Hypertension exhibited a statistically significant higher occurrence among patients with COVID-19 across all pandemic waves, which can be explained by the older age of these patients compared to the non-COVID-19 ones. Regarding pre-existing lung disease, Chong et al. reported a prevalence of less than 30% among patients with SP–SPM and COVID-19 [7]. While COPD is frequently observed in patients with SP–SPM, our dataset showed no association with the COVID-19 condition, unlike asthma (which appears to be a common comorbidity in patients with COVID-19, particularly during the third wave of the pandemic). Wang et al. [24] reported no substantial disparity between mortality rates in patients with COVID-19 with asthma and those without. Regarding the requirement for ICU admission or mechanical ventilation in patients with COVID-19 with asthma, the existing literature does not identify any discernible distinctions [25]. Our study findings may suggest that underlying pulmonary diseases alone would not significantly increase mortality in patients with SP–SPM. On the contrary, it appeared that numerous comorbidities would exacerbate the SARS-CoV-2 infection and the associated inflammatory syndrome and, thus, play an important role in the mortality increase.

In our investigation, dyspnea emerged as the most frequent symptom, followed by fatigue and cough (Supplementary Table S1). The mechanism of SP in patients with COVID-19 is far from being fully understood. Multiple hypotheses have been proposed, including delayed alveolar breach as part of a chronic inflammatory process [26] or ischemic breakdown of the alveolar wall secondary to micro-thrombi [22]. Considering that, in several studies, cough was described as a frequent symptom of SARS-CoV-2 infection and post COVID-19 syndrome [27], its increased occurrence in our dataset could be a warning regarding the patients with COVID-19. Also, dyspnea and increased respiratory drive due to SARS-CoV-2 infection might cause patient self-inflicted lung injury (P-SILI) [28] and could also be incriminated in the development of SP–SPM.

4.3. Imaging and Laboratory Findings in Patients with SP–SPM

The most common radiographic finding (as described in Supplementary Table S2) was right-sided pneumothorax, observed in 57.89% of patients, which is consistent with the results of other studies [1,3,7].

In the second pandemic wave, GGOs were observed in approximately all COVID-19 cases with the largest extent of these lesions (50% of patients exhibited GGOs covering > 50% of the lung fields). A high incidence of GGO lesions also persisted in the third wave, followed by a gradual reduction towards the fifth wave, wherein both the incidence and the extent of the lesions were reduced by half. Nevertheless, the mortality rate in the fifth wave remained high among the patients with COVID-19 compared to the non-COVID-19 cases (20.8% vs. 14.3%, respectively). This suggests that there were other contributory factors to the mortality risk in the individuals with SP–SPM beyond the extent of GGOs (which would increase the severity of COVID-19 pneumonia). One of them was found to be the presence of several comorbidities in our logistic regression analysis. Additionally, the large number of infections and subsequent overcrowding in COVID-19 wards, reduced rate of medical staff to treat patients, and nosocomial infections associated with prolonged hospitalization and mechanical ventilation could explain the persistence of increased mortality in the fifth wave.

Across the pandemic waves, the frequency of GGO lesions on chest CT scans increased among the non-COVID cases with SP–SPM (reaching from 0% in the first wave to 50% in the fifth wave). This trend might imply a potential history of SARS-CoV-2 infection in these cases and would indicate a higher risk of SP or SPM in patients with such a medical record, as was mentioned in several reports [22,29–31].

Among the patients with SP–SPM with COVID-19, the laboratory findings indicated a greater incidence of lymphopenia and increased levels of C-reactive protein, urea, and creatinine compared to the non-COVID-19 cases (Supplementary Table S3). These values were found as excessive throughout the pandemic waves, but they were most likely related to viral involvement.

4.4. Treatment Options in Patients with SP–SPM

The treatment of choice for the non-COVID-19 cases was chest tube, opposite to the COVID-19 group where the treatment of choice was conservative. We noted a slight reduction in the number of chest tubes used in the second part of the pandemic (in the fourth and fifth waves) with an increased number of patients for whom observation was decided as the most appropriate course of action. This approach can be explained by both the increased experience regarding the treatment of SP–SPM cases associated with SARS-CoV-2 infection and the recent pneumothorax management guideline that recommended a less invasive approach; according to the latest British Thoracic Society Guideline for pleural disease [32], the size of the pneumothorax is no longer a criterion for inserting a chest drain, which is now recommended for high-risk patients only.

4.5. Limitations of This Debriefing

Our study had several limitations, primarily stemming from its retrospective design. First, the absence of standardized protocols resulted in a non-uniform management of these cases, particularly during the initial waves of the pandemic. Consequently, crucial inflammatory markers in COVID-19, such as interleukin-6 and ferritin, could not be consistently determined in the ED due to a lack of reagents. CRP, procalcitonin, and D-dimers were only collected upon specific requests from the physicians, making it impossible for us to correlate the inflammatory syndrome with the occurrence of SP–SPM. Second, our hospitals did not allow routine phenotyping for each patient with COVID-19. The implementation of such phenotyping would have incurred substantial costs for an already overwhelmed healthcare system. Therefore, we considered the most prevalent national variant as the involved strain. Third, there is a possibility that some cases went undiagnosed. Some patients who presented to the hospital during the pandemic with suspected SP–SPM and tested positive for SARS-CoV-2 in the ED refused further imaging investigations and hospitalization due to distrust in the medical system and were not included in our study. Fourth, there might have been false-negative SARS-CoV-2 test results. Some patients could have been tested too early or too late in the course of their illness, leading to their erroneous inclusion in the non-COVID group of this analysis.

Despite its limitations, this analysis brought reliable evidence of no differences in mortality among the patients with SP–SPM according to the pandemic wave or severity of the virus strain. Since the emergence of the Omicron variant, severe forms of COVID-19 pneumonia have become less common. Nevertheless, we must remain vigilant regarding the heightened risk of mortality in these patients, irrespective of age. Moreover, frequent and vigilant monitoring of patients with COVID-19 should be performed in order to promptly detect the occurrence of SP. Lung ultrasound can serve as a valuable diagnostic tool at the bedside for patients with COVID-19 admitted to the ward. This approach can help avoid non-invasive ventilation or invasive mechanical ventilation in patients with SP and the associated risk of tension pneumothorax. Additionally, patients with SP–SPM and GGOs covering more than 50% of the lung surface should be considered for admission to the ICU or an intermediate care unit, depending on the hospital's policies. This level of care can ensure continuous monitoring and surveillance, which is crucial given the increased mortality risk associated with this predictor.

5. Conclusions

Over approximately three years, the risks of mortality, mechanical ventilation, and ICU admission in patients with SP–SPM were significantly dependent on the coexisting COVID-19 disease, extensive lung injury, and increased number of comorbidities, regardless of the age of the patients and the virulence of the different strains involved in a pandemic wave. Beyond the COVID-19 pandemic, these findings highlight the importance of careful observation of each SP–SPM case, accompanied by personalized and rapid intervention.

Supplementary Materials: The following supporting information can be downloaded at: https://www.mdpi.com/article/10.3390/jpm13101497/s1, Table S1: The most frequent symptoms and comorbidities observed in patients with SP–SPM. Table S2: Localization and extension of pneumothorax.; Table S3: Laboratory findings for patients with COVID-19 and non-COVID-19 cases across pandemic waves.

Author Contributions: Conceptualization, A.M.M., A.P. and D.L.; methodology, A.M.M.; software, D.L.; validation, A.M.M., A.P., C.B., A.V.S. and D.L.; formal analysis, A.C.C. and D.L.; investigation, A.M.M. and A.C.C.; resources, A.M.M., A.C.C., A.P., R.C. and A.M.; data curation, A.M.M., A.C.C. and D.L.; writing—original draft preparation, A.M.M. and A.C.C.; writing—review and editing, A.M.M., A.P., A.V.S., C.B., A.M., R.C., M.O.B., C.I.T. and D.L.; visualization, M.O.B. and C.I.T.; supervision, A.P. and D.L.; project administration, D.L. All authors have read and agreed to the published version of the manuscript.

Funding: This research received no external funding.

Institutional Review Board Statement: This study was conducted in accordance with the Declaration of Helsinki, and the protocol was approved by the Ethics Committees of the Emergency Clinical Municipal Hospital Timisoara (number I-1831/31 March 2023) and the "Pius Brinzeu" Emergency Clinical County Hospital Timisoara (number 387/22 March 2023).

Informed Consent Statement: Collected data were de-identified before conducting the statistical analysis. Considering the retrospective nature of the study as well as the importance of obtaining new important data regarding the consequences of the novel coronavirus infection, the patient's informed consent was waived.

Data Availability Statement: The datasets are not publicly available, but de-identified data may be provided upon request from Adina Maria Marza.

Acknowledgments: The authors kindly acknowledge the colleagues from the two EDs who volunteered to participate in the data collection.

Conflicts of Interest: The authors declare no conflict of interest.

Abbreviations

ARDS, acute respiratory distress syndrome; CKD, chronic kidney disease; COPD, chronic obstructive pulmonary disease; COVID-19, coronavirus disease 2019; CRP, C-reactive protein; CRT, creatinine; CT, computed tomography; DM, diabetes mellitus; ED, emergency department; EMR, electronic medical record; GGO, ground-glass opacity; GLI, glycemia; HBP, high blood pressure; Lymph, lymphocytes; MV, mechanical ventilation; OR, odds ratio; PLT, platelets; RT-PCR, reverse transcription-polymerase chain reaction; SARS-CoV-2, severe acute respiratory syndrome-coronavirus 2; SD, standard deviation; SP, spontaneous pneumothorax; SPM, spontaneous pneumomediastinum; SP–SPM, SP or SPM; SpO2, peripheral oxygen saturation on room air at hospital admittance; WBC, white blood cells.

References

1. Miró, Ò.; Llorens, P.; Jiménez, S.; Piñera, P.; Burillo-Putze, G.; Martín, A.; Martín-Sánchez, F.J.; García-Lamberetchs, E.J.; Jacob, J.; Alquézar-Arbé, A.; et al. Frequency, Risk Factors, Clinical Characteristics, and Outcomes of Spontaneous Pneumothorax in Patients with Coronavirus Disease 2019. *Chest* **2021**, *159*, 1241–1255. [CrossRef] [PubMed]
2. Martinelli, A.W.; Ingle, T.; Newman, J.; Nadeem, I.; Jackson, K.; Lane, N.D.; Melhorn, J.; Davies, H.E.; Rostron, A.J.; Adeni, A.; et al. COVID-19 and Pneumothorax: A Multicentre Retrospective Case Series. *Eur. Respir. J.* **2020**, *56*, 2002697. [CrossRef] [PubMed]
3. Marza, A.M.; Petrica, A.; Lungeanu, D.; Sutoi, D.; Mocanu, A.; Petrache, I.; Mederle, O.A. Risk Factors, Characteristics, and Outcome in Non-Ventilated Patients with Spontaneous Pneumothorax or Pneumomediastinum Associated with SARS-CoV-2 Infection. *Int. J. Gen. Med.* **2022**, *15*, 489–500. [CrossRef]
4. Taha, M.; Elahi, M.; Wahby, K.; Samavati, L. Incidence and Risk Factors of COVID-19 Associated Pneumothorax. *PLoS ONE* **2022**, *17*, e0271964. [CrossRef] [PubMed]
5. Shahsavarinia, K.; Rahvar, G.; Soleimanpour, H.; Saadati, M.; Vahedi, L.; Mahmoodpoor, A. Spontaneous Pneumomediastinum, Pneumothorax and Subcutaneous Emphysema in Critically Ill COVID-19 Patients: A Systematic Review. *Pak. J. Med. Sci.* **2022**, *38*, 730. [CrossRef]
6. Shrestha, D.B.; Sedhai, Y.R.; Budhathoki, P.; Adhikari, A.; Pokharel, N.; Dhakal, R.; Kafle, S.; Yadullahi Mir, W.A.; Acharya, R.; Kashiouris, M.G.; et al. Pulmonary Barotrauma in COVID-19: A Systematic Review and Meta-Analysis. *Ann. Med. Surg.* **2022**, *73*, 103221. [CrossRef]
7. Chong, W.H.; Saha, B.K.; Hu, K.; Chopra, A. The Incidence, Clinical Characteristics, and Outcomes of Pneumothorax in Hospitalized COVID-19 Patients: A Systematic Review. *Heart Lung* **2021**, *50*, 599–608. [CrossRef]
8. Woo, W.; Kipkorir, V.; Marza, A.M.; Hamouri, S.; Albawaih, O.; Dhali, A.; Kim, W.; Udwadia, Z.F.; Nashwan, A.J.; Shaikh, N.; et al. Prognosis of Spontaneous Pneumothorax/Pneumomediastinum in Coronavirus Disease 2019: The CoBiF Score. *J. Clin. Med.* **2022**, *11*, 7132. [CrossRef]
9. Palumbo, D.; Campochiaro, C.; Belletti, A.; Marinosci, A.; Dagna, L.; Zangrillo, A.; De Cobelli, F. Pneumothorax/Pneumomediastinum in Non-Intubated COVID-19 Patients: Differences between First and Second Italian Pandemic Wave. *Eur. J. Intern. Med.* **2021**, *88*, 144–146. [CrossRef]
10. Tacconi, F.; Rogliani, P.; Leonardis, F.; Sarmati, L.; Fabbi, E.; De Carolis, G.; La Rocca, E.; Vanni, G.; Ambrogi, V. Incidence of Pneumomediastinum in COVID-19: A Single-Center Comparison between 1st and 2nd Wave. *Respir. Investig.* **2021**, *59*, 661–665. [CrossRef]
11. Situația COVID-19 În Timișoara. Available online: https://covid19.primariatm.ro/ (accessed on 10 March 2023).
12. Infecția Cu Noul Coronavirus (SARS-CoV-2). Available online: http://www.cnscbt.ro/ (accessed on 10 March 2023).
13. Fericean, R.M.; Citu, C.; Manolescu, D.; Rosca, O.; Bratosin, F.; Tudorache, E.; Oancea, C. Characterization and Outcomes of SARS-CoV-2 Infection in Overweight and Obese Patients: A Dynamic Comparison of COVID-19 Pandemic Waves. *J. Clin. Med.* **2022**, *11*, 2916. [CrossRef]
14. Weekly Epidemiological Update on COVID-19—14 September 2021. Available online: https://www.who.int/publications/m/item/weekly-epidemiological-update-on-covid-{-}{-}-14-september-2021 (accessed on 10 March 2023).
15. Rzymski, P.; Kasianchuk, N.; Sikora, D.; Poniedziałek, B. COVID-19 Vaccinations and Rates of Infections, Hospitalizations, ICU Admissions, and Deaths in Europe during SARS-CoV-2 Omicron Wave in the First Quarter of 2022. *J. Med. Virol.* **2023**, *95*, e28131. [CrossRef] [PubMed]
16. Amodio, E.; Genovese, D.; Fallucca, A.; Ferro, P.; Sparacia, B.; D'Azzo, L.; Fertitta, A.; Maida, C.M.; Vitale, F. Clinical Severity in Different Waves of SARS-CoV-2 Infection in Sicily: A Model of Smith's "Law of Declining Virulence" from Real-World Data. *Viruses* **2022**, *15*, 125. [CrossRef] [PubMed]
17. Zawbaa, H.M.; Osama, H.; El-Gendy, A.; Saeed, H.; Harb, H.S.; Madney, Y.M.; Abdelrahman, M.; Mohsen, M.; Ali, A.M.A.; Nicola, M.; et al. Effect of Mutation and Vaccination on Spread, Severity, and Mortality of COVID-19 Disease. *J. Med. Virol.* **2022**, *94*, 197–204. [CrossRef] [PubMed]
18. Akyil, M.; Bayram, S.; Erdizci, P.; Tokgoz Akyil, F.; Ulusoy, A.; Evman, S.; Alpay, L.; Baysungur, V. The Prognostic Effect of Concomitant COVID-19 with Spontaneous Pneumothorax. *Turk. J. Thorac. Cardiovasc. Surg.* **2023**, *31*, 352–357. [CrossRef]
19. Ferreira, J.G.; Rapparini, C.; Gomes, B.M.; Pinto, L.A.C. Pneumothorax as a Late Complication of COVID-19. *Rev. Inst. Med. Trop. Sao Paulo* **2020**, *62*. [CrossRef] [PubMed]
20. Marzocchi, G.; Vassallo, A.; Monteduro, F. Spontaneous Pneumothorax as a Delayed Complication after Recovery from COVID-19. *BMJ Case Rep.* **2021**, *14*, e243578. [CrossRef]
21. Nunna, K.; Braun, A.B. Development of a Large Spontaneous Pneumothorax after Recovery from Mild COVID-19 Infection. *BMJ Case Rep.* **2021**, *14*, e238863. [CrossRef] [PubMed]
22. Abushahin, A.; Degliuomini, J.; Aronow, W.S.; Newman, T. A Case of Spontaneous Pneumothorax 21 Days After Diagnosis of Coronavirus Disease 2019 (COVID-19) Pneumonia. *Am. J. Case Rep.* **2020**, *21*, e925787-1. [CrossRef]
23. Tudora, A.; Lungeanu, D.; Pop-Moldovan, A.; Puschita, M.; Lala, R.I. Successive Waves of the COVID-19 Pandemic Had an Increasing Impact on Chronic Cardiovascular Patients in a Western Region of Romania. *Healthcare* **2023**, *11*, 1183. [CrossRef]
24. Wang, Y.; Chen, J.; Chen, W.; Liu, L.; Dong, M.; Ji, J.; Hu, D.; Zhang, N. Does Asthma Increase the Mortality of Patients with COVID-19?: A Systematic Review and Meta-Analysis. *Int. Arch. Allergy Immunol.* **2021**, *182*, 76–82. [CrossRef] [PubMed]

25. Sunjaya, A.P.; Allida, S.M.; Di Tanna, G.L.; Jenkins, C. Asthma and Risk of Infection, Hospitalization, ICU Admission and Mortality from COVID-19: Systematic Review and Meta-Analysis. *J. Asthma* **2022**, *59*, 866–879. [CrossRef] [PubMed]
26. Mocanu, A.; Lazureanu, V.; Cut, T.; Laza, R.; Musta, V.; Nicolescu, N.; Marinescu, A.; Nelson-Twakor, A.; Dumache, R.; Mederle, O. Angiocatheter Decompression on a COVID-19 Patient with Severe Pneumonia, Pneumothorax, and Subcutaneous Emphysema. *Clin. Lab.* **2022**, *68*, 2403–2412. [CrossRef] [PubMed]
27. Song, W.-J.; Hui, C.K.M.; Hull, J.H.; Birring, S.S.; McGarvey, L.; Mazzone, S.B.; Chung, K.F. Confronting COVID-19-Associated Cough and the Post-COVID Syndrome: Role of Viral Neurotropism, Neuroinflammation, and Neuroimmune Responses. *Lancet Respir. Med.* **2021**, *9*, 533–544. [CrossRef]
28. Al Armashi, A.R.; Somoza-Cano, F.J.; Patell, K.; Homeida, M.; Desai, O.; Al Zubaidi, A.; Altaqi, B.; Ravakhah, K. Spontaneous Pneumomediastinum: A Collaborative Sequelae between COVID-19 and Self-inflicted Lung Injury—A Case Report and Literature Review. *Radiol. Case Rep.* **2021**, *16*, 3655–3658. [CrossRef]
29. Wadhawan, G.; Thakkar, K.; Singh, R. Spontaneous Pneumothorax in Post COVID-19 Patients—A Case Series. *J. Surg. Res.* **2022**, *5*, 46–50. [CrossRef]
30. Kasturi, S.; Muthirevula, A.; Chinthareddy, R.R.; Lingaraju, V.C. Delayed Recurrent Spontaneous Pneumothorax Post-Recovery from COVID-19 Infection. *Indian J. Thorac. Cardiovasc. Surg.* **2021**, *37*, 551–553. [CrossRef]
31. Janssen, M.L.; van Manen, M.J.G.; Cretier, S.E.; Braunstahl, G.-J. Pneumothorax in Patients with Prior or Current COVID-19 Pneumonia. *Respir. Med. Case Rep.* **2020**, *31*, 101187. [CrossRef]
32. Roberts, M.E.; Rahman, N.M.; Maskell, N.A.; Bibby, A.C.; Blyth, K.G.; Corcoran, J.P.; Edey, A.; Evison, M.; de Fonseka, D.; Hallifax, R.; et al. British Thoracic Society Guideline for Pleural Disease. *Thorax* **2023**, *78* (Suppl. S3), S1–S42. [CrossRef]

Disclaimer/Publisher's Note: The statements, opinions and data contained in all publications are solely those of the individual author(s) and contributor(s) and not of MDPI and/or the editor(s). MDPI and/or the editor(s) disclaim responsibility for any injury to people or property resulting from any ideas, methods, instructions or products referred to in the content.

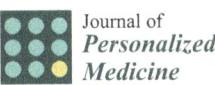

Article

PEAL Score to Predict the Mortality Risk of Cardiogenic Shock in the Emergency Department: An Observational Study

Jen-Wen Ma [1,2,3,4,†], Sung-Yuan Hu [1,2,3,4,5,*,†], Ming-Shun Hsieh [5,6,7], Yi-Chen Lee [7], Shih-Che Huang [4,8,9], Kuan-Ju Chen [1,10], Yan-Zin Chang [3,11,*] and Yi-Chun Tsai [1]

1. Department of Emergency Medicine, Taichung Veterans General Hospital, Taichung 407219, Taiwan; horseword70@gmail.com (J.-W.M.); ckz01119@gmail.com (K.-J.C.); rosa87324@gmail.com (Y.-C.T.)
2. Department of Post-Baccalaureate Medicine, College of Medicine, National Chung Hsing University, Taichung 402, Taiwan
3. Institute of Medicine, School of Medicine, Chung Shan Medical University, Taichung 40201, Taiwan
4. School of Medicine, Chung Shan Medical University, Taichung 40201, Taiwan; cucu0214@gmail.com
5. School of Medicine, National Yang Ming Chiao Tung University, Taipei 11217, Taiwan; edmingshun@gmail.com
6. Department of Emergency Medicine, Taipei Veterans General Hospital, Taoyuan Branch, Taoyuan 330, Taiwan
7. Department of Emergency Medicine, Taipei Veterans General Hospital, Taipei 11217, Taiwan; leeyichen9@yahoo.com.tw
8. Department of Emergency Medicine, Chung Shan Medical University Hospital, Taichung 40201, Taiwan
9. Lung Cancer Research Center, Chung Shan Medical University Hospital, Taichung 40201, Taiwan
10. Center for Cardiovascular Medicine, Taichung Veterans General Hospital, Taichung 407219, Taiwan
11. Department of Clinical Laboratory, Drug Testing Center, Chung Shan Medical University Hospital, Taichung 40201, Taiwan
* Correspondence: song9168@pie.com.tw (S.-Y.H.); yzc@csmu.edu.tw (Y.-Z.C.); Tel.: +886-4-23592525 (ext. 3601); +886-4-24730022 (Y.-Z.C.); Fax: +886-4-23594065 (S.-Y.H.)
† These authors contributed equally to this work.

Abstract: Background: The in-hospital mortality of cardiogenic shock (CS) remains high (28% to 45%). As a result, several studies developed prediction models to assess the mortality risk and provide guidance on treatment, including CardShock and IABP-SHOCK II scores, which performed modestly in external validation studies, reflecting the heterogeneity of the CS populations. Few articles established predictive scores of CS based on Asian people with a higher burden of comorbidities than Caucasians. We aimed to describe the clinical characteristics of a contemporary Asian population with CS, identify risk factors, and develop a predictive scoring model. Methods: A retrospective observational study was conducted between 2014 and 2019 to collect the patients who presented with all-cause CS in the emergency department of a single medical center in Taiwan. We divided patients into subgroups of CS related to acute myocardial infarction (AMI-CS) or heart failure (HF-CS). The outcome was all-cause 30-day mortality. We built the prediction model based on the hazard ratio of significant variables, and the cutoff point of each predictor was determined using the Youden index. We also assessed the discrimination ability of the risk score using the area under a receiver operating characteristic curve. Results: We enrolled 225 patients with CS. One hundred and seven patients (47.6%) were due to AMI-CS, and ninety-eight patients among them received reperfusion therapy. Forty-nine patients (21.8%) eventually died within 30 days. Fifty-three patients (23.55%) presented with platelet counts $< 155 \times 10^3/\mu L$, which were negatively associated with a 30-day mortality of CS in the restrictive cubic spline plot, even within the normal range of platelet counts. We identified four predictors: platelet counts $< 200 \times 10^3/\mu L$ (HR 2.574, 95% CI 1.379–4.805, $p = 0.003$), left ventricular ejection fraction (LVEF) $< 40\%$ (HR 2.613, 95% CI 1.020–6.692, $p = 0.045$), age > 71 years (HR 2.452, 95% CI 1.327–4.531, $p = 0.004$), and lactate > 2.7 mmol/L (HR 1.967, 95% CI 1.069–3.620, $p = 0.030$). The risk score ended with a maximum of 5 points and showed an AUC (95% CI) of 0.774 (0.705–0.843) for all patients, 0.781 (0.678–0.883), and 0.759 (0.662–0.855) for AMI-CS and HF-CS sub-groups, respectively, all $p < 0.001$. Conclusions: Based on four parameters, platelet counts, LVEF, age, and lactate (PEAL), this model showed a good predictive performance for all-cause mortality at 30 days in the all patients, AMI-CS, and HF-CS subgroups. The restrictive cubic spline

Citation: Ma, J.-W.; Hu, S.-Y.; Hsieh, M.-S.; Lee, Y.-C.; Huang, S.-C.; Chen, K.-J.; Chang, Y.-Z.; Tsai, Y.-C. PEAL Score to Predict the Mortality Risk of Cardiogenic Shock in the Emergency Department: An Observational Study. *J. Pers. Med.* **2023**, *13*, 1614. https://doi.org/10.3390/jpm13111614

Academic Editor: Ovidiu Alexandru Mederle

Received: 11 October 2023
Revised: 12 November 2023
Accepted: 14 November 2023
Published: 16 November 2023

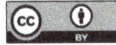

Copyright: © 2023 by the authors. Licensee MDPI, Basel, Switzerland. This article is an open access article distributed under the terms and conditions of the Creative Commons Attribution (CC BY) license (https:// creativecommons.org/licenses/by/ 4.0/).

plot showed a significantly negative correlation between initial platelet counts and 30-day mortality risk in the AMI-CS and HF-CS subgroups.

Keywords: cardiogenic shock; acute myocardial infarction; mortality risk; score; platelet counts

1. Introduction

Cardiogenic shock (CS), a heterogeneous clinical syndrome with two primary causes of acute myocardial infarction (AMI-CS) and acute-on-chronic heart failure (HF-CS), has shown increased incidence and high mortality [1–3]. Despite advances in percutaneous coronary intervention (PCI) with early revascularization and the availability of mechanical circulatory support (MCS), the improvement in CS mortality has plateaued in the past 20 years since the SHOCK (SHould we emergently revascularize Occluded Coronaries for CS) trial [2,4,5]. There has been a decline in the incidence of AMI-CS and an increase in the prevalence of decompensated heart failure (HF) with shock due to non-ischemic causes as medical therapy evolves with changes in patient characteristics and comorbidities [5,6]. In a review study of patients with CS across 16 cardiac intensive care units in North America, 30% were due to AMI-CS. In contrast, 18% and 28% were related to ischemic and non-ischemic cardiomyopathy, respectively [5,7].

In addition to various causes and diverse clinical characteristics, CS involves a continuous progression of hemodynamic abnormalities from reversible myocardial dysfunction with straightforward hypotension to intractable shock with accumulated metabolic derangements and multiple organ failure [2,8,9]. In previous clinical trials, treating all patients with CS as a single group may have led to inconclusive results concerning prognosis and response to therapy, limiting the ability to develop evidence-based therapeutic approaches, especially in HF-CS. For example, although temporary MCS devices can effectively enhance cardiac output with hemodynamic improvement, thus, extending the therapeutic time window for recovery from myocardial and end-organ damage [2,10,11], MCS application has shown a limited mortality benefit in pooled analyses and randomized trials IABP-SHOCK I and IABP-SHOCK II [11–13]. However, IABP-SHOCK II trials enrolled CS patients who were all AMI, and only 15% of patients received an intra-aortic balloon pump (IABP) before reperfusion therapy [14], resulting in lower in-hospital mortality in several studies [15–18]. Nevertheless, MCS devices can still be helpful when applied correctly in selected patients according to risk profiles, optimal MCS initiation timing, and shock severity [2,19]. A meta-analysis of thirty-three studies encompassing 5204 CS patients showed that positioning Impella before starting PCI was associated with lower short-term mortality. In contrast, older age and severe comorbidities such as diabetes mellitus (DM) significantly reduced the benefit of MCS use in CS [19].

Therefore, it is imperative to develop treatment strategies based on risk stratification and validated prognostic scores in this group with high levels of heterogeneity, particularly for the implantation of MCS devices that are resource-intensive and invasive with a risk of complications.

The prognosis and hemodynamics of CS due to non-ischemic causes are poorly understood with few evidence-based treatments [2]. Therefore, it may not be appropriate to extrapolate the characteristics of patients with AMI-CS to those with CS due to non-ischemic causes in the previous prediction systems, such as CardShock and IABP-SHOCK II risk scores, which were derived primarily from myocardial infarction complicated by CS [20,21]. In an external validation study, the two scores showed modest prognostic accuracy in patients without acute coronary syndrome (AMI) (CardShock AUC 0.648, IABP-SHOCK II AUC 0.619, $p = 0.31$), a result that reflects the complexity of this population [20–22]. These studies developed scores in Western countries with limited Asian participants. The patients with AMI in Asian countries tend to be younger and have a higher burden of comorbidities, including diabetes, hypertension, and renal failure [23,24]. As AMI treatment advances, it may limit the validity of the previously established risk scores in contemporary patients.

This study aimed to describe the clinical characteristics of patients with all-cause CS in the emergency department (ED), identify risk factors, and establish a predictive model of short-term mortality risk.

2. Materials and Methods

2.1. Study Design and Inclusion Criteria

The institutional review board of Taichung Veterans General Hospital (TCVGH), Taichung, Taiwan, approved our study (CE22240B) following the ethical guidelines of the Declaration of Helsinki. However, the patients waived the informed consent due to the retrospective design.

We conducted this retrospective observational study in a tertiary care center in Taiwan (TCVGH) that receives ~65,000 ED visits and performs PCI for 1500 cases yearly. The clinical outcomes and risk factors for 30-day mortality were evaluated in patients over 18 years of age who presented with CS to the ED between 1 January 2014 and 31 December 2019. We excluded the patients who developed CS after admission due to the uncertain time intervals between CS detection and data collection. The criteria for CS included systolic blood pressure (SBP) < 90 mmHg for 30 min despite adequate fluid resuscitation or the need for inotropes or vasopressors to maintain SBP $\geq$ 90 mmHg and clinical signs of hypoperfusion (altered mental status, cold extremities, urine output < 0.5 mL/kg/h, serum lactate $\geq$ 2.0 mmol/L). The exclusion criteria included shock of non-cardiac origin, out-of-hospital cardiac arrest (OHCA), and arrhythmia as significant causes of hypotension. For diagnostic accuracy and primary data collection without disruption by the circulatory interruption, we excluded patients with in-hospital cardiac arrest (IHCA) in the ED without obtaining laboratory data or echocardiographic evaluation.

2.2. Data Collection and Definition

We extracted the data of demographics, underlying medical conditions, clinical manifestation, first values of biochemistry before intervention on the arrival of ED, echocardiography, angiography, treatment, and outcome from the electronic medical record. AMI-CS population included patients with ST-elevation myocardial (STEMI) and non-STEMI (NSTEMI).

We calculated the estimated glomerular filtration rate (eGFR) using the chronic kidney disease epidemiology collaboration (CKD-EPI) equation. According to the etiology of CS, we divided into the AMI-CS and HF-CS subgroups. We calculated the CardShock risk scores using each parameter. The use of inotropic and vasoactive agents and the indication for endotracheal intubation were according to the clinical conditions. A 24-h on-call intervention team performed primary PCI according to the door-to-balloon time protocol. The mode of primary PCI (the target lesion only or additional PCI for non-target lesions) was according to the vascular conditions. The diagnostic accuracy was independently verified by a chart review by a board-certified cardiologist and an emergency physician.

2.3. Study Outcomes

The primary outcome of all enrolled patients was all-cause mortality at 30 days.

2.4. Statistical Analysis

We expressed categorical variables as numbers and percentages and analyzed statistical differences using the Chi-square test (χ^2 test). We expressed the continuous variables as mean and standard deviation (SD) or median and interquartile range. We used the student's t-test or Mann–Whitney test to analyze statistical differences. The variables associated with mortality in the univariate Cox proportional hazards regression analyses ($p < 0.05$) were retained to enter a stepwise Cox multivariate analysis by which the remaining variables significantly associated with mortality constitute the score parameters. The continuous variables were further dichotomized with the optimal cut-off points defined using the Youden index. A restricted cubic spline plot was fitted with a Cox proportional hazard model adjusting for covariates to examine the nonlinear relationship between platelet (PLT) counts and the risk of 30-day mortality. The scoring system was determined based on the parameters' respective hazard ratio (HR), assigning 1 or 2 points to each variable, and classified into three risk categories according to total scores. We assessed the discriminative ability of the risk prediction model in the area under the receiver operating characteristic curve (AUC) or the c-statistic. We calculated and plotted the population distribution and the mortality risk according to the cumulative points. We used the chi-square and Kaplan–Meier analyses with a pairwise log-rank test to compare the 30-day mortality rate. A two-sided $p < 0.05$ was regarded as statistically significant.

3. Results

3.1. Demographics and Clinical Characteristics

Table 1 compares the clinical characteristics of CS patients related to HF and AMI. Two hundred and twenty-five patients who presented to the ED with CS were enrolled. One hundred and fifty-nine patients (70.67%) were male, and the non-AMI causes were predominant (52.4%; $n = 118$). The mean age was 70.99 (62.52–80.8) years, and the AMI-CS subgroup was older. Regarding comorbidities, typical cardiovascular risk factors were common, and 82 patients (36.44%) had a history of coronary artery disease. Obstructive lung disease and atrial fibrillation were more prevalent in patients with HF-CS. The initial SBP was 82.86 mmHg, the diastolic blood pressure was 53.74 mmHg, and the heart rate was 89.44 beats per minute. One hundred and nine patients (48.44%) had acute pulmonary edema. More patients with AMI-CS presented conscious confusion than HF-CS (61.68% vs. 45.76%, $p = 0.024$). On average, the left ventricular ejection fraction (LVEF) was 30%, significantly higher in the AMI-CS subgroup (34% vs. 26.5%, $p = 0.001$). In general, 174 patients (77.33%) had LVEF < 40%, and 140 patients (62.22%) had moderate to severe mitral regurgitation. The mean serum lactate value was 2.99 mmol/L; more than 70% of patients had a lactate value > 2 mmol/L. Compared to HF-CS, patients with AMI-CS had higher white blood cell counts, PLT counts, CK-MB and glucose levels, and lower pH values. We found 53 patients (23.55%) with PLT counts $< 155 \times 10^3/\mu L$.

Table 1. Characteristics, clinical manifestations, laboratory data, echocardiography, shock management, reperfusion therapy, outcomes, and complications of patients with HF-CS ($n = 118$, 52.4%) and AMI-CS ($n = 107$, 47.6%).

Baseline Characteristics	All, $n = 225$ (100%)	HF-CS, $n = 118$ (52.4%)	AMI-CS, $n = 107$ (47.6%)	p-Value
Age (years)	70.99 (62.52–80.8)	68.68 (55.17–78.36)	74.16 (65.26–83.52)	0.004 **
Male	159 (70.67%)	79 (66.95%)	80 (74.77%)	0.254
Body mass index	24.02 ± 4.66	23.43 ± 4.10	24.66 ± 5.13	0.072
Coronary artery disease	82 (36.44%)	45 (38.14%)	37 (34.58%)	0.678
Prior PCI	47 (20.89%)	19 (16.10%)	28 (26.17%)	0.091
Prior CABG	24 (10.67%)	13 (11.02%)	11 (10.28%)	1.000
Diabetes mellitus	86 (38.22%)	44 (37.29%)	42 (39.25%)	0.869
Hypertension	108 (48.00%)	54 (45.76%)	54 (50.47%)	0.567
Dyslipidemia	69 (30.67%)	32 (27.12%)	37 (34.58%)	0.286
Asthma/COPD	42 (18.67%)	31 (26.27%)	11 (10.28%)	0.004 *
Old CVA	18 (8.00%)	8 (6.78%)	10 (9.35%)	0.644
Peripheral artery disease	12 (5.33%)	5 (4.24%)	7 (6.54%)	0.637
Atrial fibrillation	63 (28.00%)	49 (41.53%)	14 (13.08%)	<0.001 **
Renal insufficiency	46 (20.44%)	28 (23.73%)	18 (16.82%)	0.264
End-stage renal disease	3 (1.33%)	2 (1.69%)	1 (0.93%)	1.000
Hypothyroidism	17 (7.56%)	12 (10.17%)	5 (4.67%)	0.192

Table 1. Cont.

Baseline Characteristics	All, n = 225 (100%)	HF-CS, n = 118 (52.4%)	AMI-CS, n = 107 (47.6%)	p-Value
		Clinical presentation		
SBP (mm Hg)	82.86 ± 16.67	82.01 ± 14.72	83.80 ± 18.60	0.962
DBP (mm Hg)	53.74 ± 12.75	54.81 ± 11.61	52.56 ± 13.85	0.077
Heart rate (b.p.m.)	89.44 ± 25.25	92.79 ± 25.79	85.76 ± 24.22	0.060
Confusion	120 (53.33%)	54 (45.76%)	66 (61.68%)	0.024 *
Acute pulmonary edema	109 (48.44%)	58 (49.15%)	51 (47.66%)	0.929
		Laboratory data		
WBC counts (/μL)	11,106.71 ± 5239.41	9703.39 ± 4414.11	12,654.30 ± 5647.51	<0.001 **
Platelet counts (10^3/μL)	210.01 ± 85.85	185.58 ± 73.37	236.95 ± 90.76	<0.001 **
Hemoglobin (g/dL)	12.35 ± 2.51	12.54 ± 2.15	12.14 ± 2.85	0.232
Total bilirubin (mg/dL)	0.80 (0.5–1.6)	1.20 (0.7–2.5)	0.60 (0.4–0.9)	<0.001 **
Glucose (mg/dL)	158 (118–240)	140 (111–185)	200 (144–260)	<0.001 **
eGFR (mL/min/1.73 m2)	42.13 (24.65–64.53)	45.26 (26.45–66.29)	40.60 (20.08–63.48)	0.152
CKMB (U/L)	11.00 (7–20)	9.00 (6–15.25)	14.00 (8–31)	<0.001 **
NT-proBNP (pg/mL)	10,010 (3993–26,700)	9993 (4383–24,037)	10,400 (3809–33,250)	0.878
pH	7.34 (7.26–7.39)	7.36 (7.29–7.4)	7.33 (7.24–7.38)	0.005 **
HCO_3^- (mmol/L)	21.90 (18.8–26)	22.90 (19.5–27.3)	21.00 (18.25–24.9)	0.012 *
Lactate (mmol/L)	2.99 (1.8–5.01)	2.98 (1.79–5.89)	2.99 (1.79–4.27)	0.697
Lactate > 2 mmol/L	160 (71.11%)	83 (70.34%)	77 (71.96%)	0.904
		Echocardiography		
LVEF (%)	30.00 (20–39)	26.50 (18–37)	34.00 (25–41)	0.001 **
LVEF < 40%	174 (77.33%)	101 (85.59%)	73 (68.22%)	0.003 **
Pulmonary hypertension	98 (43.56%)	60 (50.85%)	38 (35.51%)	0.029 *
AR (moderate or severe)	66 (29.33%)	37 (31.36%)	29 (27.10%)	0.580
MR (moderate or severe)	140 (62.22%)	77 (65.25%)	63 (58.88%)	0.397
		Vasopressors		0.003 **
Dobutamine	21 (9.33%)	14 (11.86%)	7 (6.54%)	
Dopamine	160 (71.11%)	91 (77.12%)	69 (64.49%)	
Norepinephrine	40 (17.78%)	13 (11.02%)	27 (25.23%)	
Epinephrine	4 (1.78%)	0 (0%)	4 (3.74%)	
		Shock management		
Invasive MV	136 (60.44%)	61 (51.69%)	75 (70.09%)	0.007 **
IABP	55 (24.44%)	16 (13.56%)	39 (36.45%)	<0.001 **
ECMO	14 (6.22%)	6 (5.08%)	8 (7.48%)	0.642
		Outcomes/Complications		
CardShock risk score	4.52 ± 1.62	3.97 ± 1.53	5.14 ± 1.50	<0.001 **
In-hospital cardiac arrest	48 (21.33%)	20 (16.95%)	28 (26.17%)	0.128
Ventricular arrhythmias	57 (25.33%)	25 (21.19%)	32 (29.91%)	0.178
30-day mortality	49 (21.78%)	32 (27.12%)	17 (15.89%)	0.061
Length of stay (days)	13 (8–22)	11 (7–18.25)	14 (9–23)	0.004 **

Chi–squared test. Mann–Whitney U-test.* $p < 0.05$, ** $p < 0.01$, statistically significant. The continuous data are expressed as mean ± SD or median (IQR); the categorical data are expressed as number and percentage. CS related to acute myocardial infarction, AMI-CS; aortic regurgitation, AR; beats per minute, b.p.m.; coronary artery bypass graft, CABG; diastolic blood pressure, DBP; extracorporeal membrane oxygenation, ECMO; acute-on-chronic heart failure with CS, HF-CS; intra-aortic balloon pump, IABP; left ventricular ejection fraction, LVEF; mitral regurgitation, MR; percutaneous coronary intervention, PCI; systolic blood pressure, SBP; mechanical ventilation, MV.

3.2. Management and Outcomes

A higher proportion of patients with AMI-CS received mechanical ventilation (70.09% vs. 51.69%, p = 0.007). The preferred inotrope and vasopressor for shock treatment were dopamine and norepinephrine. Nine patients with AMI-CS were treated conservatively with drugs alone, while ninety-eight received reperfusion therapy. Coronary angiography showed a three-vessel disease in 43 patients and a left-main culprit lesion in 20 patients. Fifty-five patients underwent IABP, which is more common in the AMI-CS subgroup (36.45% vs. 13.56%, p < 0.001). Fifty-seven patients experienced ventricular arrhythmias, and forty-eight had an IHCA. Of the 225 patients, 49 (21.78%) died in 30 days. Compared to HF-CS, patients with AMI-CS had higher CardShock scores (5.14 ± 1.50 vs. 3.97 ± 1.53, p < 0.001) and a more extended hospital stay (14 [9–23] vs. 11 [7–18.25] days, p = 0.004), but mortality at 30 days was numerically lower (15.89% vs. 27.12%, p = 0.061).

3.3. Multivariate Cox Regression Analysis to Identify Significant Variables

As shown in Table 2, after the multivariate analysis of the Cox model, four variables remained statistically significant, including PLT counts, LVEF < 40%, age, and lactate (PEAL). A decrement of 1000 PLT counts has an incremental mortality rate of 0.8% in overall cases (HR 1.008, 95% CI 1.004–1.012, p < 0.001). The mortality rate remained significant in the analysis of subgroups, AMI-CS with HR 1.009, 95% CI 1.002–1.017, p = 0.01, and HF-CS with HR 1.006, 95% CI 1.001–1.011, p = 0.014.

Table 2. Results of the multivariate Cox regression analysis.

Variables	Cox Multivariable Model		
	Hazard Ratio	95% CI	p-Value
Platelet (counts/μL)	1.008	1.004–1.012	<0.001 **
LVEF (%)	2.67	1.05–6.80	0.040 *
Age (years)	1.02	1.00–1.05	0.018 *
Lactate (mmol/L)	1.10	1.03–1.18	0.007 **

Cox regression analysis. * p < 0.05, ** p < 0.01, statistically significant. Left ventricular ejection fraction, LVEF.

3.4. Nonlinear Relationship between Platelet Counts and 30-Day Mortality

To assess the nonlinear relationship between PLT counts and mortality, a restrictive cubic spline plot was fitted with a Cox proportional risk model with adjustments for body mass index, age, sex, heart rate, and LVEF. As shown in Figure 1, the decrease in PLT counts was significantly associated with an increased 30-day mortality risk, with an inflection point at $200 \times 10^3/\mu L$ of PLT counts. We determined the second cut-off point of PLT counts $< 155 \times 10^3/\mu L$ by the Youden index.

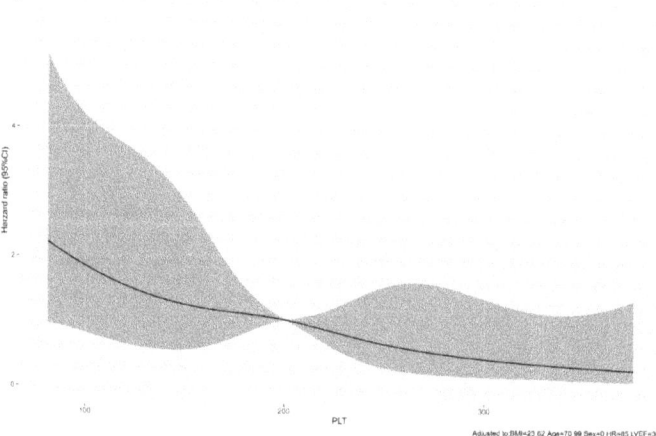

Figure 1. The restricted cubic spline plot shows hazard ratios with 95% confidence intervals for mortality in 30 days according to platelet counts. The plot was fitted with the Cox proportional hazards model, adjusting for age, sex, body mass index, heart rate, and left ventricular ejection fraction. The cut-off point of platelet counts was $200 \times 10^3/\mu L$. The shades of grey color presented the 95% confidence intervals of hazard ratios.

3.5. Determine the Cutoff Points of the Predictors and the Risk Scoring System

Age > 71 years and lactate > 2.7 mmol/L were determined as the cutoff points using the Youden index. Each predictor was assigned a score of 0 or 1 depending on the HR of the dichotomized variables, as shown in Table 3. The reflection point of $200 \times 10^3/\mu L$ in the restrictive cubic spline plot was used as the first cutoff point for PLT counts. A score of 2 was assigned for PLT counts less than $155 \times 10^3/\mu L$. We developed the PEAL score risk model (platelet, LVEF, age, and lactate) to predict the 30-day mortality risk in patients with CS in the ED, as shown in Table 4.

Table 3. Hazard ratios of dichotomized variables associated with 30-day mortality.

Variables	Hazard Ratio	95% CI	p-Value
Platelet counts < 200 ($\times 10^3/\mu L$)	2.574	1.379–4.805	0.003 **
Age > 71 (years)	2.452	1.327–4.531	0.004 **
LVEF < 40 (%)	2.613	1.020–6.692	0.045 *
Lactate > 2.7 (mmol/L)	1.967	1.069–3.620	0.030 *

Cox regression analysis. * $p < 0.05$, ** $p < 0.01$, statistically significant. Left ventricular ejection fraction, LVEF.

Table 4. Risk scoring model for the prediction of 30-day mortality in CS.

Variables		PEAL Score (Maximum 5 Points)
Platelet counts ($\times 10^3/\mu L$)	>200	0
	155–200	1
	<155	2
LVEF < 40 (%)		1
Age > 71 (years)		1
Lactate > 2.7 (mmol/L)		1

Optimal cut-off points determined by Youden index. Left ventricular ejection fraction, LVEF; Platelet, LVEF, Age, Lactate, PEAL.

3.6. Receiver Operating Characteristic Curve (ROC) of the Risk Score

Table 5 shows that this risk-scoring model has good predictive power for 30-day mortality risk in the AMI-CS and HF-CS subgroups (AUC of 0.774 for all, AUC of 0.781 for AMI-CS, and AUC of 0.759 for HF-CS), regarding the ROC curves in Figure 2.

Table 5. The area under the curve (AUC) of the receiver operating characteristic curve (ROC) for the PEAL score.

PEAL Score	AUC of ROC	95% CI	p-Value
All, n = 225	0.774	0.705–0.843	<0.001 **
AMI-CS, n = 107	0.781	0.678–0.883	<0.001 **
HF-CS, n = 118	0.759	0.662–0.855	<0.001 **

Chi-squared test. ** $p < 0.01$, statistically significant. CS related to acute myocardial infarction, AMI-CS; acute-on-chronic heart failure with CS, HF-CS.

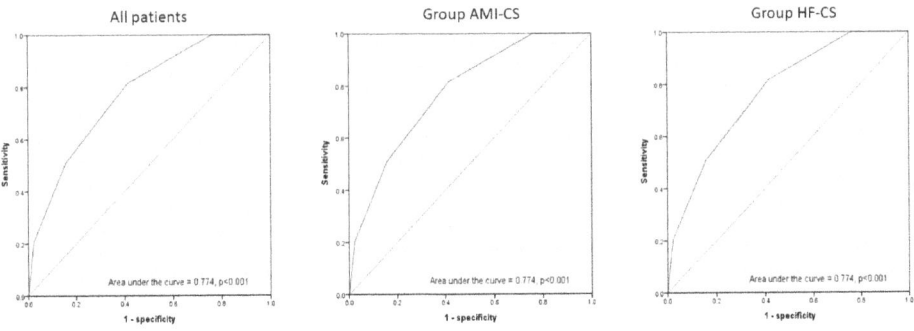

Figure 2. The receiver operating characteristic curve (ROC) of the risk score to predict mortality risk

at 30 days in all patients with CS (*n* = 225) (**A**). The ROC of the risk score to predict mortality risk at 30 days in the AMI-CS subgroup (*n* = 107) (**B**). The ROC of the risk score to predict mortality risk at 30 days in the HF-CS subgroup (*n* = 118) (**C**). The blue lines indicated the curves in the AUC of the ROC for all patients (**A**), ACS patients (**B**), and Non-ACS patients (**C**). The green lines presented the baseline in the AUC of the ROC.

3.7. Distribution of the Risk Score and Observed Mortality

Figure 3 shows the distribution of the study population and the stepwise increase in observed mortality within 30 days as the risk scores increase. There were no deaths in the 0 and 1 scores. The 30-day mortality rates for scores 2, 3, 4, and 5 were 13%, 25%, 38%, and 71%, respectively. The blue lines indicated the curves in the AUC of the ROC for all patients (A), ACS patients (B), and Non-ACS patients (C). The green lines presented the baseline in the AUC of the ROC.

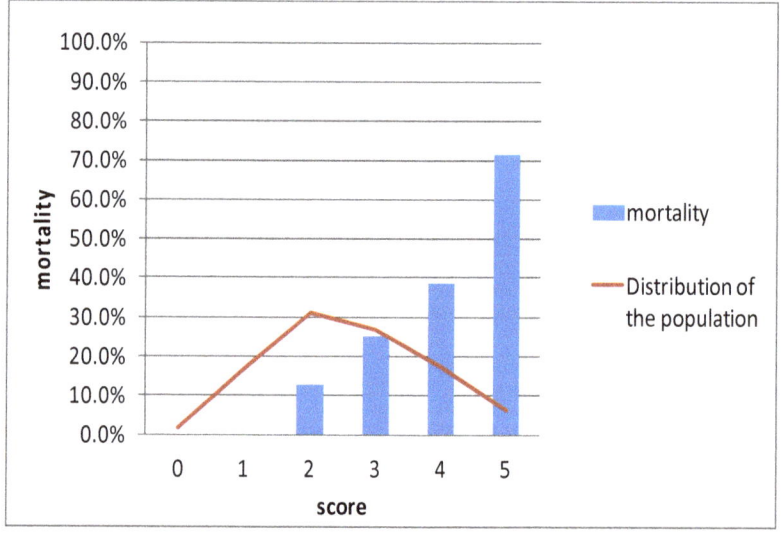

Figure 3. Distribution of the study population (red line) and mortality rate observed at 30 days (%; blue bars) across the cumulative points of the risk score.

3.8. Cumulative Mortality according to Score Categories Using the Kaplan–Meier Method

According to the risk scores, 42 patients (18.7%) were at low risk (0–1), 130 patients (57.8%) were at moderate risk (2–3), and 53 patients (23.5%) were in the high-risk group (4–5). The Kaplan–Meier survival curves showed significant differences in cumulative mortality for 30 days between the three subgroups, compared by log-rank test ($p < 0.001$ for 0–1 vs. 2–3; $p < 0.001$ for 2–3 vs. 4–5; and $p < 0.001$ for 0–1 vs. 4–5) (Figure 4).

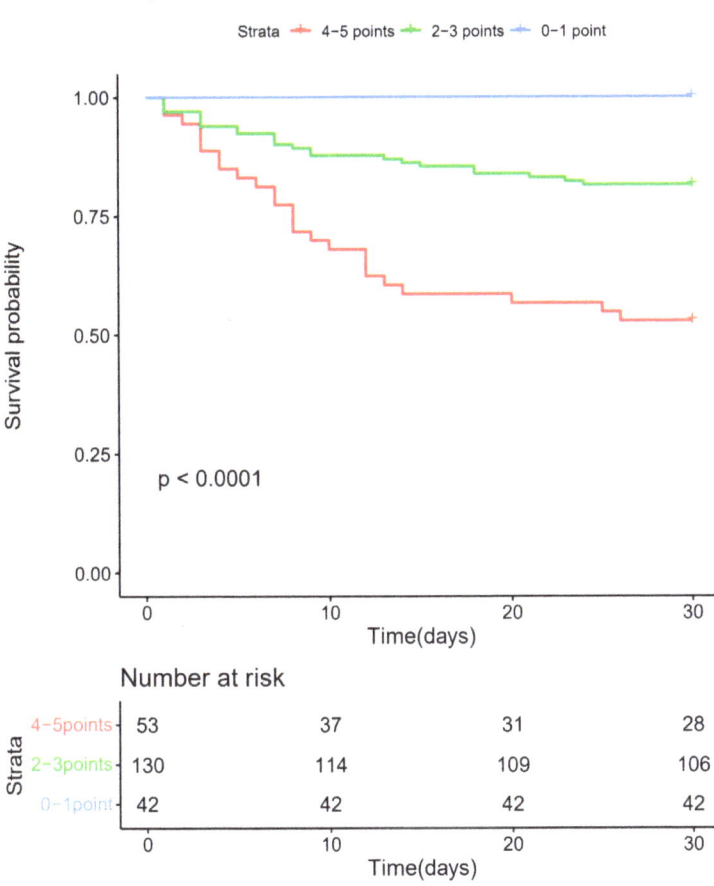

Figure 4. Kaplan–Meier survival curve for 30-day mortality according to score categories with pair-wise comparisons by log-rank test.

4. Discussion

The study described the clinical characteristics and real world practices of 225 patients with all-cause CS in the ED of a tertiary care hospital in Taiwan. With a higher proportion of patients with CS not related to AMI (HF-CS 52.4% vs. AMI-CS 47.6%), the study revealed more information on the HF-CS subgroup, which had been less addressed in the literature. Therefore, we established a predictive model of 30-day mortality for CS based on four significant variables in multivariate analyses using the Cox model, including PLT counts < $200 \times 10^3/\mu L$, LVEF < 40%, age > 71 years, and lactate > 2.7 mmol/L. The model showed good predictive power with an AUC of 0.774 with 95% CI (0.705–0.843) for all patients, 0.781 (0.678–0.883) for AMI-CS, and 0.759 (0.662–0.855) for HF-CS, all $p < 0.001$. Furthermore, the study showed that a decrement of $1000/\mu L$ in PLT counts was associated with an increment of 0.8% in cumulative 30-day mortality risk of CS, even within the normal range of PLT counts (HR 1.008, 95% CI 1.004–1.012, $p < 0.001$). This association remained significant when analyzed in the AMI-CS and HF-CS subgroups. AMI-CS had an HR of 1.009 with 95% CI 1.002–1.017, $p = 0.01$, and HF-CS had an HR of 1.006, 95% CI 1.001–1.011, $p = 0.014$. This model is the first risk score incorporating the number of PLT counts at presentation to predict short-term mortality in patients with AMI-CS and HF-CS.

The study focused on patients with CS in the ED (primary CS). At the same time, most of the criteria in the previous trials were carried out to predict the development of CS after hospital admission in patients with AMI (secondary CS) [25–29]. The recent studies have shown different trends in the incidence and mortality between primary and secondary CS. In Western countries, a stable mortality rate was observed for secondary CS (from 64.5% to 69.1%, $p = 0.731$), while the mortality rate for primary CS decreased (from 60% to 38%, $p = 0.038$). There was also a trend toward a decrease in secondary CS during hospitalization [30]. It was attributed to a timely PCI, which limits the size of the infarction and reduces subsequent complications. With the increasing population of advanced HF after AMI, CS on admission (primary CS) now accounts for most CS cases. The exclusive enrollment of primary CS cases and the exclusion of patients with OHCA and non-survivors of IHCA in the ED may have led to a lower 30-day mortality rate (21%) in this study. More importantly, mandatory health insurance and widespread hospital networks for AMI in Taiwan could reduce the time interval between the onset and coronary revascularization and decrease the mortality rate in AMI-CS by early interruption of the devastating shock spiral from isolated myocardial dysfunction to progressive multiorgan failure [8,9].

Compared to the CardShock study concerning shock severity, the study population showed comparable clinical characteristics, including age, the prevalence of comorbidities, LVEF, lactate, and eGFR, as well as a similar reperfusion rate (91% vs. 90%) in AMI-CS [20]. Three predictors in the CardShock score did not show a significant association with mortality in the study, including the etiology of AMI, the eGFR, and conscious confusion at presentation. There are some reasons for this. The study population showed a higher prevalence of chronic kidney disease (CKD) and worse mean renal function compared to the CardShock study. The mean eGFR was 42 (range of 25–65) in our study and 61 (range of 41–87) in the CardShock study. The prevalence of CKD was 20.44% in our study and 11% in the CardShock study. Consequently, using eGFR as a biomarker of end-organ dysfunction could be confounding by different baseline renal functions, particularly in areas with prevalent CKD. Furthermore, the assessment of confusion depends on the physician's subjective judgment, and the level of consciousness is susceptible to using oxygen and vasopressors or sedative medications during mechanical ventilation.

Comparing with HF-CS, AMI-CS is generally more severe with a higher SCAI shock stage despite similar hemodynamics and better LVEF [31]. In our study, AMI-CS showed higher LVEF, older, confusion, mechanical ventilation, and IABP support than those with HF-CS. Additionally, although statistically insignificant, more patients with AMI-CS experienced ventricular arrhythmias and cardiovascular collapse. Patients with AMI also showed drastic features in laboratory data, including higher white blood cell and glucose levels and more severe acidemia in arterial blood gases. Despite a more serious clinical presentation, patients with AMI-CS had a lower mortality rate than those with HF-CS, which differed from most previous studies. Timely transport and revascularization in Taiwan reduced the damaged area of the myocardium and were supposed to be the main reason for the lower mortality. Therefore, the etiology of AMI should be considered a modifiable factor rather than a constant predictor of poor outcomes in CS.

In our study, four variables showed a significant relationship with mortality in CS. However, too many predictors can be prone to overfitting and limited generalization to external populations in CS with high heterogeneity. Aging has been the most common patient-related risk factor in published prognostic scores for CS [32], possibly due to limited physiological reserve and compensatory capacity. When applying MCS in CS, older age was also significantly associated with more adverse clinical course and higher complication rates, resulting in a narrow therapeutic range for clinical physicians [19].

Lactate was a standard marker to predict the clinical outcome of CS [33,34]. Hyperlactatemia reflects impaired tissue perfusion, and cumulative cellular metabolic derangements have proven to be associated with increased mortality in the literature. In the current study, an increase of each mmol/L in lactate was associated with an adjusted HR of 1.1 for mortality at 30 days. Both older age and lactate were predictive variables in the CardShock and IABP-SHOCK II risk scores [20,21]. As a continuous variable, LVEF did not show a significant association with mortality in this study, possibly because the shock severity is related not only to reduce cardiac output and primitive LV function before the myocardial injury but also to maladaptive circulatory compensation. In the study, an LVEF < 40% was associated with increased mortality risk in CS, compatible with the results of several studies [20,35,36].

Thrombocytopenia is associated with an increased mortality rate in patients who are admitted to intensive care units [37] and in multiple cardiovascular diseases, including AMI, HF, and transcatheter aortic valve implantation (TAVI) [38–42]. In patients with AMI, studies have indicated an association between thrombocytopenia and adverse cardiovascular outcomes, including all-cause or cardiovascular death, myocardial infarction, and target lesion revascularization [39,41,43–46]. A multicenter retrospective study in 1907 patients with HFrEF (LVEF < 40%) showed higher all-cause mortality in patients combined with moderate/severe thrombocytopenia (PLT counts < $100 \times 10^3/\mu L$) compared to normal/mild thrombocytopenia (HR 1.84, 95% CI 1.33–2.56, $p < 0.001$) [39]. In a study on patients with AMI randomly assigned to unfractionated heparin or hirudin, Eikelboom et al. demonstrated a similar relationship between thrombocytopenia and adverse non-hemorrhagic outcomes in patients with AMI. They proposed that excessive PLT activation may lead to PLT consumption and the further deterioration of coronary ischemia [44]. Moreover, several studies have reported that a reduced number of PLT counts is associated with the increased mortality rate in CS with VA-ECMO and IABP institutions, with the primary mechanism involving mechanical consumption of circulating PLT counts [47–51].

However, CardShock and IABP-SHOCK II risk scores did not include PLT counts as a predictor [20,21], and there is a lack of research linking PLT counts with the prognosis of CS. A recent multicenter study in South Korea, investigating a total of 1202 patients with all-cause CS from 2014 to 2018, concluded that a decrease in PLT counts at the presentation of CS was associated with increased all-cause mortality at 30 days in the multivariate Cox model (a decrease of $1000/\mu L$ in PLT counts, HR 1.002, 95% CI 1.000–1.030, $p = 0.021$) [52], consistent with the finding in the present study, with an identical inflection point at $200 \times 10^3/\mu L$ in restrictive cubic spline plots. Furthermore, the study showed an incidence of thrombocytopenia of 20%, close to the 23% in the present study. Consequently, PLT counts could be underestimated and not adequately evaluated regarding their predictive value for the prognosis of CS.

The pathophysiological mechanisms underlying the occurrence of thrombocytopenia in CS have yet to be fully elucidated. The mean PLT volume and the PLT surface P-selectin were used as PLT activation markers in different studies and were found to be at higher levels in patients with acute decompensated HF than in stable HF [53–58]. Therefore, low PLT counts may be due to abnormal PLT activation and the subsequent destruction during the worsening status of HF. Hemodynamic instability can lead to stagnant blood flow, predisposing to PLT aggregation. In an advanced shock state, maladaptive compensatory mechanisms involving systemic inflammation, increased catecholamines, and renin–angiotensin system activation can contribute to PLT overactivation and consumption [59–62]. AMI-CS can deteriorate drastically with sharply elevated lactate levels. As the shock progresses, a decrease in PLT counts may reflect maladaptive systemic inflammation and neurohormonal compensatory responses, typical of decompensated chronic HF, in which PLT counts participate by acting as inflammatory mediators [9,63].

Based on four routinely available metrics, the current score has the advantages of being easy to calculate, allowing early prognosis prediction, and facilitating individualized therapeutic strategies from non-invasive medical treatment (Score 0–1) to maximum therapeutic options, including MCS implants for those who may have the most incredible benefits (Score 2–4) or providing palliative care for futile patients (Score 5). Due to the aging population with an increased burden of comorbidities, identifying futile groups is vital in areas with limited medical resources in the post-pandemic era.

5. Limitation

There are several limitations to be acknowledged in the study. First, this is a retrospective study of a single medical center with potentially unmeasured confounders and incomplete data; therefore, the causality between PLT counts and the outcome could not be established, and the underlying mechanism warrants further investigation. Although the diagnostic accuracy was verified by reviewing the charts, only clinical, biochemical, and echocardiographic data were universally available without providing hemodynamic measurements to clarify pure cardiogenic or mixed shock states. Concerning MCS devices, IABP was used exclusively in the study because the National Health Insurance did not cover the payment of Impella in Taiwan, which might limit the extension of study results. In addition to the limited sample size of a single database, the inclusion of patients with CS in the ED may have incurred selection bias. However, given the high heterogeneity of CS populations, it is unlikely that any single-derivation cohort will fully reflect an external population. Since the data were collected before starting any treatment, heparin-induced or mechanically disrupted thrombocytopenia with MCS could be excluded. Moreover, an extended 95% CI in the restricted cubic spline plot may indicate a more significant margin of error and a less precise estimate, partly due to the small sample size. Finally, the longitudinal follow-up on the PLT counts was lacking, which can provide more evidence of prognostic strength by relating to adverse events and hospital course.

6. Conclusions

Based on four parameters, platelet counts, LVEF, age, and lactate (PEAL), this prediction model showed a good predictive performance for all-cause mortality at 30 days in all patients and the AMI-CS and HF-CS subgroups. The restrictive cubic spline plot showed a significantly negative correlation between initial PLT counts and 30-day mortality in AMI-CS and HF-CS subgroups. The feasibility of trending serial PLT counts as clinical markers related to the severity and outcome of CS deserves further evaluation in more extensive studies.

Author Contributions: Conceptualization, J.-W.M. and S.-Y.H.; methodology, J.-W.M., S.-Y.H., M.-S.H., Y.-C.L. and K.-J.C.; data curation, J.-W.M., S.-Y.H., S.-C.H. and Y.-C.T.; writing—original draft preparation, J.-W.M. and S.-Y.H.; writing—review and editing, M.-S.H., Y.-Z.C. and S.-Y.H.; project administration, S.-Y.H. All authors have read and agreed to the published version of the manuscript.

Funding: This work was supported by grants from the Taichung Veterans General Hospital (TCVGH), Taichung, Taiwan (TCVGH-1117202C, TCVGH-1127203C, and TCVGH-T1127801), and the Taipei Veterans General Hospital, Taoyuan branch, Taoyuan, Taiwan (TYVH-10808, TYVH-10809, and TYVH-10902). The funders had no role in the study design, data collection, analysis, decision to publish, or preparation of the manuscript. No additional external funding was received for this study.

Institutional Review Board Statement: The institutional review board of Taichung Veterans General Hospital approved this study. (Study period ranged from 1 July 2021 to 30 June 2022) (IRB file number: CE22240B).

Informed Consent Statement: Patient consent was waived because this study was retrospective, observational, and anonymous.

Data Availability Statement: Readers can access the data and material supporting the study's conclusions by contacting Sung-Yuan Hu at song9168@pie.com.tw.

Acknowledgments: We thank the Clinical Informatics Research and Development Center and Biostatistics Task Force of Taichung Veterans General Hospital.

Conflicts of Interest: The authors declare no conflict of interest.

References

1. Helgestad, O.K.L.; Josiassen, J.; Hassager, C.; Jensen, L.O.; Holmvang, L.; Sørensen, A.; Frydland, M.; Lassen, A.T.; Udesen, N.L.J.; Schmidt, H.; et al. Temporal trends in incidence and patient characteristics in CS following acute myocardial infarction from 2010 to 2017: A Danish cohort study. *Eur. J. Heart Fail.* **2019**, *21*, 1370–1378. [CrossRef] [PubMed]
2. van Diepen, S.; Katz, J.N.; Albert, N.M.; Henry, T.D.; Jacobs, A.K.; Kapur, N.K.; Kilic, A.; Menon, V.; Ohman, E.M.; Sweitzer, N.K.; et al. Contemporary Management of CS: A Scientific Statement From the American Heart Association. *Circulation* **2017**, *136*, e232–e268. [CrossRef] [PubMed]
3. Thiele, H.; Ohman, E.M.; de Waha-Thiele, S.; Zeymer, U.; Desch, S. Management of CS complicating myocardial infarction: An update 2019. *Eur. Heart J.* **2019**, *40*, 2671–2683. [CrossRef] [PubMed]
4. Vahdatpour, C.; Collins, D.; Goldberg, S. CS. *J. Am. Heart Assoc.* **2019**, *8*, e011991. [CrossRef]
5. Berg, D.D.; Bohula, E.A.; Morrow, D.A. Epidemiology and causes of CS. *Curr. Opin. Crit. Care.* **2021**, *27*, 401–408. [CrossRef]
6. Chioncel, O.; Parissis, J.; Mebazaa, A.; Thiele, H.; Desch, S.; Bauersachs, J.; Harjola, V.P.; Antohi, E.L.; Arrigo, M.; Ben Gal, T.; et al. Epidemiology, pathophysiology and contemporary management of CS—A position statement from the Heart Failure Association of the European Society of Cardiology. *Eur. J. Heart Fail.* **2020**, *22*, 1315–1341. [CrossRef]
7. Berg, D.D.; Bohula, E.A.; van Diepen, S.; Katz, J.N.; Alviar, C.L.; Baird-Zars, V.M.; Barnett, C.F.; Barsness, G.W.; Burke, J.A.; Cremer, P.C.; et al. Epidemiology of Shock in Contemporary Cardiac Intensive Care Units. *Circ. Cardiovasc. Qual. Outcomes* **2019**, *12*, e005618. [CrossRef]
8. Reynolds, H.R.; Hochman, J.S. CS: Current concepts and improving outcomes. *Circulation* **2008**, *117*, 686–697. [CrossRef]
9. Jones, T.L.; Nakamura, K.; McCabe, J.M. CS: Evolving definitions and future directions in management. *Open Heart* **2019**, *6*, e000960. [CrossRef]
10. Thiele, H.; Jobs, A.; Ouweneel, D.M.; Henriques, J.P.S.; Seyfarth, M.; Desch, S.; Eitel, I.; Pöss, J.; Fuernau, G.; de Waha, S. Percutaneous short-term active mechanical support devices in CS: A systematic review and collaborative meta-analysis of randomized trials. *Eur. Heart J.* **2017**, *38*, 3523–3531. [CrossRef]
11. Thiele, H.; Zeymer, U.; Neumann, F.J.; Ferenc, M.; Olbrich, H.G.; Hausleiter, J.; Richardt, G.; Hennersdorf, M.; Empen, K.; Fuernau, G.; et al. Intraaortic balloon support for myocardial infarction with CS. *N. Engl. J. Med.* **2012**, *367*, 1287–1296. [CrossRef] [PubMed]
12. Sjauw, K.D.; Engström, A.E.; Vis, M.M.; van der Schaaf, R.J.; Baan, J., Jr.; Koch, K.T.; de Winter, R.J.; Piek, J.J.; Tijssen, J.G.; Henriques, J.P. A systematic review and meta-analysis of intra-aortic balloon pump therapy in ST-elevation myocardial infarction: Should we change the guidelines? *Eur. Heart J.* **2009**, *30*, 459–468. [CrossRef] [PubMed]
13. Prondzinsky, R.; Lemm, H.; Swyter, M.; Wegener, N.; Unverzagt, S.; Carter, J.M.; Russ, M.; Schlitt, A.; Buerke, U.; Christoph, A.; et al. Intra-aortic balloon counterpulsation in patients with acute myocardial infarction complicated by CS: The prospective, randomized IABP SHOCK Trial for attenuation of multiorgan dysfunction syndrome. *Crit. Care Med.* **2010**, *38*, 152–160. [CrossRef]
14. Thiele, H.; Zeymer, U.; Neumann, F.J.; Ferenc, M.; Olbrich, H.G.; Hausleiter, J.; de Waha, A.; Richardt, G.; Hennersdorf, M.; Empen, K.; et al. Intra-aortic balloon counterpulsation in acute myocardial infarction complicated by CS (IABP-SHOCK II): Final 12 month results of a randomised, open-label trial. *Lancet* **2013**, *382*, 1638–1645. [CrossRef] [PubMed]
15. Kapur, N.K.; Paruchuri, V.; Urbano-Morales, J.A.; Mackey, E.E.; Daly, G.H.; Qiao, X.; Pandian, N.; Perides, G.; Karas, R.H. Mechanically unloading the left ventricle before coronary reperfusion reduces left ventricular wall stress and myocardial infarct size. *Circulation* **2013**, *128*, 328–336. [CrossRef] [PubMed]
16. Abdel-Wahab, M.; Saad, M.; Kynast, J.; Geist, V.; Sherif, M.A.; Richardt, G.; Toelg, R. Comparison of hospital mortality with intra-aortic balloon counterpulsation insertion before versus after primary percutaneous coronary intervention for CS complicating acute myocardial infarction. *Am. J. Cardiol.* **2010**, *105*, 967–971. [CrossRef]
17. Schwarz, B.; Abdel-Wahab, M.; Robinson, D.R.; Richardt, G. Predictors of mortality in patients with CS treated with primary percutaneous coronary intervention and intra-aortic balloon counterpulsation. *Med. Klin. Intensivmed. Notfmed.* **2016**, *111*, 715–722. [CrossRef]
18. Davierwala, P.M.; Leontyev, S.; Verevkin, A.; Rastan, A.J.; Mohr, M.; Bakhtiary, F.; Misfeld, M.; Mohr, F.W. Temporal Trends in Predictors of Early and Late Mortality After Emergency Coronary Artery Bypass Grafting for CS Complicating Acute Myocardial Infarction. *Circulation* **2016**, *134*, 1224–1237. [CrossRef]
19. Panuccio, G.; Neri, G.; Macrì, L.M.; Salerno, N.; De Rosa, S.; Torella, D. Use of Impella device in cardiogenic shock and its clinical outcomes: A systematic review and meta-analysis. *Int. J. Cardiol. Heart Vasc.* **2022**, *40*, 101007.
20. Harjola, V.P.; Lassus, J.; Sionis, A.; Køber, L.; Tarvasmäki, T.; Spinar, J.; Parissis, J.; Banaszewski, M.; Silva-Cardoso, J.; Carubelli, V.; et al. Clinical picture and risk prediction of short-term mortality in CS. *Eur. J. Heart Fail.* **2015**, *17*, 501–509. [CrossRef]
21. Pöss, J.; Köster, J.; Fuernau, G.; Eitel, I.; de Waha, S.; Ouarrak, T.; Lassus, J.; Harjola, V.P.; Zeymer, U.; Thiele, H.; et al. Risk Stratification for Patients in CS After Acute Myocardial Infarction. *J. Am. Coll. Cardiol.* **2017**, *69*, 1913–1920. [CrossRef] [PubMed]
22. Rivas-Lasarte, M.; Sans-Roselló, J.; Collado-Lledó, E.; González-Fernández, V.; Noriega, F.J.; Hernández-Pérez, F.J.; Fernández-Martínez, J.; Ariza, A.; Lidón, R.M.; Viana-Tejedor, A.; et al. External validation and comparison of the CardShock and IABP-SHOCK II risk scores in real-world CS patients. *Eur. Heart J. Acute Cardiovasc. Care* **2021**, *10*, 16–24. [CrossRef] [PubMed]
23. Selvarajah, S.; Fong, A.Y.; Selvaraj, G.; Haniff, J.; Uiterwaal, C.S.; Bots, M.L. An Asian validation of the TIMI risk score for ST-segment elevation myocardial infarction. *PLoS ONE* **2012**, *7*, e40249. [CrossRef]

24. Zuhdi, A.S.; Ahmad, W.A.; Zaki, R.A.; Mariapun, J.; Ali, R.M.; Sari, N.M.; Ismail, M.D.; Kui Hian, S. Acute coronary syndrome in the elderly: The Malaysian National Cardiovascular Disease Database-Acute Coronary Syndrome registry. *Singapore Med. J.* **2016**, *57*, 191–197. [CrossRef] [PubMed]
25. Babaev, A.; Frederick, P.D.; Pasta, D.J.; Every, N.; Sichrovsky, T.; Hochman, J.S.; NRMI Investigators. Trends in management and outcomes of patients with acute myocardial infarction complicated by CS. *JAMA* **2005**, *294*, 448–454. [CrossRef]
26. Menon, V.; Hochman, J.S. Management of CS complicating acute myocardial infarction. *Heart* **2002**, *88*, 531–537. [CrossRef] [PubMed]
27. Dziewierz, A.; Siudak, Z.; Rakowski, T.; Dubiel, J.S.; Dudek, D. Predictors and in-hospital outcomes of CS on admission in patients with acute coronary syndromes admitted to hospitals without on-site invasive facilities. *Acute Card. Care* **2010**, *12*, 3–9. [CrossRef]
28. Hasdai, D.; Califf, R.M.; Thompson, T.D.; Hochman, J.S.; Ohman, E.M.; Pfisterer, M.; Bates, E.R.; Vahanian, A.; Armstrong, P.W.; Criger, D.A.; et al. Predictors of CS after thrombolytic therapy for acute myocardial infarction. *J. Am. Coll. Cardiol.* **2000**, *35*, 136–143. [CrossRef]
29. Jarai, R.; Huber, K.; Bogaerts, K.; Sinnaeve, P.R.; Ezekowitz, J.; Ross, A.M.; Zeymer, U.; Armstrong, P.W.; Van de Werf, F.J.; ASSENT-4 PCI investigators. Prediction of CS using plasma B-type natriuretic peptide and the N-terminal fragment of its pro-hormone [corrected] concentrations in ST elevation myocardial infarction: An analysis from the ASSENT-4 Percutaneous Coronary Intervention Trial. *Crit. Care Med.* **2010**, *38*, 1793–1801. [CrossRef]
30. Aissaoui, N.; Puymirat, E.; Delmas, C.; Ortuno, S.; Durand, E.; Bataille, V.; Drouet, E.; Bonello, L.; Bonnefoy-Cudraz, E.; Lesmeles, G.; et al. Trends in CS complicating acute myocardial infarction. *Eur. J. Heart Fail.* **2020**, *22*, 664–672. [CrossRef]
31. Thayer, K.L.; Zweck, E.; Ayouty, M.; Garan, A.R.; Hernandez-Montfort, J.; Mahr, C.; Morine, K.J.; Newman, S.; Jorde, L.; Haywood, J.L.; et al. Invasive Hemodynamic Assessment and Classification of In-Hospital Mortality Risk Among Patients With CS. *Circ. Heart Fail.* **2020**, *13*, e007099. [CrossRef] [PubMed]
32. Acharya, D. Predictors of Outcomes in Myocardial Infarction and CS. *Cardiol. Rev.* **2018**, *26*, 255–266. [CrossRef] [PubMed]
33. Fuernau, G.; Desch, S.; de Waha-Thiele, S.; Eitel, I.; Neumann, F.J.; Hennersdorf, M.; Felix, S.B.; Fach, A.; Böhm, M.; Pöss, J.; et al. Arterial Lactate in CS: Prognostic Value of Clearance Versus Single Values. *JACC Cardiovasc. Interv.* **2020**, *13*, 2208–2216. [CrossRef]
34. Lindholm, M.G.; Hongisto, M.; Lassus, J.; Spinar, J.; Parissis, J.; Banaszewski, M.; Silva-Cardoso, J.; Carubelli, V.; Salvatore, D.; Sionis, A.; et al. Serum Lactate and A Relative Change in Lactate as Predictors of Mortality in Patients With CS—Results from the Cardshock Study. *Shock* **2020**, *53*, 43–49. [CrossRef]
35. Aissaoui, N.; Riant, E.; Lefèvre, G.; Delmas, C.; Bonello, L.; Henry, P.; Bonnefoy, E.; Schiele, F.; Ferrières, J.; Simon, T.; et al. Long-term clinical outcomes in patients with CS according to left ventricular function: The French registry of Acute ST-elevation and non-ST-elevation Myocardial Infarction (FAST-MI) programme. *Arch. Cardiovasc. Dis.* **2018**, *111*, 678–685. [CrossRef] [PubMed]
36. Liu, Y.; Zhu, J.; Tan, H.Q.; Liang, Y.; Liu, L.S.; Li, Y.; China CREATE Investigation Group. Predictors of short term mortality in patients with acute ST-elevation myocardial infarction complicated by CS. *Zhonghua Xin Xue Guan Bing Za Zhi* **2010**, *38*, 695–701. [PubMed]
37. Zarychanski, R.; Houston, D.S. Assessing thrombocytopenia in the intensive care unit: The past, present, and future. *Hematology Am. Soc. Hematol. Educ. Program.* **2017**, *2017*, 660–666. [CrossRef]
38. Vanderschueren, S.; De Weerdt, A.; Malbrain, M.; Vankersschaever, D.; Frans, E.; Wilmer, A.; Bobbaers, H. Thrombocytopenia and prognosis in intensive care. *Crit. Care Med.* **2000**, *28*, 1871–1876. [CrossRef]
39. Mojadidi, M.K.; Galeas, J.N.; Goodman-Meza, D.; Eshtehardi, P.; Msaouel, P.; Kelesidis, I.; Zaman, M.O.; Winoker, J.S.; Roberts, S.C.; Christia, P.; et al. Thrombocytopaenia as a Prognostic Indicator in Heart Failure with Reduced Ejection Fraction. *Heart Lung Circ.* **2016**, *25*, 568–575. [CrossRef]
40. Gore, J.M.; Spencer, F.A.; Gurfinkel, E.P.; López-Sendón, J.; Steg, P.G.; Granger, C.B.; FitzGerald, G.; Agnelli, G.; GRACE Investigators. Thrombocytopenia in patients with an acute coronary syndrome (from the Global Registry of Acute Coronary Events [GRACE]). *Am. J. Cardiol.* **2009**, *103*, 175–180. [CrossRef]
41. Yadav, M.; Généreux, P.; Giustino, G.; Madhavan, M.V.; Brener, S.J.; Mintz, G.; Caixeta, A.; Xu, K.; Mehran, R.; Stone, G.W. Effect of Baseline Thrombocytopenia on Ischemic Outcomes in Patients With Acute Coronary Syndromes Who Undergo Percutaneous Coronary Intervention. *Can. J. Cardiol.* **2016**, *32*, 226–233. [CrossRef] [PubMed]
42. Dvir, D.; Généreux, P.; Barbash, I.M.; Kodali, S.; Ben-Dor, I.; Williams, M.; Torguson, R.; Kirtane, A.J.; Minha, S.; Badr, S.; et al. Acquired thrombocytopenia after transcatheter aortic valve replacement: Clinical correlates and association with outcomes. *Eur. Heart J.* **2014**, *35*, 2663–2671. [CrossRef] [PubMed]
43. Roy, S.K.; Howard, E.W.; Panza, J.A.; Cooper, H.A. Clinical implications of thrombocytopenia among patients undergoing intra-aortic balloon pump counterpulsation in the coronary care unit. *Clin. Cardiol.* **2010**, *33*, 30–35. [CrossRef] [PubMed]
44. Eikelboom, J.W.; Anand, S.S.; Mehta, S.R.; Weitz, J.I.; Yi, C.; Yusuf, S. Prognostic significance of thrombocytopenia during hirudin and heparin therapy in acute coronary syndrome without ST elevation: Organization to Assess Strategies for Ischemic Syndromes (OASIS-2) study. *Circulation* **2001**, *103*, 643–650. [CrossRef]
45. Liu, R.; Liu, J.; Yang, J.; Gao, Z.; Zhao, X.; Chen, J.; Qiao, S.; Gao, R.; Wang, Q.; Yang, H.; et al. Association of thrombocytopenia with in-hospital outcome in patients with acute ST-segment elevated myocardial infarction. *Platelets* **2019**, *30*, 844–853. [CrossRef]

46. Rubinfeld, G.D.; Smilowitz, N.R.; Berger, J.S.; Newman, J.D. Association of Thrombocytopenia, Revascularization, and In-Hospital Outcomes in Patients with Acute Myocardial Infarction. *Am. J. Med.* **2019**, *132*, 942–948.e5. [CrossRef]
47. Wang, L.; Shao, J.; Shao, C.; Wang, H.; Jia, M.; Hou, X. The Relative Early Decrease in Platelet Count Is Associated With Mortality in Post-cardiotomy Patients Undergoing Venoarterial Extracorporeal Membrane Oxygenation. *Front. Med.* **2021**, *8*, 733946. [CrossRef]
48. Jiritano, F.; Serraino, G.F.; Ten Cate, H.; Fina, D.; Matteucci, M.; Mastroroberto, P.; Lorusso, R. Platelets and extra-corporeal membrane oxygenation in adult patients: A systematic review and meta-analysis. *Intensive Care Med.* **2020**, *46*, 1154–1169. [CrossRef]
49. Wang, L.; Yang, F.; Wang, X.; Xie, H.; Fan, E.; Ogino, M.; Brodie, D.; Wang, H.; Hou, X. Predicting mortality in patients undergoing VA-ECMO after coronary artery bypass grafting: The REMEMBER score. *Crit. Care* **2019**, *23*, 11. [CrossRef]
50. Takano, A.M.; Iwata, H.; Miyosawa, K.; Kimura, A.; Mukaida, H.; Osawa, S.; Kubota, K.; Doi, S.; Funamizu, T.; Takasu, K.; et al. Reduced Number of Platelets During Intra-Aortic Balloon Pumping Counterpulsation Predicts Higher Cardiovascular Mortality After Device Removal in Association with Systemic Inflammation. *Int. Heart J.* **2020**, *61*, 89–95. [CrossRef]
51. Gemmell, C.H.; Ramirez, S.M.; Yeo, E.L.; Sefton, M.V. Platelet activation in whole blood by artificial surfaces: Identification of platelet-derived microparticles and activated platelet binding to leukocytes as material-induced activation events. *J. Lab. Clin. Med.* **1995**, *125*, 276–287. [PubMed]
52. Lee, H.H.; Hong, S.J.; Ahn, C.M.; Yang, J.H.; Gwon, H.C.; Kim, J.S.; Kim, B.K.; Ko, Y.G.; Choi, D.; Hong, M.K.; et al. Clinical Implications of Thrombocytopenia at CS Presentation: Data from a Multicenter Registry. *Yonsei Med. J.* **2020**, *61*, 851–859. [CrossRef] [PubMed]
53. Huczek, Z.; Kochman, J.; Filipiak, K.J.; Horszczaruk, G.J.; Grabowski, M.; Piatkowski, R.; Wilczynska, J.; Zielinski, A.; Meier, B.; Opolski, G. Mean platelet volume on admission predicts impaired reperfusion and long-term mortality in acute myocardial infarction treated with primary percutaneous coronary intervention. *J. Am. Coll. Cardiol.* **2005**, *46*, 284–290. [CrossRef] [PubMed]
54. Kandis, H.; Ozhan, H.; Ordu, S.; Erden, I.; Caglar, O.; Basar, C.; Yalcin, S.; Alemdar, R.; Aydin, M. The prognostic value of mean platelet volume in decompensated heart failure. *Emerg. Med. J.* **2011**, *28*, 575–578. [CrossRef] [PubMed]
55. Chung, I.; Choudhury, A.; Lip, G.Y. Platelet activation in acute, decompensated congestive heart failure. *Thromb. Res.* **2007**, *120*, 709–713. [CrossRef]
56. Gibbs, C.R.; Blann, A.D.; Watson, R.D.; Lip, G.Y. Abnormalities of hemorheological, endothelial, and platelet function in patients with chronic heart failure in sinus rhythm: Effects of angiotensin-converting enzyme inhibitor and beta-blocker therapy. *Circulation* **2001**, *103*, 1746–1751. [CrossRef]
57. O'Connor, C.M.; Gurbel, P.A.; Serebruany, V.L. Usefulness of soluble and surface-bound P-selectin in detecting heightened platelet activity in patients with congestive heart failure. *Am. J. Cardiol.* **1999**, *83*, 1345–1349. [CrossRef]
58. Stumpf, C.; Lehner, C.; Eskafi, S.; Raaz, D.; Yilmaz, A.; Ropers, S.; Schmeisser, A.; Ludwig, J.; Daniel, W.G.; Garlichs, C.D. Enhanced levels of CD154 (CD40 ligand) on platelets in patients with chronic heart failure. *Eur. J. Heart Fail.* **2003**, *5*, 629–637. [CrossRef]
59. Jafri, S.M.; Ozawa, T.; Mammen, E.; Levine, T.B.; Johnson, C.; Goldstein, S. Platelet function, thrombin and fibrinolytic activity in patients with heart failure. *Eur. Heart J.* **1993**, *14*, 205–212. [CrossRef]
60. Anfossi, G.; Trovati, M. Role of catecholamines in platelet function: Pathophysiological and clinical significance. *Eur. J. Clin. Invest.* **1996**, *26*, 353–370. [CrossRef]
61. Larsson, P.T.; Schwieler, J.H.; Wallén, N.H. Platelet activation during angiotensin II infusion in healthy volunteers. *Blood Coagul. Fibrinolysis* **2000**, *11*, 61–69. [CrossRef] [PubMed]
62. Gando, S.; Wada, T. Disseminated intravascular coagulation in cardiac arrest and resuscitation. *J. Thromb. Haemost.* **2019**, *17*, 1205–1216. [CrossRef] [PubMed]
63. Kalra, S.; Ranard, L.S.; Memon, S.; Rao, P.; Garan, A.R.; Masoumi, A.; O'Neill, W.; Kapur, N.K.; Karmpaliotis, D.; Fried, J.A.; et al. Risk Prediction in CS: Current State of Knowledge, Challenges and Opportunities. *J. Card. Fail.* **2021**, *27*, 1099–1110. [CrossRef] [PubMed]

Disclaimer/Publisher's Note: The statements, opinions and data contained in all publications are solely those of the individual author(s) and contributor(s) and not of MDPI and/or the editor(s). MDPI and/or the editor(s) disclaim responsibility for any injury to people or property resulting from any ideas, methods, instructions or products referred to in the content.

MDPI
St. Alban-Anlage 66
4052 Basel
Switzerland
www.mdpi.com

Journal of Personalized Medicine Editorial Office
E-mail: jpm@mdpi.com
www.mdpi.com/journal/jpm

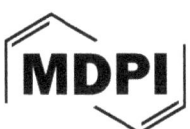

Disclaimer/Publisher's Note: The statements, opinions and data contained in all publications are solely those of the individual author(s) and contributor(s) and not of MDPI and/or the editor(s). MDPI and/or the editor(s) disclaim responsibility for any injury to people or property resulting from any ideas, methods, instructions or products referred to in the content.

www.ingramcontent.com/pod-product-compliance
Lightning Source LLC
LaVergne TN
LVHW070658100526
838202LV00013B/995